HEALTH PROMOTING UNIVERSITIES

Advancing Wellbeing through a Systems Approach

Edited by Vicki Squires, Chad London, and Matt Dolf

Written by health promoting university leaders, practitioners, and scholars, *Health Promoting Universities* presents approaches and strategies to advance health and wellbeing on higher education campuses and beyond.

Amid global challenges like climate change, systemic racism, and the COVID-19 pandemic, the complexity of higher education's role in addressing human health and wellbeing is evident. *Health Promoting Universities* explores how post-secondary education can address interconnected wellbeing challenges through collaborative leadership at organizational, provincial/state, national, and international levels.

With contributions from health promoting university leaders from Canada, the United Kingdom, and the United States, this collection reflects on research findings and emergent insights in taking a systems and settings approach to promote health and wellbeing. The authors advocate for prioritizing authentic, collaborative, and altruistic leadership to secure the systemic change necessary to sustain and promote the health of the planet and its citizens. The book examines systems-wide health promotion within post-secondary campuses, emphasizing higher education's role as an incubator to design and implement community-led processes and leadership strategies to enhance wellbeing. By engaging in knowledge mobilization practices that include the community, the book invites leaders, practitioners, and researchers to use these approaches to lead wellbeing efforts beyond the physical boundaries of their campuses.

Drawing on the collective knowledge of the authors in leading health promotion on campuses and beyond, *Health Promoting Universities* ultimately seeks to answer the question, how can higher education improve people's wellbeing, create healthy campus communities, and ensure a healthy planet?

VICKI SQUIRES is the associate dean of research, graduate support, and international initiatives in the College of Education at the University of Saskatchewan.

CHAD LONDON is the provost and vice-president, academic, and a professor of health and physical education at Mount Royal University.

MATT DOLF is the director for the Office of Wellbeing Strategy at the University of British Columbia and co-chair of the Canadian and International Health Promoting Campuses Networks.

Health Promoting Universities

Advancing Wellbeing through a Systems Approach

EDITED BY VICKI SQUIRES, CHAD LONDON, AND MATT DOLF

UNIVERSITY OF TORONTO PRESS
Toronto Buffalo London

ISBN 978-1-4875-4676-2 (cloth)   ISBN 978-1-4875-4791-2 (EPUB)
ISBN 978-1-4875-4788-2 (paper)   ISBN 978-1-4875-4897-1 (PDF)

Library and Archives Canada Cataloguing in Publication

Title: Health promoting universities : advancing wellbeing through a systems
   approach / edited by Vicki Squires, Chad London, and Matt Dolf.
Names: Squires, Vicki, editor. | London, Chad, editor. | Dolf, Matt, editor.
Description: Includes bibliographical references and index.
Identifiers: Canadiana (print) 20250132389 | Canadiana (ebook) 20250132427 |
   ISBN 9781487546762 (cloth) | ISBN 9781487547882 (paper) |
   ISBN 9781487548971 (PDF) | ISBN 9781487547912 (EPUB)
Subjects: LCSH: Universities and colleges—Health promotion services. |
   LCSH: College students—Health and hygiene. | LCSH: Health education. |
   LCSH: Health promotion.
Classification: LCC LB3497 .H43 2025 | DDC 378.1/971—dc23

Cover illustration and design by Sebastian Frye

We wish to acknowledge the land on which the University of Toronto Press
operates. This land is the traditional territory of the Wendat, the Anishnaabeg,
the Haudenosaunee, the Métis, and the Mississaugas of the Credit First Nation.

This book has been published with the help of a grant from the Federation
for the Humanities and Social Sciences, through the Awards to Scholarly
Publications Program, using funds provided by the Social Sciences and
Humanities Research Council of Canada.

University of Toronto Press acknowledges the financial support of the
Government of Canada, the Canada Council for the Arts, and the Ontario Arts
Council, an agency of the Government of Ontario, for its publishing activities.

Canada Council   Conseil des Arts
for the Arts   du Canada

ONTARIO ARTS COUNCIL
CONSEIL DES ARTS DE L'ONTARIO
an Ontario government agency
un organisme du gouvernement de l'Ontario

Funded by the   Financé par le
Government   gouvernement
of Canada   du Canada

Canadä

Contents

Conclusion: The Future of Health Promotion: Moving from Local and
National to Global Wellbeing   257

HEALTH PROMOTING UNIVERSITIES

Introduction: The Health Promotion Initiative

CHAD LONDON

This book grew from an initial research study regarding the implementation of the Okanagan Charter (2015) at several Canadian universities. As editors of this volume, we met with colleagues across Canada, the United States, and the United Kingdom, we discussed our progress in health promotion efforts on campuses and our shared passion for this work as a framework to improve wellbeing on campuses; these efforts then translate to enhanced wellbeing in the broader communities as our students become citizens and eventually leaders in society. By engaging others on our campuses and beyond, we can amplify our health promotion efforts and empower campuses through systems and settings approaches to improve health and wellbeing globally. To that end, we hope that this book will serve as a text for classes in health promotion, in systems and settings approaches, and in leadership and change management to address complex and multifaceted issues that are impacting us. We especially hope that campus senior leaders refer to this book so that they will consider the crucial nature of leadership support for health promotion and identify key mechanisms to anchor this work. Further, we believe that this book can be used as a resource for students, faculty, staff, and local communities who are passionate about building better places and spaces so that we may protect the health of humankind.

This chapter outlines the main threads that are woven throughout this edited book, including the role higher education institutions play in promoting health and wellbeing, and the systems approaches available to health promoting universities. An overview is provided of the chapters and their organization.

The impact of wicked challenges like climate change, systemic racism, and the COVID-19 global pandemic underscores the increasing complexities of attempts to enhance human health and wellbeing. When wellbeing is defined as a "positive state experienced by individuals and societies," this encompasses quality of life and the ability of people and societies to contribute to the world with a sense of purpose (WHO, 2021, p. 10), and never has the focus on wellbeing been more urgent than now (as noted by the United Nations when it released its Sustainable Development Goals [SDGs]; UN, 2022). While individual and societal health have far-ranging determinants, post-secondary education has a key role in addressing interconnected wellbeing challenges, and an opportunity to demonstrate effective leadership in using a systems approach to promote health and wellbeing within university campuses at organizational, provincial/state, national, and international levels. There are clear connections between the mandates of institutions of higher education and the imperative to enhance health and wellbeing. Universities are considered "health promoting" when they make efforts to promote wellbeing for the individuals within their institutions and the communities they serve across their mandates of teaching, research, and community service.

If universities have such opportunities, why are students, faculty, and staff reporting significant personal challenges in mental, physical, social, and emotional health (Cordaro, 2020; Entz et al., 2017; Herman, 2017; Lattie et al., 2019)? Beyond the contextual factors that may affect people's wellbeing, as historically siloed and loosely connected organizations, universities are not ideally structured to advance a systems- and settings-based, holistic approach to promote wellbeing. Universities have been described as loosely coupled institutions whose governance resembles "organized anarchy" (Austin & Jones, 2016). While there is some weakening of disciplinary and departmentalized structures in other countries, the roles of departments and disciplines in the governance of Canadian and American universities remain strong (Eastman et al., 2022). Many calls for higher education reform focus on the need to dismantle the silos and ensure that governance processes allow for innovation and nimbleness (Eastman et al., 2022).

The hierarchical and bureaucratic governance structures in post-secondary education institutions can limit collaboration and collaborative leadership, both of which are key aspects of systems approaches to advancing wellbeing. Regardless of these barriers, there are promising examples across the globe of institutions that are successfully overcoming these challenges.

Campuses can be incubators for investigating and implementing effective processes and leadership strategies to facilitate wellbeing. Further, engaging in knowledge mobilization practices that include the community and beyond, leaders, practitioners, and researchers can leverage these approaches to lead health promotion and wellbeing efforts beyond the physical spaces of university campuses. While there are exemplars of health promotion leadership in Canada and internationally, capitalizing on these successes and building a broad network of health promotion champions and leaders has proven more difficult to achieve. The goal of this book is to highlight work from pre-eminent and emergent scholars in this space to leverage our collective knowledge in leading health promotion on campuses and beyond, answering the question: How can higher education improve human and ecological health and wellbeing?

This edited book features authors that comprise a multinational team of researchers and practitioners who are health promoting campus leaders from Canada, the UK, and the US, and who collectively reflect on research findings and emergent understandings for how to use a systems and settings approach to promote health and wellbeing. The first section of the book includes chapter 1 by Mark Dooris and Matt Dolf, which lays the foundations of what is meant by promoting wellbeing and health promotion in campus contexts, including an explanation of systems- and settings-based approaches. This chapter sets out the underpinning conceptual frameworks and current context of the health promoting universities movement, detailing the development and calls to action of the Okanagan Charter (Okanagan Charter, 2015). The chapter summarizes the current state of global, regional, and national networks that have been mobilizing the tenets of the Charter.

The second section explores the infrastructure and processes related to the role of leadership for health promotion, explaining the unique and complex context of universities and colleges, the role of governance and policies, and the type of leadership required to move the health promotion agenda from adoption to implementation and evaluation. It begins with chapter 2 from Vicki Squires, Chad London, and Olena Shakhova on collaborative leadership in the university context that outlines various models of leadership, including the promising potential for collaborative leadership strategies and tactics for facilitating health promotion efforts in universities. The well-known adage that "what gets measured, gets treasured" is applied to the post-secondary setting in chapter 3 by Guy Faulkner, Caroline Wu, Kelly Wunderlich, and Michael Fang, who present a rationale for developing shared measurement tools for gathering information on the health and wellbeing of its community. The process in developing the Canadian Campus Wellbeing Survey (CCWS; www.ccws-becc.ca), a framework for a post-secondary health surveillance tool in Canada, is described, and key lessons learned are presented for how the CCWS data has been used by institutions and researchers.

The third section includes a variety of chapters that explore components of health promotion work on campuses. Although each chapter focuses on one facet of a broader system, the authors identify how these facets connect to building a holistic approach to health and wellbeing. Chapter 4 from Heather Foulds and Leah Ferguson is focused on supporting Indigenous Peoples' wellbeing, including a description of the diverse wellness needs of Indigenous Peoples, the types of supports that are found on many university campuses, and an assessment of the extent to which wellbeing initiatives are supporting Indigenous students, staff, and faculty. Chapter 5 by Maha Kumaran and Suresh Kalagnanam describes the emerging focus of universities on addressing equity, diversity, and inclusion. A definition of EDI is presented and examples of EDI programs, policies, practices, and initiatives are explored. The authors conclude by describing how principles of inclusion and belonging can be incorporated into a systems approach to wellbeing. The final chapter in this section, chapter 6, is authored by Ainsley Carry, a senior university leader with executive experience in taking responsibility for student affairs at universities in Canada and the US. Dr. Carry makes the case for the imperative that universities have in placing student health and wellbeing at the core of student affairs work. The challenges that students are facing are not contained to individuals or small groups of students; rather, they have broad societal implications that universities have the opportunity to meaningfully impact.

The final section concludes the book with five chapters that highlight key understandings, identify potential pathways forward, and emphasize the need for immediate action. It begins with Chad London and Tanya Forneris describing in chapter 7 how academics and academic units can play significant roles in health promotion on their campuses through teaching, research, and community engagement. Chapter 8 from Sara Kozicky, Vanessa Cunningham, Min-Jung Kim, Sam Laban, and Philip Loring explains the impact of food insecurity as a major public health issue, and how university students are particularly vulnerable. This chapter explores how Canadian universities are promoting food-secure campus communities by attending to complexity, innovation, and leadership, informed by the Okanagan Charter. Crystal Hutchinson, Natasha Malloff, and Alicia Hibbert in Chapter 9 describe how workplace health promotion has expanded from a focus on the physical environment to including health literacy and psychosocial factors such as organizational culture and psychological support. Examples of how a workplace perspective can advance health promotion actions are shared from universities and colleges across the world. Chapter 10 from C. Oliver Tacto provides an overview of how US colleges are creating healthy settings by designing campuses where students, faculty, and staff can live, learn, work, and experience college in a meaningful way. This chapter explores the benefits and outcomes of using a systems approach to apply health promoting principles by applying concepts of built environment, university urbanization, and sustainability. Chapter 11, the final chapter leading to the book's conclusion, is written by Chad London and Vicki Squires and highlights the key learnings and challenges of the first ten Canadian universities that signed onto the Okanagan Charter and began implementing and evaluating their commitments to the charter. Best practices are shared from those universities that are leading the way in delivering a systems approach to campus wellbeing.

Vicki Squires concludes the book by noting how advocacy coalitions can facilitate change to the university landscape on a global scale and pointing out hopeful trends and potential opportunities for furthering the goal of human health. Collectively, the contents of this book will propose priorities for harnessing and nurturing authentic, collaborative, and altruistic leadership to secure the systemic change necessary to sustain and promote the health of the planet and its citizens.

This book addresses how and why universities can move towards whole campus health promotion. Several chapters examine essential pieces of this approach including leadership structures, the work of academic units and human resources units, student leadership, and equity, diversity, and inclusion principles. Other chapters explore what is meant by a systems approach and emphasize that the achievement of health promotion on campuses requires collaborative approaches within the university and with broader communities. We must build bridges across the traditional silos of higher education to approach wellbeing with an emphasis on promotion rather than intervention. We emphasize that we must shift thinking of wellbeing away from belonging solely within a medical model and instead view health broadly where everyone's efforts have an impact.

REFERENCES

Austin, I., & Jones, G.A. (2016). *Governance of higher education: Global perspectives, theories, and practices.* Routledge.

Cordaro, M. (2020). Pouring from an empty cup: The case for compassion fatigue in higher education. *Building Healthy Academic Communities Journal, 4*(2), 17–28. https://doi.org/10.18061/bhac.v4i2.7618

Eastman, J., Jones, G.A., Trottier, C., & Begin-Caouette, O. (2022). *University governance in Canada: Navigating complexity.* McGill-Queen's University Press.

Entz, M., Slater, J., & Desmarais, A.A. (2017). Student food insecurity at the University of Manitoba. *Canadian Food Studies, 4*(1), 139–59. https://doi.org/10.15353/cfs-rcea.v4i1.204

Herman, K.M. (2017). How did we get so sedentary? Sedentary behaviours among Canadian adults. *Alberta Centre for Active Living, 28*(4), 1–5. Retrieved from https://www.centre4activeliving.ca/media/filer_public/21/cc/21ccbb90-7210-4d43-973a-1ce5e70d542d/2017-apr-sedentary.pdf

Lattie, E.G., Adkins, E.C., Winquist, N., Stiles-Shields, C., Wafford, Q.E., & Graham, A.K. (2019). Digital mental health interventions for depression, anxiety, and enhancement of psychological wellbeing among college students: Systematic review. *Journal of Medical Internet Research, 21*(7), e12869. https://doi.org/10.2196/12869.

Okanagan Charter: An International Charter for Health Promoting Universities and Colleges. (2015). *Okanagan Charter.* Kelowna, BC: Author. Retrieved from http://internationalhealthycampuses2015.sites.olt.ubc.ca/files/2016/01/Okanagan-Charter-January13v2.pdf

United Nations (UN). (2022). The Sustainable Development Goals Report 2022.

World Health Organization (WHO). (2021). Health Promotion Glossary of Terms 2021.

1 Laying the Foundations for the Health Promoting Universities Movement

MATT DOLF AND MARK DOORIS

Note: we use the term "universities" to represent all universities, colleges, and institutions in the post-secondary or higher education sector. Terminology for health promotion in higher education varies depending on regional contexts. Most Spanish-speaking, European, and Asian countries use "universities"; Canada and the US use "universities and colleges" or "campuses"; while other countries prefer "tertiary education" or "higher education."

Introduction

Health promotion offers a framework to mobilize large-scale whole system change for the wellbeing of people, places, and the planet. The Geneva Charter for Wellbeing (WHO, 2021) "underlines the urgency of creating sustainable 'wellbeing societies,' committed to achieving equitable health now and for future generations without breaching ecological limits" (p. 1), suggesting that the role of health promotion is to catalyze and support a flourishing future through a whole-of-society approach by:

- Ensuring that people and communities are enabled to take control of their health and lead fulfilling lives with a sense of meaning and purpose, in harmony with Nature, through education, culturally relevant health literacy, meaningful empowerment and engagement.
- Enabling, mediating, and advocating for a unifying approach to creating wellbeing societies by shaping the determinants of health across settings.
- Ensuring that promotive, preventive, curative, rehabilitative and palliative health and social services are high quality, affordable, accessible and acceptable and are provided according to needs, especially for those often left behind. (p. 4)

This book focuses on universities and colleges as settings for health promotion. Higher education is not a health sector – although many universities do contain faculties of health and medicine – and yet it is a setting that significantly shapes opportunities for positive human and ecological impact and can maximize these opportunities through a systemic "health in all policies" approach. These higher education institutions are well positioned to act as living laboratories and agents of change within the broader society for several reasons. Building on prior contributions by Dooris (2022), a commitment by health promoting universities (HPUs) to promote health and wellbeing can maximize opportunities to:

- positively impact the health and wellbeing of students, faculty, and staff through their core activities and specific interventions;
- build on the Health Promoting Schools movement and "join up" across the education timeline;
- benefit the local community through citizen engagement, community service, and co-created research;
- improve human and ecological health through the design and stewardship of the significant building stock and land base located on campuses, as well as influencing the travel to and from surrounding areas;
- contribute to the long-term health improvement of the population through education, research, and knowledge exchange;
- enhance a university's core business, in terms of key priorities such as achievement, performance, productivity, and reputation; and
- generate health, justice, equity, diversity, inclusion, and sustainability in families, neighbourhoods, and society through their potential to "future-shape" students, staff, and faculty as local and global citizens.

The authors of this chapter are current and recent co-chairs of the International Health Promoting University Campuses Network, as well as of the HPU networks in Canada and the UK. We have also been architects of developing HPU approaches within the University of Central Lancashire (UK) and the University of British Columbia (Canada). This experience has given us first-hand insights into the foundational elements of the HPUs movement, which will be outlined in this chapter. These elements are not universally agreed upon, however, and the field continues to develop, both in terms of theory and its application by practitioners in higher education settings. We believe that understanding and applying these key ingredients give us the best chance of enacting the ambitious and holistic vision for HPUs set out in the Okanagan Charter's "Shared Aspirations" (2015):

> Health Promoting Universities and Colleges transform the health and sustainability of our current and future societies, strengthen communities and contribute to the wellbeing of people, places and the planet. Health promoting universities and colleges infuse health into everyday operations, business practices and academic mandates. By doing so, health promoting universities and colleges enhance the success of our institutions; create campus cultures of compassion, wellbeing, equity and social justice; improve the health of the people who live, learn, work, play and love on our campuses; and strengthen the ecological, social and economic sustainability of our communities and wider society. (p. 2)

Like the Geneva Charter for Wellbeing, the Okanagan Charter reflects a growing consensus that health and sustainability are essentially interconnected (Orme & Dooris, 2010). This consensus holds that the wellbeing of people cannot be separated from the wellbeing of the planet. Both of these concepts can be used to provide an overarching conceptual and implementation framework for promoting wellbeing, and different institutions tend to choose one or the other depending on perceived resonance and traction at a particular point in time (Dooris, 1998). For the purposes of this chapter and book, we have chosen to emphasize health as the overarching theme, while also actively seeking to integrate sustainability and a focus on planetary health.

Context

The wellbeing of individuals, communities, societies, and our planet as a whole requires urgent attention and innovative joined-up approaches now more than at any time in history. Despite the significant improvements in population health and life expectancy achieved globally since the millennium, progress has slowed markedly since 2015 in relation to Sustainable Development Goal (SDG) indicators such as maternal mortality, under-five/neonatal mortality, premature mortality from major non-communicable diseases, and suicide and road traffic mortality. Additionally, there are alarming trends in areas such as air pollution, obesity, and mental health, and there continue to be entrenched inequalities in access to health-related services, exposure to health risks, and mortality rates (WHO, 2023).

According to the latest report from the Intergovernmental Panel on Climate Change (IPCC), the earth's climate is changing rapidly, and emergency measures are urgently needed to stave off the severe climate-related impacts (Contribution of Working Group II, 2022). The IPCC report also concludes that climate change is adversely affecting our physical and mental health in many ways, including trauma from climate events, increasing temperatures, displacement and loss of livelihoods, and increased exposure to heat and smoke. A paradigm shift is needed in how societies use and mobilize resources to restore human and ecological balance and health.

The COVID-19 pandemic directly or indirectly claimed fifteen million lives in its first two years, highlighting the importance of combining health care, education, prevention, and promotion measures to effectively restore civil society (UN, 2022). Believed to be of zoonotic origin, COVID-19 has highlighted the exploitative character of our relationship with nature "driven by an unsustainable food system linked to habitat destruction and biodiversity decline" (de León et al., 2021, p. 827) and has also amplified existing injustices. The extreme wealth gap between societies' richest and poorest exacerbates health inequities; indeed, almost 10 per cent of the world's population still live in extreme poverty and struggle to meet basic needs like health, education, and access to water and sanitation (UN, 2022).

Further, centuries of colonialism and systemic racism continue to cause deep harm, especially to Indigenous people, Black people, people of colour, and other equity-deserving groups. These global systemic threats negatively impact human mental, physical, and social health, as well as the health of our flora and fauna. Effective solutions must harness systems thinking and connect across silos, weaving together actions on health, sustainability, wellbeing, equity, justice, and Indigenous rights – requiring all sectors of civilization to be mobilized.

For millennia, Indigenous peoples have taught that human and ecological wellbeing are inseparable and that we should use nature as our guide to inspire healthy, reciprocal, and sustainable solutions. Unfortunately, universities have relied too long on colonial and reductionist views to shape how we think and act. To care for the health of our people and of our planet, we must build holistic, systems-based solutions drawing on the knowledge and relationships with our whole community. Indigenous scholars, elders, and knowledge holders have been at the forefront of advocating for this approach. They have also proven over millennia that they have been the most capable of caretaking our lands in harmony with people. According to the global assessment report on biodiversity and ecosystem services, "Nature managed by Indigenous peoples and local communities is under increasing pressure. Nature is generally declining less rapidly in Indigenous peoples' land than in other lands, but is nevertheless declining, as is the knowledge of how to manage it" (IPBES, 2019, p. 14). The HPU field is still at the beginning of its journey to recognize and create opportunities for this knowledge to inform the health and wellbeing movement in academia.

The Health Promoting Universities Movement

Starting in the mid-1990s with the universities of Lancaster and Central Lancashire in the UK writing the first HPU guidance in collaboration with the WHO, the HPUs movement has grown to become a strong network of activity across the globe (Dooris, 2022; Meier et al., 2007; Squires & London, 2021; Suárez-Reyes & Van den Broucke, 2016; Waterworth & Thorpe, 2017).

The Okanagan Charter clearly articulates a vision, calls to action, and principles for universities to engage with (2015):

Vision

Health promoting universities and colleges transform the health and sustainability of our current and future societies, strengthen communities, and contribute to the wellbeing of people, places, and the planet.

Calls to Action

1 Embed health into all aspects of campus culture, across the administration, operations, and academic mandates.
2 Lead health promotion action and collaboration locally and globally.

Principles

1 Use settings and whole system approaches
2 Ensure comprehensive and campus-wide approaches
3 Use participatory approaches and engage the voice of students and others
4 Develop trans-disciplinary collaboration and cross-sector partnerships
5 Promote research, innovation, and evidence-informed action
6 Build on strengths
7 Value local and indigenous communities' contexts, and priorities
8 Act on a universal responsibility (pp. 2–10)

Universities are still relatively new at embodying a broad health promotion and wellbeing agenda, and their approach often remains limited in scope (Dooris et al., 2021; Squires & London, 2021). Some focus on the student experience, some prioritize a human resources and staff wellbeing perspective, and most struggle to invest financial and staff resources to get beyond a crisis-prevention focus of risk management and treating symptoms through health care services and health education. These universities miss out on the long-term benefits of embedding and applying all the principles of the Okanagan Charter, to scaffold a true HPU approach.

This section outlines some key characteristics of HPUs and highlights some of the foundational conferences, publications, and networks that guide the movement. Table 1.1 provides a timeline summary from Dooris, which has been updated with recent developments (2022, p. 153).

Ottawa Charter for Health Promotion, 1986

The Ottawa Charter is the seminal document that set out the blueprint for health promotion. It was created as part of the first WHO International Conference on health promotion held in Ottawa, Canada (WHO, 1986). The Ottawa Charter was also a call to action to achieve "health for all" by the year 2000 and beyond. It sets out the prerequisites for health, as well as three strategies (to enable, mediate, and advocate) and five action areas (build healthy public policy, create supportive environments, strengthen community action, develop personal skills, and reorient health services) for health promotion. Importantly, it suggested that "Health is created and lived by people within the settings of their everyday life; where they learn, work, play and love" (p. 4) – the statement that launched the healthy settings movement, of which Health Promoting Universities is now an integral part.

Bangkok Charter for Health Promotion in a Globalized World, 2005

The Bangkok Charter was developed at the 6th World Health Organization (WHO) Global Conference on Health Promotion held in Bangkok, Thailand (WHO, 2005). It built on the Ottawa Charter by identifying strategies and commitments to address the determinants of health in a globalized world with an emphasis on health equity. It called on all sectors of society to embed the promotion of health for all as a central commitment.

Edmonton Charter for Health Promoting Universities and Institutions of Higher Education, 2006

The Edmonton Charter was an outcome of the 2005 International Conference of Health Promoting Universities hosted by the University of Alberta in Edmonton, Canada (WHO, 2006). Its purpose is to identify

Table 1.1. Health Promoting Universities Milestones: Timeline of Key Publications, Conferences, and Networks

Year	HPU Milestone
1986	Ottawa Charter for Health Promotion
1994/5	First HPU initiatives established at universities of Lancaster and Central Lancashire, UK
1995	German HPU network established
1996	International HPU Conference, Lancaster, UK
1998	WHO publishes "HPUs: Concept, Experience & Framework for Action"
2003	I International HPU Congress, Ibero-American network established
2005	II International HPU Congress and Edmonton Charter
2006	UK and Spanish HPU networks established
2007	Ibero-American HPU network expanded to include Spain and Portugal
2009	Austrian and Swiss HPU networks established
2014	ASEAN HPU network established
2015	VII International HPU Congress and Okanagan Charter, New Zealand HPU network established
2016	International HPU steering group and Canadian HPU network established
2018	Irish HPU network established
2019	International HPU Symposium, Rotorua, New Zealand
2020	USA HPU network established
2022	International HPU Symposium, Canada (virtual)

what it means to be an HPU and to act as a resource for dialogue and to influence decision makers in higher education settings. It was the first widely taken up Charter guiding health promotion for higher education.

Okanagan Charter: An International Charter for Health Promoting Universities & Colleges, 2015

Ten years after the Edmonton Charter, researchers, practitioners, administrators, students, and policymakers from forty-two countries informed the development of the Okanagan Charter, an outcome of the international conference in its name held on the Okanagan campus of the University of British Columbia in Kelowna, Canada (Okanagan Charter, 2015). The Okanagan Charter emphasized the integration of systemic and ecological approaches to health promotion, grounded on concepts of social determinants of health, health in all policies, and settings. It was also designed to be concise and action oriented with flexibility for global application (Black & Stanton, 2016). The Okanagan

Charter has accelerated the HPUs movement by providing a common framework for action, rooted in concepts of health promotion, sustainability, equity, and Indigenous contexts and priorities. Numerous countries have developed national networks that provide a formal mechanism for HPU leadership to adopt and commit to implementing the Okanagan Charter.

The Geneva Charter for Wellbeing, 2021

The Geneva Charter is the output of the 10th Global Conference on Health Promotion, building on the original Ottawa Charter (WHO, 2021). It calls for urgent action to set the foundation for "wellbeing societies," focusing on equitable health for all and staying within ecological limits. It also calls for coordinated societal action across five areas consistent with the 2030 Agenda for Sustainable Development in order to "steward a flourishing future."

HPU Networks

The Health Promoting Universities (HPUs) movement has matured significantly and taken root across the globe. Currently, there are at least fifteen national, regional, and language-based networks involving approximately forty countries and hundreds of universities and colleges. The German network was the first to be established in 1995. In the 2000s, the Ibero-American network (RIUPS) was established, linked to developments within Spain, Portugal, and several countries in Latin America, with national networks also emerging in the United Kingdom, Austria, and Switzerland. Subsequently, the ASEAN (Association of Southeast Asian Nations) network has been formed, with multiple other countries such as Canada, China, Ireland, New Zealand, and the USA forming national networks, and individual universities in countries such as India, Turkey, Bulgaria seeking to stimulate developments.

The creation of the Okanagan Charter led to an increase in collaboration between these networks and an acceleration of the formation of new networks. In 2015, the International Health Promoting Campuses Network was formed by representatives of HPU networks around the globe. Its aim is to advance the Okanagan Charter internationally, thereby inspiring and catalyzing further action towards the creation of health promoting universities and colleges. Key focus areas include network building and development, future conferences, and charter communication, activation, and mobilization (International Health Promoting Campuses Network, n.d.).

Concepts and Emerging Directions

The field of HPUs and its application are emergent. Indeed, even our understanding and usage of key terms such as "health," "health promotion," "wellbeing," and "sustainability" differ widely. This section reviews key concepts that all researchers and practitioners should be aware of: healthy settings approach, whole university/systems approach, and finally salutogenic and regenerative sustainability approaches.

Healthy Settings Approach

This quote by Norman and Reist (2022) nicely illustrates what a settings-based approach looks like: "If the frogs in a pond behave strangely, our first reaction would not be to punish them or treat them. Instinctively, we'd wonder what was going on in the pond" (p. 6). Universities should therefore ask themselves if they are putting adequate resources into treating individuals (the frogs) through supports such as student health services or employee health benefits as well as putting resources into changing the university system and culture (the pond) by dedicating time, resources, and leadership to engage community in developing and implementing policies and campus master plans with a health and wellbeing lens.

A healthy settings approach applied to HPUs requires the following actions:

• ensuring a focus on people, place, and planet;
• understanding that the university itself is a setting that directly and indirectly impacts health and wellbeing
• and integrating health promotion within the culture, ethos, structures, processes, and routine life of the university as an institution.

Drawing on settings theory, a health promoting university should have five primary characteristics (Dooris, 2022):

1 A shift of focus towards a salutogenic view concerned not only with preventing and addressing illness, but with wellbeing and what makes people thrive and flourish (Antonovsky, 1996) – fostering health potentials inherent in the university setting and strengthening the resources that can empower people to increase control over the determinants of health (Kickbush, 1996).
2 Adopting an ecological model. It appreciates that health is multilayered and determined by a complex interaction of personal, social, behavioural, and environmental factors, and it addresses

human health within the framework of ecosystem health (Hancock, 2015). Recognizing the interplay between structure and agency, it appreciates that different stakeholders have different degrees of access to and control over the determinants of their health and wellbeing.

3 Viewing the university as a dynamic complex system, acknowledging interconnectedness and synergy between its component parts, and recognizing that it is connected to the world around it (Dooris, 2001; Naaldenberg et al., 2009).

4 Adopting a comprehensive holistic change focus, drawing on learning from organization and community development and using multiple, interconnected interventions to embed health within the university's culture, ethos, structures, processes, and routine life (Dooris, 2009).

5 Appreciating that universities, like many other settings, do not have health as their main mission or raison d'être, and that it is therefore essential to advocate for health in terms of impact on or outflow from core business (Dooris et al., 2012).

It is also important to reflect on the position that universities occupy in what can be termed the "ecosystem of settings":

• they are educational settings forming part of the wider educational system and pathway;
• they are workplaces for multiple academic and non-academic staff;
• they prepare many students for employment and roles in diverse workplaces;
• they often represent "cities" within "cities" – large multi-component settings within their "place";
• they manage a significant land base and building stock, impacting the surrounding flora and fauna;
• they are one of multiple interconnected settings that university populations move in and out of in their daily lives;
• and they are places where transitions – into, through, and out of university – can be of particular importance, times when students are at their most vulnerable, particularly in terms of mental wellbeing.

Whole University/Systems Approach

There is a broad consensus on the benefits of taking whole university and whole system approaches as called for in the principles of the Okanagan

Charter (Dooris et al., 2020). A whole university approach connects and harnesses the multiple stakeholders and multiple components of an institution into a cohesive whole. A whole system approach understands the university as part of the wider higher education system, influenced by external policy and regulations, and locates the university within its context/place, connecting with multiple sectors and external service providers to ensure a joined-up and coherent program.

The UK HPU network drew on the early work of Baric/Barić (1993, 1994) and its membership to produce a model for applying a healthy settings approach to universities (see figure 1.1). This depicts how underpinning values (e.g., equity, engagement, sustainability) and influences from within both higher education and public health support action across three focus areas:

1 Create learning, working, and living environments that support and sustain the health and wellbeing of the university population, and help people flourish.
2 Integrate health and sustainable development within the university's core business of learning, research, and knowledge exchange.
3 Connect with and contribute to the wellbeing, resilience, and sustainability of local, regional, national, and global communities.

These all lead to an arrow pointing outwards labelled "Deliverables and Impacts."

A whole university approach is also supported by the following complementary strategies (Dooris et al., 2022):

- Anticipating and responding to higher education and public health drivers;
- Securing "top–down" leadership while also engaging "bottom–up" stakeholder engagement and participation;
- Combining long-term organization development and change with high-visibility project work; and
- Balancing a pathogenic focus on addressing needs and problems with a salutogenic focus on harnessing a university's strengths, assets, and potentials in order to support the wellbeing and flourishing of students, staff, and the wider community.

Salutogenic and Regenerative Sustainability Approaches

As highlighted in the introduction, health and sustainability are strongly interconnected. Health promotion and regenerative sustainability are

Figure 1.1. Healthy Universities – A model for conceptualizing and applying the healthy settings approach to higher education (adapted from Dooris et al., 2010)

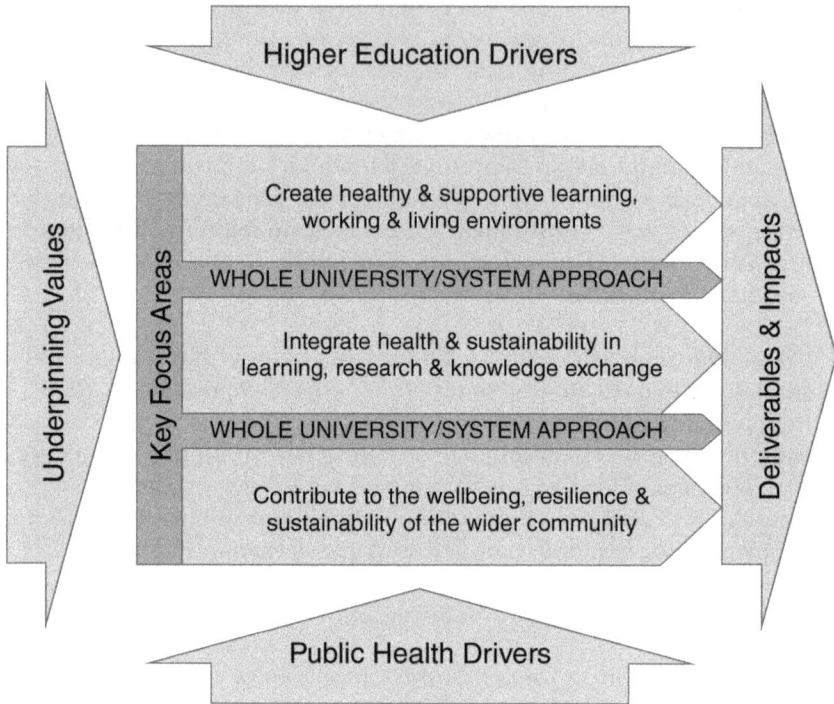

both useful theoretical frameworks that provide us with underlying concepts and principles to effectively improve conditions of health and sustainability. Both look beyond lifestyle influences, highlighting the intersection of environmental, social, and economic determinants. In their operations, universities have for many years implemented preventative health interventions and environmental sustainability management systems – with health promotion and sustainability largely being viewed as separate domains despite the growing convergence of agendas and emphasis on co-benefits (Orme & Dooris, 2010). However, the Okanagan Charter signalled the importance of moving towards a more integrated and salutogenic approach that focuses on the wellbeing of people, places, and the planet.

As noted in the "healthy settings approach" above, the salutogenic orientation is a key characteristic of the settings approach as applied to universities. Many of the health topics that universities seek to address – for example, substance abuse, mental illness, and sedentary behaviour – tend to have been constructed as problems and treated as ill health. These topics could be reframed as promoting healthy substance use, mental health, and physical activity. While it is obviously necessary to take seriously and address the challenges that they present, numerous authors, such as Dooris et al. (2022) and Waterworth and Thorpe (2017), have highlighted the importance and benefits of taking a salutogenic orientation with its focus on assets and strengths, and what makes people and places flourish. Waterworth and Thorpe (2017) have also pointed out the link to prioritizing Indigenous knowledge and experience in this regard.

Like salutogenesis – with its shift of focus to embrace not only illness but wellbeing and what makes people thrive – regenerative sustainability (Brown, 2016; Robinson & Cole, 2015) moves beyond the traditional concern of "reducing the negatives" to consider how we can achieve net positive" impacts for both people and ecosystems. "Regenerative sustainability" advances commonly used concepts and implementation strategies of "sustainability" to emphasize that we also need to restore what has been lost. This is an important distinction given that the earth is currently in a state of dangerous overshoot beyond several safe ecological thresholds and must be brought back into balance (Lyle, 1996; Rockstrom et al., 2009).

Proponents of regenerative sustainability also argue that university settings can employ principles rooted in net-positive change, systems thinking, place- and nature-based design, and community engagement to support human and ecological wellbeing both on and off campus (Cole, 2011; Dolf, 2017; Mang & Reed, 2011). By bringing together the common perspectives that flow from a commitment to salutogenesis, health promotion, and regenerative sustainability, we can raise our aspirations so that our campus design, operational management, research focus, and curricular orientation promote the wellbeing and flourishing of people, place, and planet.

Reflections on Applying Theory to Practice at Our Own Institutions

The University of British Columbia (UBC)

Founded in 1915, UBC is one of the largest public universities in Canada, comprising 71,000 students, 19,000 faculty and staff, 20,000 community residents on university lands, 500 buildings, and two main campuses: Vancouver Point Grey, on 1,000 acres on the traditional, ancestral, and unceded territory of the Musqueam people; and Okanagan, on 500 acres on the unceded territory of the Syilx Okanagan Nation. Going back as far as the launch of UBC's Student Health Service in 1929, there have been pockets of leadership within student services, human resources, and academia, but not a whole of university commitment and structure. UBC Wellbeing was formalized as a collective priority in 2014 to make the university a better place to live, work, learn, and play through a systems-wide approach to embedding health and wellbeing across our campuses. UBC takes a collaborative leadership approach to health promotion and sustainability, seeking to embed wellbeing as a priority in policy, academia, and operations for the whole university community.

Key to success has been:

- Embedding wellbeing across the institution as part of a cultural shift is done through ongoing dialogue with students, faculty, staff, community members, and senior leadership. At all levels, we explore the question: How can UBC become a health and wellbeing promoting university where all people, places, and communities can flourish?
- Convening conversations and sharing best practices with campuses across Canada and internationally.
- Building on and partnering with other system-wide strategic initiatives, including sustainability, equity and inclusion, campus planning, and Indigeneity.
- Formal adoption of the Okanagan Charter in 2016 by the university executive along with ongoing investments to create strategic supports for faculties, administrative units, and our community to facilitate UBC-wide action on wellbeing.
  - Wellbeing noted as a priority within UBC's Strategic Plan (University of British Columbia, 2018), in particular: Core Area – People and Places: Creating vibrant, sustainable environments that enhance wellbeing and excellence for people at UBC and beyond. (p. 37)
  - Strategy 3 – Thriving Communities: Support the ongoing development of sustainable, healthy and connected campuses and communities. (p. 42)
  - The ensuing UBC Wellbeing and Thrive at UBC programs are system-wide efforts to make the university a better place to live, work and learn. Our focus on mental health is integral to our success as an institution and as a source of influence for positive change in

society. UBC's Wellbeing Strategic Plan will channel university-wide effort and ensure continued focus. (p. 40)

- The development of UBC's Wellbeing Strategic Framework, created through community and stakeholder engagement to mobilize priority areas for action in line with an HPU approach.
- Strategic direction is provided by a UBC Wellbeing advisory committee made up of senior administrators, academics, elected student leaders, as well as strategic leadership in the areas of student affairs, human resources, health promotion, sustainability, equity, campus planning, and Indigenous engagement.
- Coordination, implementation, planning, communication, and engagement is facilitated by a "strategic support team" drawing on staff across both the Vancouver and Okanagan campuses from health promotion units in student affairs, human resources, and an Office of Wellbeing Strategy.
- Taking a regenerative (or salutogenic) approach to shift from a harm-reduction lens to aspire to net-positive outcomes. UBC's goal is to enable people to leave campus better equipped than when they first arrived and to carry the skills, values, and priorities that the university helps them to foster into the next phase of their lives, thus affecting longer-term societal and ecological wellbeing.

This collaborative, integrated approach across such a large and complex organization has been both a strength and a challenge. On the positive side, recognition of wellbeing as a collective priority has increased dramatically. In most community engagement consultations, wellbeing consistently emerges as a top priority to inform new plans and policies. Senior leaders are embedding specific commitments to promote health and wellbeing within their portfolio or unit-level plans and commitments. Community-led initiatives pop up like mushrooms in faculties, classrooms, research projects, and off-campus projects with our neighbouring cities. At the same time, the diffusion of activity and responsibility can make it challenging to demonstrate impact, support many community priorities in a coordinated way, and keep leadership informed and engaged. The backbone organizational structure of UBC Wellbeing is therefore constantly evolving to support effective distributed systemic change in line with the principles of the Okanagan Charter.

Going forward, we increasingly recognize the need for new approaches to systemic change in the face of multiple crises – most notably climate change, anti-racism, Indigenous reconciliation and decolonization, and COVID-19. These simultaneous crises mean that we can no longer focus on any one priority at a time. These issues are fundamentally connected, and they all need to be addressed through systems- and settings-based approaches together. Our siloed administrative and research structures are not well equipped to deal with this complexity. Some promising ways we are looking at to innovate our HPU approach include centring Indigenous knowledge, strengthening alignment to sustainability and equity initiatives, and applying organizational change concepts like "collective impact," "multi-solving," and "collaborative leadership."

University of Central Lancashire

The University of Central Lancashire collaborated with the WHO to organize a symposium entitled *Settings-Based Health Promotion* back in 1993, which provided an entry point for securing senior executive support and commitment. This led to the appointment of a coordinator in 1995 to set up a new health promoting university initiative. Since then, the initiative has, perhaps inevitably, gone through ups and downs, navigating its way within a changing landscape influenced by external funding and regulatory cycles, changes in leadership, and shifting institutional priorities.

The following have been key to success:

- A concern not only to identify and respond to needs, but also to map what is in place to support wellbeing across the university (whether or not it uses the terminology of "health");
- Find appropriate windows of opportunity and identify senior-level leaders with understanding, passion, and influence;
- Harness, connect, and mobilize different parts of the university and knit them together into a coherent whole organization program;
- Forge strong links with parallel agendas such as civic engagement; equality, diversity and inclusion; and sustainability, biodiversity, and climate action – prioritizing thematic areas that can illustrate the connections between human and planetary health, such as food and travel; and
- Embed a joined-up commitment to health, wellbeing, and sustainability into the university's strategic planning and policy.

In relation to the last point, the University of Central Lancashire published its new seven-year Strategic Plan in 2021 (University of Central

Lancashire, 2021). In the lead-up to this, we worked hard to ensure that it included a firm commitment to sustainability, and to the health and wellbeing of students, staff, and local communities, resulting in the inclusion of the following statements:

> Sustaining and enhancing the wellbeing of people, places & the planet are amongst the most important challenges we face today. (p. 23)
>
> Our unwavering commitment to sustainability, health & wellbeing will become the benchmark for the UK university community. (p. 23)

We are particularly pleased with the strength of these statements, the ambition this represents, and the clearly articulated concern to connect the health and wellbeing of people, places, and the planet. Alongside this, the Sub Strategy on Future-Proofing Our University (University of Central Lancashire, 2022) further reinforces the connections between health, wellbeing, fairness, sustainability, biodiversity and climate action – and makes explicit reference to the Okanagan Charter and to the healthy universities approach and the University of Central Lancashire's leadership role over many years:

> We will sustain and enhance the wellbeing of people, places and the planet, recognising that they are interconnected and interdependent. We will protect and improve health, while also tackling the climate and ecological emergencies, promoting biodiversity, and supporting a just transition to a greener future. (p. 2)
>
> We have long pioneered the "Healthy Universities" approach and have provided leadership to this movement nationally and internationally over many years. Encapsulated in the 2015 Okanagan International Charter for Health Promoting Universities and Colleges, the approach is underpinned by "whole university" and "whole system" perspectives and seeks to create an organisational culture and learning, working and living environments that support wellbeing – thereby enhancing performance and productivity. Working in collaboration with the Students' Union and partner organisations, we will harness this trailblazing history and implement evidence-informed actions to promote the health and wellbeing of students, staff, and our wider communities. (p. 5)

As we look to the future, we are hopeful that this strategic-level commitment will provide a valuable basis for us to advocate for strengthened governance and reporting structures and mediate for continued investment.

Conclusion

In this chapter, we have laid the groundwork for the HPUs movement. The Ottawa Charter set out the principles of health promotion, the Edmonton Charter provided the first health promotion guidance specific to university settings, and the Okanagan Charter added a focus on ecology, equity, and Indigenous priorities in higher education along with new calls to action that have accelerated the recognition of HPU campuses and networks.

These health promotion charters advance the notion of the civic university – that HPUs have a future-shaping and capacity-building role in driving cultural, economic, and social development in ways that allow both people and the planet to flourish. They are well-positioned to promote knowledge and action on human rights, health, sustainable development, democracy, and peace and justice in support of the UN Sustainable Development Goals.

Other chapters in this book build on this foundation with research and case studies related to the implementation of HPU initiatives in higher education settings. We hope you are inspired to use this book as a teaching tool for your university classes; to share with a member of your university executive; to inspire discussion themes for a session with your community of practice; and to strengthen working relationships with other university partners leading systems and settings-based work in health, sustainability, campus planning, or justice, equity, diversity, and inclusion – to name a few.

The societal challenges we face are enormous, and universities have a vital role to play in driving collective, innovative, and transformative action.

REFERENCES

Antonovsky, A. (1996). The salutogenic model as a theory to guide health promotion? *Health Promotion International, 11*(1), 11–18. https://doi.org /10.1093/heapro/11.1.11

Baric, L. (1993). The settings approach–Implications for policy and strategy. *Journal of the Institute of Health Education, 31*(1), 17–24. https://doi.org/10.10 80/03073289.1993.10805782

Barić, L. (1994). *Health promotion and health education in practice: Module 2 – The organisational model.* Barns.

Black, T., & Stanton, A. (2016, 4 February). *Final report on the development of the Okanagan Charter: An international charter for health promoting universities & colleges.* doi:http://dx.doi.org/10.14288/1.0372504

Brown, M. (2016). *FutuREstorative: Working towards a new sustainability*. RIBA Publishing.

Cole, R.J. (2011). Regenerative design and development: Current theory and practice. *Building Research & Information, 40*(1), 1–6. https://doi.org/10.1080/09613218.2012.617516

https://www.ipcc.ch/report/ar6/wg2/downloads/report/IPCC_AR6_WGII_FullReport.pdf

de León, E.A., Shriwise, A., Tomson, Gö., Morton, S., Lemos, D.S., Menne, B., & Dooris, M. (2021). Beyond building back better: Imagining a future for human and planetary health. *The Lancet Planetary Health, 5*(11), e827–e839. https://doi.org/10.1016/S2542-5196(21)00262-X.

Dolf, M. (2017). *A life cycle assessment of the environmental impacts of small to medium sports events* [PhD dissertation, University of British Columbia]. https://open.library.ubc.ca/collections/ubctheses/24/items/1.0362385

Dooris, M. (1998). Healthy cities and Local Agenda 21. *Health Promotion International, 14*(4), 365–75. https://doi.org/10.1093/heapro/14.4.365

Dooris, M. (2001). The "Health Promoting University": A critical exploration of theory and practice. *Health Education, 101*(2), 51–60. https://doi.org/10.1108/09654280110384108

Dooris, M. (2009). Holistic and sustainable health improvement: The contribution of the settings-based approach to health promotion. *Perspectives in Public Health, 129*(1), 29–36. https://doi.org/10.1177/1757913908098881.

Dooris, M. (2022). Health-promoting higher education. In Kokko, S., & Baybutt, M. (Eds.), *Handbook of settings-based health promotion* (pp. 151–65). Springer International Publishing. https://doi.org/10.1007/978-3-030-95856-5_8

Dooris, M., Cawood, J., Doherty, S., & Powell, S. (2010). *Healthy universities: Concept, model and framework for applying the healthy settings approach within higher education in England. Final project report*. RSPH. http://www.healthyuniversities.ac.uk/wp-content/uploads/2016/10/HU-Final_Report-FINAL_v21.pdf

Dooris, M., Doherty, S., Cawood, J., & Powell, S. (2012). The healthy universities approach: Adding value to the higher education sector. In Scriven, A., & Hodgins, M. (Eds.), *Health promotion settings: Principles and practice*. Sage.

Dooris, M., Doherty, S., & Orme, J. (2022). Applying salutogenesis in higher education. In Mittelmark,, M.B. Bauer, G.F., Vaandrager, L., Pelikan, J.M., Sagy, S., Eriksson, M., Lindström, B., & Meier Magistretti, C. (Eds.), *The handbook of salutogenesis* (pp. 307–19). Springer International Publishing. https://doi.org/10.1007/978-3-030-79515-3_30.

Dooris, M., Powell, S., & Farrier, A. (2020). Conceptualizing the 'whole university' approach: An international qualitative study. *Health Promotion International, 35*(4), 730–40. https://doi.org/10.1093/heapro/daz072.

Dooris, M., Powell, S., Parkin, D., & Farrier, A. (2021). Health promoting universities: Effective leadership for health, wellbeing and sustainability. *Health Education, 121*(3), 295–310. https://doi.org/10.1108/HE-12-2020-0121

Hancock, T. (2015). Population health promotion 2.0: An eco-social approach to public health in the Anthropocene. *Canadian Journal of Public Health, 106*(4), e252–e255. https://doi.org/10.17269/cjph.106.5161.

International Health Promoting Campuses Network. (n.d.). *International Health Promoting Campuses Network.* IHPCN. Retrieved 7 August 2022 from https://www.healthpromotingcampuses.org

IPBES. (2019). Summary for policymakers of the global assessment report on biodiversity and ecosystem services. IPBES secretariat. https://doi.org/10.5281/zenodo.3553579

Kickbush, I. (1996). Tribute to Aaron Antonovsky – 'What creates health.' *Health Promotion International, 11*(1), 5–6. https://doi.org/10.1093/heapro/11.1.5

Lyle, J.T. (1996). *Regenerative design for sustainable development.* John Wiley and Sons. http://ca.wiley.com/WileyCDA/WileyTitle/productCd-0471178438.html

Mang, P., & Reed, B. (2011). Designing from place: A regenerative framework and methodology. *Building Research & Information, 40*(1), 23–38. https://doi.org/10.1080/09613218.2012.621341

Meier, S., Stock, C., & Krämer, A. (2007). The contribution of health discussion groups with students to campus health promotion. *Health Promotion International, 22*(1), 28–36. https://doi.org/10.1093/heapro/dal041.

Naaldenberg, J., Vaandrager, L., Koelen, M., Wagemakers, A.-M., Saan, H., & de Hoog, K. (2009). Elaborating on systems thinking in health promotion practice. *Global Health Promotion, 16*(1), 39–47. https://doi.org/10.1177/1757975908100749.

Norman, T., & Reist, D. (2022). *Understanding substance use: A health promotion perspective.* HeretoHelp. https://www.heretohelp.bc.ca/infosheet/understanding-substance-use-a-health-promotion-perspective#top

Okanagan Charter: An International Charter for Health Promoting Universities and Colleges. (2015). *Okanagan Charter.* Kelowna, BC: Author. Retrieved from http://internationalhealthycampuses2015.sites.olt.ubc.ca/files/2016/01/Okanagan-Charter-January13v2.pdf

Orme, J., & Dooris, M. (2010). Integrating health and sustainability: The higher education sector as a timely catalyst. *Health Education Research, 25*(3), 425–37. https://doi.org/10.1093/her/cyq020.

Robinson, J., & Cole, R. J. (2015). Theoretical underpinnings of regenerative sustainability. *Building Research & Information, 43*(2), 133–43. https://doi.org/10.1080/09613218.2014.979082

Rockstrom, J., Steffen, W., Noone, K., Persson, A., Chapin, F.S., Lambin, E.F., Lenton, T.M., Scheffer, M., Folke, C., Schellnhuber, H.J., Nykvist, B., de Wit, C.A., Hughes, T., van der Leeuw, S., Rodhe, H., Sorlin, S., Snyder,

P.K., Costanza, R., Svedin, U., … Foley, J.A. (2009). A safe operating space for humanity. *Nature, 461*(7263), 472–5. https://doi.org/10.1038/461472a.

Squires, V., & London, C. (2021). The Okanagan Charter: Evolution of health promotion in Canadian higher education. *Canadian Journal of Higher Education / Revue canadienne d'enseignement Supérieur, 51*(3), 100–14. https://doi.org/10.47678/cjhe.vi0.189109

Suárez-Reyes, M., & Van den Broucke, S. (2016). Implementing the Health Promoting University approach in culturally different contexts: A systematic review. *Global Health Promotion, 23*(1 suppl), 46–56. https://doi.org/10.1177/1757975915623933.

United Nations (UN). (2022). *The Sustainable Development Goals Report 2022.*

University of British Columbia. (2018). *Shaping UBC's next century: Strategic Plan 2018–2028.* https://strategicplan.ubc.ca/wp-content/uploads/2019/09/2018_UBC_Strategic_Plan_Full-20180425.pdf

University of Central Lancashire. (2021). *Strategic Plan 2021–2028.* https://www.uclan.ac.uk/about-us/strategic-plan-2021-2028

University of Central Lancashire. (2022). *Strategic Plan 2021–2028 sub strategy sustainability. Priority 6: Future-uroofing our University.* https://www.uclan.ac.uk/assets/sustainability/sustainability-strategy.pdf

Waterworth, C., & Thorpe, A. (2017). Applying the Okanagan Charter in Aotearoa New Zealand. *Journal of the Australian & New Zealand Student Services Association, 49*, 49–61.

World Health Organization (WHO) (Ed.). (1986). *Ottawa Charter for Health Promotion.* https://www.who.int/teams/health-promotion/enhanced-wellbeing/first-global-conference

World Health Organization (WHO) (Ed.). (2005). *The Bangkok Charter for Health Promotion in a Globalized World.* https://www.who.int/teams/health-promotion/enhanced-wellbeing/sixth-global-conference/the-bangkok-charter

World Health Organization (WHO). (2006). *The Edmonton Charter for Health Promoting Universities and Institutions of Higher Education.* World Health Organization. https://healthycampuses.ca/wp-content/uploads/2015/01/2005_Edmonton_Charter_HPU.pdf

World Health Organization (WHO) (Ed.). (2021). *The Geneva Charter for Wellbeing.* https://www.who.int/publications/m/item/the-geneva-charter-for-wellbeing

World Health Organization (WHO) (Ed.). (2023). World health statistics 2023: Monitoring health for the SDGs, sustainable development goals.

2 Collaborative Leadership and Its Role in Whole Systems Approaches

VICKI SQUIRES, CHAD LONDON, AND OLENA SHAKHOVA

Current Context for Campus Leaders

Challenges that higher education institutions face today necessitate innovative approaches to leadership. An unpredictable financial environment, an increase in international partnerships, a need for new business frameworks, implementation of innovations and technologies, as well as changing demographics are some of the emergent issues that require new leadership solutions within the higher education sector (Kezar & Holcombe, 2017). Furthermore, there is pressure to progress from evaluating the outputs to measuring the impact of the practices across the entire institution and its core mandates of teaching, learning, and research (Jones & Harvey, 2017). Another crucial element that educational systems aspire to today is preparing students to effectively operate in a technology-driven multicultural society. Additionally, since the crucial competencies for future occupations are most likely to be collaboration and problem-solving skills, universities need to change their traditional models to ensure that students can be competitive in the workforce (O'Shea, 2021).

Moreover, the COVID-19 pandemic highlighted the crucial importance of health and wellbeing (Babb et al., 2022; Fruehwirth et al., 2021; Gestsdottir et al., 2021; Son et al., 2020). While the impacts on physical health due to COVID-19 were evident, the toll on mental health has been extraordinary (Carr et al., 2022; Charles et al., 2021; Wilson et al., 2021). Stress and depression were exacerbated by worries over financial wellbeing and the anxiety around the impacts of the pandemic on work and families (Browning et al., 2021; Hoyt et al., 2021; Schiff et al., 2022; Ulrich et al., 2021); additionally, the loss of or severely limited social connections with friends and family have contributed to a dramatic increase in reports of mental health issues (Leal Filho et al., 2021; Wang et al., 2020; Yorguner et al., 2021). Students from some demographic groups such as lesbian, gay, bisexual, and transgender communities may have faced even more pronounced challenges (Gonzales et al., 2020). These evolving challenges for post-secondary organizations are adding significant new pressures and require campuses to adapt to emergent conditions. According to Burns and Mooney (2018), a collaborative leadership approach supports a more nimble and responsive organization that is capable of adaptation. Furthermore, Van Wart (2013) contended that collaborative leadership is particularly well suited as a model for leading systems approaches to resolving the complex issues such as health promotion and wellbeing that are evident locally and globally.

This chapter describes shared leadership as an overarching theory and then examines in more depth collaborative leadership by exploring definitions of this approach and delineating it from other shared leadership approaches, describing its intended outcomes, different models, challenges of implementation, and conditions for its development in universities. The chapter ends with an example of a collaborative leadership model implemented to advance health promotion at one Canadian university.

Shared Leadership

The idea of multiple leaders was referred to as early as Follett's (1924) work, according to D'Innocenzo et al. (2016). However, the body of research literature on shared leadership has mostly evolved since the mid-1990s with a substantial debate on types of shared leadership emerging in the 2010s (D'Innocenzo et al., 2016). One prominent definition that has been taken up in multiple spaces is that offered by Pearce and Conger (2003). Shared leadership is a "dynamic, interactive influence process among individuals in groups for which the objective is to lead one another to the achievement of group or organizational goals or both. This influence process often involves peer, or lateral, influence and at other times involves upward or downward hierarchical influence" (p. 1). Some researchers including Kezar and Holcombe (2017) used the umbrella term "shared leadership" to encompass all forms of leadership where authority and power are shared in various ways. According to Kezar and Holcombe (2017), shared leadership is characterized by the involvement of a greater number of individuals, the interchange of leaders and followers, the use of several perspectives and expertise of different team members, and cooperation across the institution. Dampson et al. (2018) contended that multiple terms and models of shared leadership are very close in meaning and can be used interchangeably.

However, several researchers have tried to delineate the nuances among the models of shared leadership.

While shared leadership involves the engagement of different individuals in decision-making, it does not mean that the group is leaderless. It means that various team members display leadership behaviours and become leaders at different times, allowing everyone opportunities to be both a leader and a follower (Lawrence, 2017). Depending on the situation, different skills and knowledge might be needed, and accordingly, different individuals emerge as leaders. Moreover, Eckel and Kezar (2016) characterized shared leadership as a complex web of leadership with vertical and horizontal connections.

Importantly, Eckel and Kezar (2016) emphasized that shared governance systems are common in universities, but shared leadership is not. In shared governance, authority for certain topics or functions is delegated to specific bodies, but with shared leadership there is delegated authority for leading specific initiatives. Pearce et al. (2018) contended that shared governance was underpinned by scepticism, gatekeeping, and compliance, and was reactive, whereas shared leadership was founded on trust, shared decision making, commitment, and was proactive. Pearce et al. (2018) emphasized the need to move from shared governance to shared leadership.

According to Eckel and Kezar (2016), there are several strong advantages of a shared leadership model. First, the "rate and pace of decision making has increased" (p. 181) and senior executive leaders are accessing a larger network of leaders with expertise across a breadth of topics. Second, a shared leadership model enhances the capacity of the organization to address a larger, more complex, and more diverse agenda. Third, expanded leadership helps ensure that a diversity of perspectives is considered in understanding and addressing an issue. Lastly, a shared leadership model better serves the larger, more diverse, and more complex higher education institutions of the twenty-first century (Eckel & Kezar, 2016).

To provide more delineation, Kezar and Holcombe (2017) described three major models of shared leadership. In the first model, called co-leadership or pooled leadership, leadership is usually shared only between two co-leaders or small groups of individuals at the top of the institutional hierarchy. In this model, the roles of leaders are clearly differentiated and specialized. The second model, team leadership, is about the involvement of people with "the most relevant expertise ... at the most appropriate moment" (Kezar & Holcombe, 2017, p. 7). Leadership is shared both vertically and horizontally based on the pertinent expertise of team members. In the third model, known as distributed leadership, leadership is shared across organizations or organizational boundaries. Kezar and Holcombe (2017) described distributed leadership as a model in which different people at various levels "cross organizational boundaries" (p. 7) to affect a decision-making process during certain projects or times.

Other researchers have weighed in on the state of shared leadership theory and explored the many nuances among the related terms (D'Innocenzo et al., 2016: Ulhøi & Müller, 2014; Zhu et al., 2016). D'Innocenzo et al. (2016) identified that "the literature has become quite disjointed with a proliferation of nomenclature and conceptualizations" (p. 1965). Moreover, Ulhøi and Müller (2014) compared the various definitions for shared leadership and distributed leadership as evident in the literature, and then presented a further delineation of fourteen different concepts of collective forms of leadership described in the literature. While it is beyond the scope of this chapter to explore the differences among the concepts, a description of distributed leadership and a comparison to collaborative leadership will illustrate why collaborative leadership models are more applicable to the complexities of higher education institutional leadership and to the collective work required in addressing the complex problems we face today.

Distributed Leadership

One specific model of shared leadership is distributed leadership. While this model has been explored extensively within the context of primary and secondary education (cf. Hallinger & Heck, 2010; Spillane, 2012; Spillane et al., 2004), its application to post-secondary contexts is less common. However, researchers including Avissar et al. (2017), Floyd and Fung (2017), Jones et al. (2017), O'Shea (2021), and Vuori (2019) have illustrated the application of distributed leadership models in higher education.

In describing the model, O'Shea (2021) stated that distributed leadership is a practice in which educators in formal and non-formal management positions are given more independence in decision-making. Jones et al. (2017) noted that distributed leadership is underpinned by a collective and inclusive philosophy. This statement was supported by other researchers including Awadh (2018). According to Awadh, the value of this leadership approach lies within an opportunity for team members to see different viewpoints regardless of their ethnicity, race, culture, or socio-economic status. He also stressed that this model should create a favourable environment for teamwork, promote the engagement of all members, and, as a result, provide the institution with a variety of perspectives so that problems can be examined from multiple angles to generate possible solutions.

Because of this teamwork approach, distributed leadership is one of the tools that can contribute to the long-term implementation of whole systems approaches, such as sustainability in universities (Avissar et al., 2017). According to Avissar et al. (2017), this concept creates a change in the institutional internal culture that allows the promotion of more environment-related initiatives. Distributed leadership encourages the development of different structures that later become institutionalized and integrate sustainability into the institution as a whole (Avissar et al., 2017).

Avissar et al. (2017) shared this perspective on distributed leadership by mentioning that, within this model, leadership is a practice "shared between leaders, followers, and a situation" (p. 522). Moreover, Avissar et al. (2017) contended that distributed leadership consists of three distinguishing elements, which include emergent property, the openness of boundaries, and leadership according to expertise. Emergent property refers to the participation of groups in the leadership process and their interactions with each other. The openness of boundaries describes the blurring of boundaries that allows different individuals to emerge as leaders. Thus, leaders are emergent based on expertise that is relevant to the issue, and they work with other groups across boundaries.

In addition, Floyd and Fung (2017) highlighted the importance of creating meaningful relationships and involving more stakeholders in leadership. They stated that the goal is to have "more hands-on leadership, guidance, support and advice to individual academic colleagues, as well as to allow more staff to contribute to college-wide decision-making processes" (p. 1500). Similarly, Jones et al.'s (2017) research findings emphasized the need to develop an inclusive participatory approach where academic, administrative, professional, and executive staff work collaboratively within a network to develop systematic, multifaceted leadership.

Some of these elements were reflected in the distributed leadership description provided by Jones et al. (2017), who identified the foundations for distributed leadership as engagement of people, the organization of supportive processes, the arrangement of professional development and networking opportunities, and the presence of resources. They defined four main dimensions of this concept, which included "a context of trust; a culture of respect; recognition of the need to change from a single hierarchical decision-making process to an approach combining top-down, middle-out, bottom-up methods; and collaborative relationships" (p. 199). O'Shea (2021) also emphasized empowerment through decision-making as one of the main elements of distributed leadership because individuals will have some influence and control over their own work. While many of these same elements are part of a collaborative leadership model, there are nuanced differences that are further described in the next section.

Defining Collaborative Leadership

DeWitt (2018), writing from the perspective of primary and secondary education, defined collaborative leadership as the "purposeful actions that we take as leaders to enhance the instruction of teachers, build deep relationships with all stakeholders through understanding self-efficacy, and build collective efficacy to deepen our learning together" (p.10). A similar viewpoint was expressed by Bishop et al. (2017), who described collaborative leadership as shared power where participants are "exploring together, dwelling together, struggling together, and creating together" (p. 70).

Jones and Harvey (2017) claimed that universities today need leadership that is founded on collaboration and not authority or positions. Collaborative leadership, founded on cooperation and teamwork, allows for overcoming challenges that are created by the needs of a modern technology-driven society of the twenty-first century (Kezar & Holcombe, 2017). Van Wart (2013) also posited that collaborative leadership is well suited as a framework for leading systems. Specifically, a collaborative leadership structure assists with boundary crossing and dismantling silos. This structural challenge was emphasized by Burns and Mooney (2018), who noted that "numerous semi-autonomous academic, administrative, and staff structures characterized by relatively highly educated, creative individuals make the higher education environment particularly susceptible to 'silo' thinking which limits the communication and interaction across areas necessary for optimal success" (p. 61). Thus, finding effective mechanisms and using leadership approaches to work across boundaries is essential if we are to address considerable global challenges.

At the same time, it is important to mention that one of the crucial parts of collaborative leadership is the engagement of people who represent diverse backgrounds. Lawrence (2017) discussed the benefits of global collaboration, which allows exploring different opinions and expertise that might not exist in one's local culture. Furthermore, he stated that "when we value all contributions, and embrace diversity, the collaborative team is strengthened" (p. 93). Kezar and Holcombe (2017) posited that certain groups, such as women or racial and ethnic minorities, often show an interest in adopting a collaborative leadership approach, which leads to increasing workplace diversity.

Moreover, different authors also provided various characteristics of the collaborative leadership model. The collaboration and consideration of different viewpoints that Kezar and Holcombe (2017) described as critical to shared leadership are enhanced in a model of collaborative leadership as described by Lawrence (2017). Lawrence emphasized that collaborative leadership included "shared vision and values, interdependence and shared responsibility, mutual respect, empathy and willingness to be vulnerable, ambiguity, effective communication, and synergy" (p. 91). Interestingly, VanVector (2012) noted that most definitions include elements pertaining to coordination of a task, working synergistically, and engaging in mutually established work processes. The interactions and engagement foster motivation and lead to collective outcomes that outweigh the sum of individual contributions (VanVector, 2012). Kouzes and Posner (2007) added that collaboration is so crucial to organizational and leadership success that collaborative relationships must be prioritized and supported.

These collaborative relationships are supported and nurtured through strong communication strategies; "collaborative communication strategies involve an unimpeded, continual cycle of information flowing freely among the members of a team and organization" (VanVector, 2012, p. 555). According to VanVector (2012), developing a robust and collaborative communication strategy must be prioritized. This framework supports opportunities to create an ongoing dialogue and prioritizes two-way communication because the effectiveness of the communication strategy is measured through the feedback loop. VanVector (2012) noted that "communicating collaboratively must become a perpetual cycle of interactivity among multiple stakeholders to ensure communication channels remain unimpeded" (p. 560).

VanVector (2012) posited that "collaborative leadership is a unique style of leadership that is styled as a transformational style of leadership" (p. 561) where multiple groups and individuals work towards a common goal. Input is sought from multiple individuals for the purposes of decision-making; critical to inviting this input is the development of trust (Burns & Mooney, 2018). The climate of trust removes constraints, and colleagues are able to freely innovate and problem solve together (Burns & Mooney, 2018). Burns and Mooney (2018) contended that collaborative leaders are "curators of talent who motivate" (p. 59); they minimize power differentials and empower others to contribute. Furthermore, Burns and Mooney (2018) contended that collaborative leaders are excellent at boundary crossing and working with diverse groups. They are ready to face complex challenges even when the way forward is unclear and there may be disagreement on the best approach. As well, they are skilled at focusing attention during the collaborative process even when it appears messy and unfocused.

Jappinen (2014) also identified that, as organizational complexity expands, so must the leaders develop a better understanding of the complex human dynamics within organizations. Leaders need to establish the environment to best facilitate these interactions by ensuring that there is "collective, personal, moral and social responsibility; supportive and shared attitudes; high moral standards; approval of jointly agreed-upon practices; finishing one's obligations; proactive attitudes; and long-term activities" (Jappinen, 2014, p. 11). Jappinen's (2014) study emphasized effective decision-making processes that support this collective work and enhance collective impact. Specifically, possible solutions are developed through the promotion of exploring alternate solutions, investigating the contributing and underlying issues, allowing for intuition, examining unexpected results, and making incremental decisions that move organizations towards the end goals (Jappinen, 2014).

Several authors posited that the collaborative leadership model addresses a primary weakness of the silo-based structure of the contemporary post-secondary institution, namely, the "inability of the institution to take full advantage of skills and expertise presently on campus" (Burns & Mooney, 2018, p. 62). By setting up the conditions for effective communication, decision-making, and relationship building, universities can invite fulsome exploration of solutions from multiple perspectives and types of expertise across campuses. Now that the description of shared leadership as a broad term has been articulated, and the nuances of collaborative leadership and distributed leadership have been described, we present in the next section the critiques of these types of leadership models. Understanding the critiques helps leaders proactively address these issues, resulting in a stronger application and implementation of the models.

Critiques of Shared and Collaborative Leadership

Youngs (2017) stated that distributed and collaborative leadership models are claimed to be leadership approaches that can bridge the divide between professional and academic staff groups, a dualistic positioning that arose through practices implemented because of the influence of New Public Management, an approach that privileged performance indicators and global competition; however, Youngs contended that these leadership models may instead maintain this duality and reaffirm these structures and interests. He added that distributing leadership can become a functional tool to distribute the workload and activities across all employees rather than meaningful distribution of influence and authority in decision-making. Furthermore, those who have budgetary authority hold a disproportionate degree of influence in decision-making, and if participants are invited to provide advice rather than authentically engage in decision-making, there is an illusion of shared leadership (Youngs, 2017). Erosion of trust and emergence of scepticism will be a result.

Additionally, collaborative leaders may need to further develop their skills to be effective. O'Leary et al. (2010) noted that professional development should focus on cultivating skills and capacities such as "convening a network with the right members, structuring governance processes, engaging in collaborative practice using the skills of negotiation, facilitation, and conflict management, designing processes for public engagement, evaluating progress toward outcomes, and ensuring that the network operates in a transparent and accountable fashion" (p. 586). Developing these skills will take time and mentorship. This challenge is exacerbated when most of the leaders of academic units have engaged in minimal professional development or deeper learning regarding leadership and have been appointed to the leadership position by virtue of their academic expertise in a specific field (Austin & Jones, 2016).

Lastly, as stated previously, shared governance models, which are predominant in higher education, are not necessarily aligned with shared leadership models (Eckel & Kesar, 2016); in shared governance models, authority for specific functions is delegated to a body whose membership is clearly defined. These governance bodies are constituted through by-laws and policies adopted by the institution (Austin & Jones, 2016). These structures may be further entrenched through legislative acts that established the post-secondary institutions. These structural boundaries may be difficult to penetrate, even when representatives from the various governing bodies may be participating in collaborative leadership teams that focus on an institutional priority. In the following section, possible strategies to establish a successful collaborative leadership structure will be explored as potential ways to ameliorate these aforementioned challenges.

Models for Implementing Collaborative Leadership

Several researchers proposed defined models and aligned frameworks that can contribute to the effective implementation of this concept. For example, Lawrence (2017) described three major theoretical frameworks that can underpin collaborative leadership at universities. These frameworks are transformative learning, experiential learning, and feminist theory. By transformative learning, the author implied a need to make a shift from a hierarchical notion of leadership to a culture of collaboration. However, to do that it is important to start with the individual transformation of a leader to be open to the creation of this collaborative culture in the organization. A leader needs to make a change from seeing oneself as an individual to being a part of the group. Through the second framework of experiential learning, team members are encouraged to share their experiences and reflect on them. Such learning takes the form of a collaborative activity, where everyone is seen as potential teachers and learners (Lawrence, 2017). The third framework, feminist theory, challenges patriarchy and hierarchical leadership models that often oppress numerous groups such as women, people of colour, individuals with disabilities, and 2SLGBTQ+ people. Collaborative leadership that uses this framework provides team members with a "more inclusive and equitable strategy for leading" (Lawrence, 2017, p. 91).

Interestingly, Burns and Mooney (2018) extended the model of collaborative leadership by describing transcollegial leadership within the context of higher education. Briefly defined, transcollegial leadership is "the process involved in leaders systematically, but informally, relating to persons and groups of equivalent authority in different areas of an institution of higher education for the advancement of its mission, not for personal gain" (Burns & Mooney, 2018, p. 63). They posited that implementation of such a model can deepen and sustain collaborative processes and lead to strong institutional outcomes.

After making efforts to implement a collaborative leadership approach, it is important to evaluate measures undertaken to foster this concept on campus. Thus, understanding which model of collaborative leadership the university is going to use, which theoretical framework underpins it, and how to assess the effectiveness of this model's implementation can help universities execute collaborative leadership in a way that strengthens its positive effects.

Effects of Collaborative Leadership

The positive outcomes of collaboration and collaborative leadership are stressed by all the authors who researched this concept. This leadership approach affects all the stakeholders involved in the decision-making process and, thereby, individuals affected by these decisions. Some of the parties whose roles and operations will undergo significant but positive changes due to the implementation of collaborative leadership on campus are senior management, faculty and staff, and students. For all constituents, a collaborative leadership structure is conducive to fostering a sense of belonging, which in turn enhances commitment to the organization and its priorities (Burns & Mooney, 2018).

Importantly, senior leaders can see "increased satisfaction among team members, stronger group cohesion, increased confidence, trust, and social integration, more constructive interaction style, better coordination of activities, and higher task reliability" (Kezar & Holcombe, 2017, p. 8). Additionally, collaboration promotes a culture on campus that fosters innovation (O'Shea, 2021; Vuori, 2019). According to Vuori (2019), this approach also decreases the perceived gap between the administrative and teaching staff, which positively affects the operations of the entire institution. For example, the teaching staff becomes more empowered (O'Shea, 2021) leading to enhanced innovation in pedagogy and changes in the curriculum. Because of the increased sense of empowerment, university members are better linked to a common goal, which makes them more engaged in the activities of the institution (Awadh, 2018). The impact may also extend beyond the campus boundaries. Vuori (2019) claimed that collaborative leadership encourages the creation of partnerships with local employers and can help increase students' employment rates.

Working with internal and external partners is also beneficial in addressing global challenges such as sustainability. After the adoption of the 2030 UN Sustainable Development Agenda, there was an increase in research that focused on the importance of the education sector in solving sustainability-related challenges that the world is currently facing (Žalėnienėa & Pereira, 2021). Since collaborative leadership encourages partnerships and joint efforts among different departments, it is possible to create a holistic sustainability discourse on campus.

Another stakeholder that undoubtedly receives benefits from the implementation of collaborative leadership on campus is employees, namely, faculty and staff. First and foremost, this leadership approach positively affects their health and wellbeing (Vuori, 2019). It is also important to stress that the increase in job satisfaction among educators results from collaborative leadership, according to O'Shea (2021). DeWitt (2018) contended that it also allows educators to improve self-efficacy and create collective efficacy. Awadh (2018) supported this contention, adding that collaborative leadership allows them to increase their abilities in achieving educational goals, and enhances motivation, empowerment, performance, and a sense of responsibility. Through the exchange of knowledge and joint efforts in troubleshooting, faculty and staff can become more confident in their ability to motivate their students (Awadh, 2018). These benefits realized by faculty and staff will also positively affect students' engagement and hence their performance.

Other benefits that students receive due to collaborative leadership include a change from being passive receivers of information to active learners (Vuori, 2019), which aligns with Lawrence's (2017) second frame of experiential learning; by being invested in the process of decision-making, students enhance their self-efficacy and motivation. Because of being more engaged in their education, students are more involved in creating a learning environment where they can develop and test new ideas (O'Shea, 2021). Thus, when implemented successfully, collaborative leadership positively affects all stakeholders involved in the decision-making process and the beneficiaries of these decisions.

Moreover, Humphreys (2013) believed that collaborative leadership had reputational and operational benefits for higher education institutions. He posited that the implementation of this model of leadership will help to

1 develop greater understanding of our enterprise among the public, policymakers, students, parents, and members of the media in order to garner the financial and regulatory support we need to maintain healthy institutions;
2 increase the efficiency with which we maintain the quality of our operations; and
3 develop more effective ways to actually educate a far wider proportion of the society to meet twenty-first-century demands. (Humphreys, 2013, p. 2)

Collaboration across the institution improves outcomes for internal constituents and can also promote better understanding and build upon relationships with external constituents.

Challenges in Implementing Collaborative Leadership

The engagement of an increased number of stakeholders will inevitably lead to certain challenges. Many authors indicated that the implementation of collaborative leadership might be a difficult experience, especially at the beginning of this process. For example, as stated by Lawrence (2017), fostering collaborative leadership means accepting and being willing to live with ambiguities and uncertainties. This environment can become a barrier, especially for leaders who are used to being in control. Besides having to change a familiar model of decision-making, senior leadership also has to overcome another challenge – accountability. Even though leadership functions are distributed among employees in a collaborative leadership model, senior leaders are the ones who are ultimately responsible for these decisions (Floyd & Fung, 2017). These barriers and the difficulties in the prediction of outcomes can put additional pressure on university governance, as pointed out by Lawrence (2017).

However, even when leaders agree to share a decision-making process, faculty, staff, and students may hold a sceptical view of leadership and may not trust the process; furthermore, they may see their involvement in leadership as unnecessary and unrewarding (Avissar et al., 2017). For this reason, they might view collaboration as a waste of time that is not worthy of their efforts. It is important to stress that collaborative leadership might not remedy all the problems that an institution faces. Avissar et al. (2017) stated that a group may not be able to fully achieve the organization's initial plans and the group will not be sustainable; changes in personnel and changes in campus leadership add to this challenge. VanVector's (2012) study of collaborative leadership within a health care setting uncovered the negative impacts that inter-organizational barriers and intra-organizational silos can have on effective decision-making; this critique can be applied to higher education institutions as well. Working collaboratively to dismantle those barriers would also be beneficial in massaging the strategy and improving results.

Even if employees decide to engage in leadership activities, the involvement of many stakeholders in decision-making can lead to contradictory messages from the university, crossed lines of communication, and opposition to the organizational value systems (Floyd & Fung, 2017). Kezar and Holcombe (2017) shared this viewpoint by stating that collaborative leadership can contribute to the creation of different views on organizational values, such as shared governance, institutional and professional autonomy, and academic freedom. It can also result in the emergence of different interests and agendas due to the involvement of many stakeholders, which causes decision-making to slow down. The time taken for collaborative decision-making can be challenging, especially in times of crises where direction is urgently needed (Austin & Jones, 2016).

Another potential negative consequence of collaborative leadership is groupthink (Kezar & Holcombe, 2017), which is a phenomenon that occurs when team members choose unanimity over an objective estimation of the situation (Akhmad et al., 2021). It is also important to mention that since the foundation of collaborative leadership is communication, there are cases where shared decision-making can be more difficult, if not impossible, due to barriers which may be related to "language, culture, education, or mental capacity and external factors like the state of emergency or the availability of alternative sources of information" (Giuliani et al., 2019). Therefore, while this leadership approach does have many benefits, it is important to consider the challenges that stakeholders can face while implementing it. Being prepared to face these barriers is crucial for the university's governance team to react to them promptly, and, thus, ensure that the positive effects of collaborative leadership can be realized.

Conditions for Fostering Collaborative Leadership in Universities

To incorporate collaborative leadership effectively in the university's operations, there is a need to create a certain environment. Many researchers shared similar viewpoints on the elements that contribute to the creation of this environment. First, the university needs to establish a culture that would promote the importance of collaboration (Jones et al., 2012). As stated by Lawrence (2017), collaborative leadership is not only about working together, but it is also about putting joint efforts into the creation of "a new culture that values collective learning and decision-making" (p. 94). Second, to establish such a culture there is a need for support from university governance that would encourage team members to cooperate. This statement was supported by researchers DeWitt (2018), Jones et al. (2017), and Kezar and Holcombe (2017), who claimed the need for support across vertical or hierarchical structures. The university's senior leaders should be the ones who help faculty and staff let go of the "need to be the sole expert" (Lawrence, 2017, p. 93). Kezar and Holcombe (2017) explained that "it is critical for vertical leaders to establish support structures and delegate authority so that the team is empowered to think and act creatively to solve the problem" (p. 22). Third, it is crucial to have a shared purpose, goal, and vision (DeWitt, 2018; Kezar & Holcombe, 2017).

After ensuring there are supportive leaders who are invested in establishing a culture of collaboration and shared vision, it is crucial to nurture relationships. One of the essential criteria for collaborative leadership is a powerful team where every individual is valued (Awadh, 2018). Lawrence (2017) highlighted the importance of creating connections that go beyond collegial, to relationships where team members get to know each other as individuals and cultivate trust. Since employees are often not used to shared decision-making, it might take time and members may need to engage in more professional development before the process has clarity and members adapt (Lawrence, 2017). Jones et al. (2017) also emphasized that it is important to implement professional development training since some employees might lack skills in teamwork and experience in leadership positions.

Another element that plays a significant role in ensuring collaborative leadership can work successfully to implement agreed-upon initiatives is resources. Floyd and Fung (2017) stated that for institutions to overcome certain challenges, it is essential first to understand the availability of resources and then to allocate them in a way that would allow leaders to collaboratively establish certain initiatives; this sentiment is reiterated by DeWitt (2018) and Jones et al. (2017). Moreover, when team members are encouraged to participate in decision-making, they will develop stronger commitment and will bring more resources and engagement to the task (Wu & Cormican, 2021). Therefore, it is essential to understand what kind of resources each team member has and allocate them appropriately to advance the social capital of the team. Furthermore, the dedication of human and financial resources to a strategy elevates that work and indicates to the campus that the work is among the high priorities identified by the governing bodies.

After an institution decides on a model to incorporate collaborative leadership and then works to establish the conditions necessary to embed collaborative leadership in its daily operations, it is important to continue to promote this approach among university employees. According to DeWitt (2018), to promote collaboration, all leaders from various organizational levels and units should become involved in the leadership growth cycle that consists of stages of goal setting, understanding current realities, evidence gathering, and action steps. O'Shea (2021) claimed that one of the ways to promote collaborative leadership is to raise awareness about the positive effects of this approach.

Collaborative leadership is a promising model that may support the higher education sector in overcoming barriers caused by the challenges that are arising in the technology-driven and increasingly complex globalized society of the twenty-first century. However, to overcome these constraints, university leaders should understand the model and theoretical frameworks underpinning the model, possible challenges of its implementation, and conditions needed to consider during its execution. In this way, university governance will create an institutional culture that values the contribution of different stakeholders, resulting in a positive impact on all constituents of higher education campuses. The following section explains a real example from our work on health promotion efforts.

Putting the Collaborative Leadership Work in Perspective: Why Does This Matter?

Interestingly, in our study exploring the implementation of the Okanagan Charter at the first ten signatory campuses in Canada, leadership emerged as a crucial and foundational piece of the process; the full findings of the study will be described in another chapter later in this book. We identified that much of the University of British Columbia's successful implementation of the Charter was attributed to the implementation of a collaborative leadership approach. Wellbeing champions from that campus labelled the leadership structure specifically as collaborative leadership and noted that the model first emerged on their campus to support the implementation of a holistic sustainability strategy for the campus. The processes and practices established to further sustainability priorities across the campus were adopted by the health promotion team members so that wellbeing and health promotion initiatives would be embedded across the organizational boundaries and be evident to all members of the campus.

Notably, there is a dedicated team of administrative professionals who support the initiative. These team members coordinate the communication strategies, serve as liaisons with academic and other administrative units, and organize opportunities to bring interested constituents together and harness their engagement and attachment with the aligned activities. There are champions on campus who are instrumental promoters of the wellbeing initiatives and programs. Importantly, the president was seen as being the ultimate champion of the work; he used every opportunity to highlight the ongoing concerns regarding mental health issues. He emphasized that everyone should strive to achieve work-life balance throughout his public-facing engagements. The president was part of a high-level steering committee that oversaw the work of the support teams and the multi-stakeholder working groups. While the pinnacle of the hierarchy remained the president in terms of setting priorities, there were leaders at multiple levels of the organization who led particular groups or initiatives.

In addition to the formal leaders on campus, the health promotion group provided students, faculty, and staff with opportunities for authentic engagement as members, and furthermore, students led or were core members of some of the initiatives. Smaller groups facilitated core activities and innovative programs. Then, the whole group met once or twice a year to engage in dialogue regarding the progress that was made and future actions. Membership in this group included people who held key formal leadership positions, emergent leaders from all levels of the organization, and people with expertise relevant to specific projects or goals; even though membership changed over time, the collaborative environment was conducive to ensuring the work continued despite some turnover in team members. Importantly, milestones and goals were developed during these conversations so that everyone understood the direction of the group and the framework or roadmap for achieving those well-articulated goals. The members of the group also were tasked with spreading awareness beyond the boundaries of the group to others in their units; a website dedicated to health promotion ensured that the campus members could discover the details of the priorities and the aligned actions and milestones. Even people outside of the organization can access the extensive information easily. Thus, the health promotion strategy is well-articulated, transparent, and supported by a collaborative network of formal and informal leaders across the campus.

Interestingly, the structure supporting UBC Wellbeing was described by Dooris (2022) in his work examining health promoting higher education; UBC was one of three cases he presented in that chapter. Dooris (2022) noted that there were connections among senior executive leaders, unit leaders, and student leaders through the steering committee, and the Strategic Support Team assisted with the organization, coordination, and implementation of the initiatives. This model exemplified the elements of the "whole university" approach as described by Dooris et al. (2019). Dooris et al. (2019) presented a conceptual framework for this approach, highlighting that universities must "knit together disparate areas of activity and bridge silos" (p. 731) and that there was a need to "balance top-down leadership and direction with bottom-up engagement, ownership and action" (p. 731). A collaborative leadership model reflects the notions described by Dooris and his colleagues.

The criticality of appropriate leadership structures is highlighted in this one example. This leadership structure was widely recognized across campus as a collaborative leadership model and labelled as such. The joined-up approach of leadership at multiple levels of the organization ensures that everyone's voices are heard and that pockets of expertise are leveraged to build a joined-up approach for addressing complex and emergent problems.

Conclusion

Collaborative leadership is a promising approach that can be applied at higher education institutions to further cross-institutional goals such as a health promotion strategy or a sustainability plan. This approach is especially beneficial when leading complex systems and engaging in systemic change. The shared governance systems in higher education may prove challenging to navigate when trying to establish a shared leadership model for cross-institutional work. However, the complexities and challenges of higher education in the twenty-first century may be better addressed by collaborative models drawing in expertise to share perspectives and galvanize strengths.

REFERENCES

Akhmad, M., Chang, S., & Deguchi, H. (2021). Closed-mindedness and insulation in groupthink: Their effects and the devil's advocacy as a preventive measure. *Journal of Computational Social Science, 4*, 455–78. https://doi.org/10.1007/s42001-020-00083-8

Austin, I., & Jones, G. (2016). *Governance of higher education: Global perspectives, theories, and practices.* Routledge.

Avissar, I., Alkaher, I., & Gan, D. (2017). The role of distributed leadership in mainstreaming environmental sustainability into campus life in an

Israeli teaching college: A case study. *International Journal of Sustainability in Higher Education, 19*(3), 518–46. https://doi.org/10.1108/IJSHE -07-2017-0105

Awadh, M. (2018). The effects of collective leadership on student achievement and teacher instruction. *Open Journal of Leadership, 7*(4), 1–16. https://doi .org/10.4236/ojl.2018.74015

Babb, S.J., Rufino, K.A., & Johnson, R.M. (2022). Assessing the effects of the COVID-19 pandemic on nontraditional students' mental health and wellbeing. *Adult Education Quarterly, 72*(2), 140–57. https://doi.org/10.1177 /07417136211027508

Bishop, K., Weigler, W., Lloyd, T., & Beare, D. (2017). Fostering collaborative leadership through playbuilding. *New Directions for Adult and Continuing Education, 156*, 65–75. https://doi.org/10.1002/ace.20260

Browning, M., Larson, L.R., Sharaievska, I., Rigolon, A., McAnirlin, O., Mullenbach, L., ... & Alvarez, H.O. (2021). Psychological impacts from COVID-19 among university students: Risk factors across seven states in the United States. *PloS ONE, 16*(1), e0245327. https://doi.org/10.1371/journal .pone.0245327

Burns, D.J., & Mooney, D. (2018). Transcollegial leadership: A new paradigm for leadership. *International Journal of Educational Management, 32*(1), 57–70. https://doi.org/10.1108/IJEM-05-2016-0114.

Carr, E., Davis, K., Bergin-Cartwright, G., Lavelle, G., Leightley, D., Oetzmann, C., ... & Hotopf, M. (2022). Mental health among UK university staff and postgraduate students in the early stages of the COVID-19 pandemic. *Occupational and Environmental Science, 79*(4), 259–67. https://doi. org/10.1136/oemed-2021-107667

Charles, N.E., Strong, S.J., Burns, L.C., Bullerjahn, M.R., & Serafine, K.M. (2021). Increased mood disorder symptoms, perceived stress, and alcohol use among college students during the COVID-19 pandemic. *Psychiatry Research, 296*, 113706. https://doi.org/10.1016/j.psychres.2021.113706

Dampson, D.G., Havor, F.M., & Laryea, P. (2018). Distributed leadership an instrument for school improvement: The study of public senior high schools in Ghana. *Journal of Education and e-Learning Research, 5*(2), 79–85. https:// doi.org/10.20448/journal.509.2018.52.79.85

DeWitt, P. M. (2018). What is collaborative leadership? In P.M. DeWitt (Ed.), *School climate: Leading with collective efficacy* (pp. 9–34). Corwin.

D'Innocenzo, L., Mathieu, J.E., & Kukenberger, M.R. (2016). A meta-analysis of different forms of shared leadership – Team performance relations. *Journal of Management, 42*(7), 1964–91. https://doi.org/10.1177/0149206314525205

Dooris, M. (2022). Health-promoting higher education. In S. Kokko & M. Baybutt (Eds.), *Handbook of settings-based health promotion* (pp. 151–65). Springer.

Dooris, M., Powell, S., & Farrier, A. (2019). Conceptualizing the 'whole university approach: An international qualitative study. *Health Promotion International, 35*, 730–740. https://doi.org/10.1093/heapro/daz072

Eckel, P.D., & Kezar, A. (2016). The intersecting authority of boards, presidents, and faculty: Toward shared leadership. In MN. Bastedo, P. G. Albach, & P. . Gumport (Eds.), *American higher education in the twenty-first century: Social, political, and economic challenges* (pp. 155–87). Johns Hopkins University Press.

Floyd, A., & Fung, D. (2017). Focusing the kaleidoscope: Exploring distributed leadership in an English university. *Studies in Higher Education, 42*(8), 1488–1503. https://doi.org/10.1080/03075079.2015.1110692

Fruehwirth, J.C., Biswas, S., & Perreira, K.M. (2021). The COVID-19 pandemic and mental health of first-year college students: Examining the effect of COVID-19 stressors using longitudinal data. *PLoS ONE, 16*(3), e024799. https://doi.org/10.1371/journal.pone.024799

Gestsdottir, S., Gisladottir, T., Stefansdottir, R., Johannsson, E., Jakobsdottir, G., & Rognvaldsdottir, V. (2021). Health and wellbeing of university students before and during COVID-19 pandemic: A gender comparison. *PLoS ONE, 16*(12), e0261346. https://doi.org/10.1371/journal.pone.0261346

Gonzales, G., de Molab, E.L., Gavulic, K.A., McKay, T., & Purcell, C. (2020). Mental health needs among lesbian, gay, bisexual, and transgender college students during the COVID-19 pandemic. *Journal of Adolescent Health, 67*, 645–8. https://doi.org/10.1016/j.jadohealth.2020.08.006

Giuliani, E., Melegari, G., Carrieri, F., & Barbieri, A. (2019). Overview of the main challenges in shared decision making in a multicultural and diverse society in the intensive and critical care setting. *Journal of Evaluation in Clinical Practice, 26*, 520–3. https://doi.org/10.1111/jep.13300

Hallinger, P., & Heck, R.H. (2010). Leadership for learning: Does collaborative leadership make a difference in school improvement? *Educational Management Administration and Leadership, 38*(6), 654–78. https://doi.org/10.1177/1741143210379060

Hoyt, L.T., Cohen, A.K., Dull, B., Castro, E.M., & Yazdani, N. (2021). "Constant stress has become the new normal": Stress and anxiety inequalities among U.S. college students in the time of COVID-19. *Journal of Adolescent Health, 68*(2), 270–6. https://doi.org/10.1016/j.jadohealth.2020.10.030.

Humphreys, D. (2013). Deploying collaborative leadership to reinvent higher education for the twenty-first century. *Peer Review, 15*(1), 4–6.

Jappinen, A. (2014). Collaborative educational leadership: The emergence of human interactional sense-making process as a complex system. *Complicity: An International Journal of Complexity in Education, 11*(2), 65–85. https://doi.org/10.29173/cmplct22978

Jones, S., & Harvey, M. (2017). A distributed leadership change process model for higher education. *Journal of Higher Educational Policy and*

Management, 39(2), 126–39. http://dx.doi.org/10.1080/1360080X.2017
.1276661

Jones, S., Harvey, M., Hamilton, J., Bevacqua, J., & Egea, K. (2017).
Demonstrating the impact of a distributed leadership approach in higher
education. *Journal of Higher Educational Policy and Management, 39*(2), 197–211.
http://dx.doi.org/10.1080/1360080X.2017.1276567

Jones, S., Lefoeb, G., Harvey, M., & Ryland, K. (2012). Distributed leadership:
A collaborative framework for academics, executives and professionals in
higher education. *Journal of Higher Education Policy and Management, 34*(1),
67–78. https://doi.org/10.1080/1360080X.2012.642334

Kezar, J., & Holcombe, E.M. (2017). *Shared leadership in higher education:
Important lessons from research and practice.* American Council on Education.
https://www.acenet.edu/Documents/Shared-Leadership-in-Higher
-Education.pdf

Kouzes, J.M., & Posner, B.Z. (2007). *The leadership challenge* (4th ed.). Wiley.

Lawrence, R.L. (2017). Understanding collaborative leadership in theory and
practice. *New directions for adult and continuing education, 156*, 89–96. https://
doi.org/10.1002/ace.20262

Leal Filho, W., Wall, T., Rayman-Bacchus, L., Mifsud, M., Pritchard,
D.J., Lovren, V O., & Balogun, A.L. (2021). Impacts of COVID-19 and social
isolation on academic staff and students at universities: A cross-sectional
study. *BMC Public Health, 21*(1), 1–19. https://doi.org/10.1186/s12889-021
-11040-z.

O'Leary, R., Blomgren Bingham, L., & Choi, Y. (2010). Teaching collaborative
leadership: Ideas and lessons for the field. *Journal of Public Affairs, Education,
16*(4), 565–92. https://doi.org/10.1080/15236803.2010.12001615

O'Shea, C. (2021). Distributed leadership and innovative teaching practices.
International Journal of Educational Research Open, 2, 1–12. https://doi.org
/10.1016/j.ijedro.2021.100088

Pearce, C.L., & Conger, J.A. (2003). All those years ago: The historical
underpinnings of shared leaders. In C.L. Pearce & J.A. Conger (Eds.), *Shared
leadership: Reframing the hows and whys of leadership* (pp. 1–18). Sage.

Pearce, C.L., Wood, B.G., & Wassenaar, C.L. (2018). The future of leadership
in public universities: Is shared leadership the answer? *Public Administration
Review, 78*(4), 640–4. https://doi.org/10.1111/puar.12938

Schiff, M., Pat-Horenczyk, R., & Benbenishty, R. (2022). University students
coping with COVID-19 challenges: Do they need help? *Journal of American
College Health*, 1-9. https://doi.org/10.1080/07448481.2022.2048838.

Son, C., Hegde, S., Smith, A., Wang, X., & Sasangohar, F. (2020). Effects of
COVID-19 on college students' mental health in the United States: Interview
survey study. *Journal of Medical Internet Research, 22*(9), 1–14. https://doi.org
/10.2196/21279.

Spillane, J. (2012) *Distributed leadership.* Jossey-Bass.

Spillane, J., Halverson, R., & Diamond, J. (2004). Towards a theory of leadership practice: A distributed perspective. *Journal of Curriculum Studies, 36*(1), 3–34. https://doi.org/10.1080/0022027032000106726

Ulhøi, J.P., & Müller, S. (2014). Mapping the landscape of shared leadership: A review and synthesis. *International Journal of Leadership Studies, 8*(2), 66–87.

Ulrich, A.K., Full, K.M., Cheng, B., Gravagna, K., Nederhoff, D., & Basta, NE. (2021). Stress, anxiety, and sleep among college and university students during the COVID-19 pandemic. *Journal of American College Health, 71*(5), 1323–7. https://doi.org/10.1080/07448481.2021.1928143

VanVector, J. D. (2012). Collaborative leadership model in the management of health care. *Journal of Business Research, 65*, 555–61. https://doi.org/10.1016/j.busres.2011.02.021

Van Wart, M. (2013). Lessons from leadership theory and the contemporary challenges of leaders. *Public Administration Review, 73*(4), 553– 65. https://doi.org/10.1111/puar.12069

Vuori, J. (2019). Distributed leadership in the construction of a new higher education campus and community. *Educational Management Administration and Leadership, 47*(2), 224–40. https://doi.org/10.1177/1741143217725322

Wang, X., Hegde, S., Son, C., Keller, B., Smith, A., & Sasangohar, F. (2020). Investigating mental health of US college students during the COVID-19 pandemic: Cross-sectional survey study. *Journal of Medical Internet Research, 22*(9), e22817. 1-11. https://doi.org/10.2196/22817.

Wilson, O.W., Holland, KE., Elliott, L. D., Duffey, M. & Bopp, M. (2021). The impact of the COVID-19 pandemic on US college students' physical activity and mental health. *Journal of Physical Activity and Health, 18*, 272–8. https://doi.org/10.1123/jpah.2020-0325.

Wu, Q., & Cormican, K. (2021). Shared leadership and team effectiveness: An investigation of whether and when in engineering design teams. *Frontiers in Psychology, 11*, 1–12. https://doi.org/10.3389/fpsyg.2020.569198.

Yorguner, N., Serkut Bulut, N., & Akvardar, Y. (2021). An analysis of the psychosocial challenges faced by the university students during COVID-19 pandemic and the students' knowledge, attitudes and practices toward the disease. *Archives of Neuropsychiatry, 58*(1), 3–10. https://doi.org/10.29399/npa.27503.

Youngs, H. (2017). A critical exploration of collaborative and distributed leadership in higher education: Developing an alternative ontology through leadership-as-practice. *Journal of Higher Education Policy and Management, 39*(2), 140–54. https://doi.org/10.1080/1360080X.2017.1276662

Žalėnienėa, I., & Pereira, P. (2021). Higher education for sustainability: A global perspective. *Geography and Sustainability, 2*(2), 99–106. https://doi.org/10.1016/j.geosus.2021.05.001

Zhu, J., Liao, Z., Yam, K.C., & Johnson, R.E. (2016). Shared leadership: A state-of-the-art review and future research agenda. *Journal of Organizational Behavior, 39*, 834–52. https://doi.org/10.1002/job.2296

3 What Gets Treasured, Gets Measured? Considering the Role of a Common Health and Wellbeing Assessment Tool for Canadian Post-secondary Settings

GUY FAULKNER, CAROLINE WU, KELLY WUNDERLICH, AND MICHAEL FANG

The Post-secondary Campus as a Critical Setting for Health Promotion

Over two million young adults attend post-secondary institutions in Canada (Statistics Canada, 2020). In these institutions, the majority of the student body consists of individuals whom some academics have conceptualized as "emerging adults" (Arnett, 2019). First introduced by Arnett in the early 2000s, the theory of emerging adulthood proposes individuals between the ages of eighteen to roughly twenty-five experience a stressful and unstable transitional period that consists of an ever-changing social environment (Arnett, 2000, 2006). For example, many individuals experience varying degrees of changes to their living arrangements, relationships, education environments, and responsibilities during this time. This transitional period presents an opportunity for individuals to learn more about themselves but can also be a time when they are exposed to stressful experiences and new responsibilities. While Arnett's (2006) perspective on emerging adulthood considers it a psychosocial transition period, there is a case for this period also being a distinct biological life-history phase (Hochberg & Konner, 2020). For example, emerging adulthood is associated with patterns of structural and functional brain development distinct from those observed in adolescence (Taber-Thomas & Pérez-Edgar, 2015). Given the collective evidence that brain development and maturation continue beyond adolescence into young adulthood, Hochberg and Konner (2020) go as far as suggesting "emerging adults require protection because they are still *both learning and maturing*" (p. 9).

Emerging adulthood is clearly a period of great change, responsibility, and growth. This developmental period is also associated with fluctuations in physical and mental health. Weight gain and changes in other cardiometabolic risk factors are common among students (Vadeboncoeur et al., 2015). Substance use may be most tolerated or even promoted during emerging adulthood (Sussman & Arnett, 2014), while evidence suggests this population faces an even greater risk of experiencing poor mental health (Pedrelli et al., 2015). The post-secondary campus becomes, for Hochberg and Konner's (2020) notion of protection, a critical setting for health promotion. There is potential for exposing university and college students to sustained health messaging through already established knowledge exchange methods and messengers. There are subsidized facilities, programs, and staffing commonly available to support intervention work. In other words, we can intervene (Kwan & Faulkner, 2010).

Canadian colleges and universities are becoming increasingly committed to fostering student health and wellness through programming and services for emerging adults. The 2015 International Conference on Health Promoting Universities and Colleges in Kelowna, British Columbia, established the Okanagan Charter, with key calls to action: "1. To embed health into all aspects of campus culture, across the administration, operations and academic mandates. [and] 2. To lead health promotion action and collaboration locally and globally" (International Conference on Health Promoting Universities & Colleges, 2015, p. 3). A traditional aphorism posits that "what gets measured gets done" – that measuring indicators of performance, for example, focuses attention and resources on meeting goals associated with a given indicator. What is perhaps more pertinent is that measurement reflects the value an institution places on a given indicator – that what is treasured, gets measured. If wellbeing is an institutional priority, then a mechanism for its measurement and tracking over time is required that is tailored for the emerging adult population.

The primary purpose of this chapter is to describe the need for, and the process of developing, a post-secondary wellbeing assessment mechanism in Canada, known as the Canadian Campus Wellbeing Survey (CCWS; www.ccws-becc.ca). Implementation of the CCWS will be described with some discussion of how the CCWS data are being used by institutions. Finally, current and future challenges and opportunities inherent to an undertaking like the CCWS will be presented.

The Need for a National Post-secondary Wellbeing Measurement Mechanism

Evidence-based decisions need to be anchored in meaningful data. To intervene on the health and wellbeing of students, there is a need for a robust mechanism assessing the prevalence and correlates of mental health at a local level. In turn, this information can guide intervention prioritization, selection, and implementation (Cameron et al., 2007). Ongoing evaluation completes the cycle to assess the impact of intervention activities and inform future initiatives. A crucial element to such a mechanism is a shared measurement tool that allows comparison across institutions and across time. Increasing the number of institutions sharing a common surveillance system is important for several reasons (Faulkner et al., 2019). First, by reaching a greater number of institutions, collected data enable opportunities to examine priority health issues affecting the broader Canadian post-secondary population, explore differences between geographic regions, and provide a basis for making comparisons between prevalence and progress to national and provincial norms. Second, if institutions share a common surveillance tool, then it becomes possible to determine over time the institutions that are successful in changing mental health indicators of interest. This information might identify promising policies or strategies associated with such change, which can then be disseminated nationally.

There are many student health and wellbeing surveys competing for space at post-secondary institutions. At an international level, the World Health Organization's World Mental Health International College Student Survey (WMH-ICS) is a needs assessment self-report survey designed for post-secondary institutions to collect data on mental, substance, and behavioural disorders among institutions (Cuijpers et al., 2019). The survey generates data that can estimate the prevalence of mental disorders, consequences of these disorders, help-seeking patterns of these disorders, and barriers to treatment. Post-survey, each participating country consortium receives a dataset of their country's data, and a cross-national file is built with consenting country consortiums. Over their post-secondary career, follow-up surveys are provided to the same participating students (first-year students at baseline) to allow data collection and monitoring of mental health prevalence, and incidence over time.

Using the WMH-ICS, Auerbach et al. (2018) estimated the prevalence of mental disorders among first-year college students between 2014 and 2017 in nineteen post-secondary institutions from eight countries. Correlates of positive screening for mental disorders in students were identified, including being older age, of female sex, no religious affiliation, low secondary school ranking, and non-heterosexual identification and behaviour. A study by McLafferty et al. (2021) used data from WMH-ICS to identify rates of depression, anxiety, suicidal behaviour, and main stressors at post-secondary institutions in Ireland during the COVID-19 pandemic. They reported increased rates of depression, decreased rates of anxiety, no difference in suicidal behaviour, and identified social isolation as a main stressor for post-secondary students.

The WMH-ICS focuses on screening for mental disorders and does not currently assess a broader spectrum of health behaviours (e.g., physical activity) or indicators (e.g., food security). In the absence of a coordinated Canadian system for collecting health data prior to 2020, some colleges and universities have been subscribing to the National College Health Assessment service of the American College Health Association (NCHA-ACHA). This survey does include a broad range of health and wellbeing measures assessing alcohol, tobacco, and other drug use, sexual health, weight, nutrition, exercise, mental health, personal safety, and violence. Using NCHA data collected at one Canadian institution, Kwan et al. (2016) found that students with the highest likelihood of engaging in multiple health-risk behaviours (cannabis use, smoking, binge drinking, poor diet, physical inactivity, and insufficient sleep) reported poorer mental health. In another study drawing on NCHA data from eight Canadian post-secondary institutions, Kwan et al. (2013) highlighted the need for more concentrated health promotion campaigns, specifically targeting sleep, fruit and vegetables intake, and greater participation in physical activity.

While the NCHA instrument was completely revised in 2019, perhaps based on its limitations (Rahn et al., 2016), concerns remain about using an instrument that is not aligned with existing Canadian health survey measures or health guidelines. An example is the difference in physical activity guidelines between Canada and the United States. Canada has moved to a 24-Hour Movement approach where the whole day matters (Ross et al., 2020). Consequently, measures of physical activity, sedentary behaviour, and sleep duration are required to assess the prevalence of Canadian students meeting the guidelines. The NCHA tool does not currently assess the volume of sedentary behaviour. Being able to compare findings with other Canadian surveys such as the Canadian Community Health Survey (CCHS) may also be beneficial, but this requires harmonized measures. An example is Health Canada's development and launch of the Canadian Postsecondary Education Alcohol and Drug use Survey (CPADS; https://health-infobase.canada.ca/alcohol/cpads/) in 2019. This survey contributes to Health Canada's substance use surveillance strategy and provides an in-depth assessment of alcohol and substance use among students at post-secondary institutions. This includes data on what substances are used, how much, and how frequently, as well as the students' experience of harms associated with substance use. The CCWS uses the same core measures for binge drinking, cannabis use, smoking, and vaping to allow cross-comparisons between the two surveys.

Finally, the administration of the NCHA is neither comprehensive nor coordinated with Canadian research or data, thereby limiting opportunities for institutional comparisons and to identify best practices. The NCHA is restricted to individual-level behaviours based on the cycle that each institution subscribes to and is not as flexible for different institutional-level comparisons (e.g., other universities or colleges; research-intensive universities; rural or urban institutions). For example, we may want to understand what programs and policies are associated with healthier student-level profiles. If institutions from across Canada adopt a common surveillance tool, it becomes possible to determine over time which institutions are successful in changing health behaviours of interest. In turn, this information might identify promising policies or strategies associated with such change, which can subsequently be implemented at other institutions. This also provides the capacity for quasi-experimental and natural experiments at the local, provincial, or national levels (Leatherdale, 2019).

Therefore, the long-term goal of the CCWS is to develop a comprehensive surveillance system that will enable post-secondary institutional leaders and health services to a) identify population-level estimates of health behaviour and wellbeing; b) identify intervention priorities at their institutions; and c) evaluate intervention implementation. The CCWS is primarily considered a quality assurance and improvement activity undertaken by institutions. To develop benchmarks for comparison, a research database has also been created that aggregates and securely stores all collected data. Individual researchers can also seek access to de-identified data to address hypothesis-driven research questions.

For example, in response to the development of new Canadian 24-Hour Movement guidelines for adults (see Ross et al., 2020), Weatherson et al. (2021) examined post-secondary student adherence to the guidelines and its associations with sociodemographic factors and mental health using data from the first cycle of the CCWS. Only 9.9 per cent of students (females 10.4%; males 9.2%) were currently achieving four components of the 24-Hour Movement guidelines. Notably, students who reported higher psychological wellbeing were more likely to meet the guidelines. Extending this work, Porter et al. (2023) examined data from the 2020 cycle of the CCWS, and reported that students with chronic health conditions and disabilities had significantly lower odds of meeting the movement guidelines than their peers. Disparities in guideline adherence were most pronounced among those with multimorbidity, developmental, and physical disabilities (Porter et al., 2023). The CCWS now provides one mechanism for monitoring adherence to the guidelines among Canadian post-secondary students (Weatherson et al., 2021).

The Development of the Canadian Campus Wellbeing Survey

Support from the Rossy Foundation, a Montreal-based philanthropic foundation, was integral to supporting the development of the CCWS. Stakeholders across Canada, including institutional leaders, service providers, and students, were consulted in 2018 on the need for the CCWS and the priority indicators for measurement at a student level (see Faulkner et al., 2019, for further details). To ensure the CCWS met the needs of its intended users, we conducted a Delphi survey with knowledge users from the Canadian Health Promoting Universities and Colleges Network (https://www.chpcn.ca) to develop a consensus framework regarding mental health priorities (i.e., what mental health constructs to measure and how), analysis needs, and preferred feedback report content and structure. A final in-person panel meeting of thirty knowledge users from across Canada met to confirm a consensus framework on what indicators should be assessed in the student-level survey.

An expert panel of Canadian researchers in epidemiology was then convened to create the student-level survey instrument. The Positive Health Surveillance Indicator Framework from the Public Health Agency of Canada is the basis of the survey instrument (https://health-infobase. canada.ca/positive-mental-health/). This panel identified validated and reliable measures of positive mental health, and multiple risk and protective factors including connectedness, social and emotional skills, academic performance, safety, sleep, physical activity, food security, and substance use. The student-level survey is a modular design with a core survey that takes students at participating institutions fifteen to twenty minutes to complete. With a commitment to inclusive practice, the CCWS also gives voice to the many Canadian students traditionally excluded from surveys of its type using best practices in assessing gender identity, Indigeneity, and sexual orientation, for example.

After finalizing the survey in the spring of 2019, focus groups were conducted to ensure appropriateness, comprehensiveness, and student comprehension of the CCWS. To assess reliability, a convenience sample of two hundred students completed the CCWS twice one week apart in early 2019. A technical report describing the results of this process is available at www.ccws-becc.ca. In parallel, work started on developing the surveillance infrastructure to be housed at the University of British Columbia in collaboration with the Planning and Institutional Research Office of the UBC Office of the Provost and Vice-President, of Academics. After piloting the CCWS at three institutions in the fall of 2019, the BC Ministry of Advanced Education supported the deployment of the CCWS to all BC institutions in the winter of 2020. Coordinating consortiums for deployment is important – the value of the CCWS lies in being able to make relevant comparisons between similar institutions (geography, enrolment, type of institution, etc.). Accordingly, the CCWS was deployed in the fall of 2020 in the Atlantic region, and Saskatchewan institutions in the spring of 2021. In 2021 an important development, the creation of an employee version of the CCWS, now allows post-secondary institutions to adopt a whole campus approach to wellbeing (Wunderlich et al., 2022). The CCWS is available in French or English to any post-secondary institution for a fee, and approximately eighty-nine institutions have participated as of December 2024. The next section outlines some of the key elements in implementing the CCWS.

Implementing the CCWS

Evaluation itself is a complex process and involves a range of actors to be successful. Stakeholder engagement is essential to the mechanism as the CCWS team is guided by the Technical Advisory Committee (TAC) and Data Access Committee (DAC). Both committees are composed of representatives from post-secondary institutions that are participating, or have previously participated, in the CCWS, as well as researchers and members at large as required. The role of the TAC is to advise the CCWS team in supporting the successful administration of the survey following the CCWS service agreement. This includes having the DAC uphold the principles, policies, and procedures through which access to CCWS data is sought and granted. The DAC is responsible for reviewing applications to access the CCWS research database and determining if they meet the requirements of the Data Access Policy, primarily that institutions or individuals who participated are not identifiable.

At an institutional level, staff time must be dedicated to both preparing to participate in the CCWS and disseminating results in order to make changes. This includes collaborating as needed to select optional additional modules and up to five institution-specific questions that help to assess institutional priorities, engaging leadership to champion and promote the survey, connecting with the institution's ethics review board (if applicable) to get the necessary permission to participate, and marketing to help socialize the survey among the student population over time. Fostering connections with different stakeholders at the institution helps to ensure that, once the results from the survey are returned to the institution, data can be used to inform practices, policies, and other actions. The network of actors at participating institutions, including those who engage with the CCWS committees, is essential to creating a successful evaluation mechanism.

The CCWS was developed to be flexible based on the needs of participating institutions. This includes providing two survey distribution methods that both ensure participating students are not identified, offering both an English and French version of the survey, allowing institutions to choose how long their survey is available, the number of reminders sent, and their sampling frame (i.e., random sampling so that they can reduce survey burden if conducting multiple surveys around the same time, or census if they are a small institution), and using a modular system where institutions can customize their survey by including optional additional modules or up to five institution-specific questions in addition to the core survey. This flexibility requires institutions to determine what suits them best, which furthers the need for intra-institutional communication and coordination when preparing to participate.

A vital feature of the CCWS is an improved feedback mechanism where institutions have timely access to visual representations of their data and normative references, and the capacity to customize analyses. This also allows for easy filtering and dissemination of data to stakeholders, as the institutional coordinator can provide filtered reports based on demographics, or on specific health outcomes, to different partners. As of 2022, the CCWS uses Tableau (www.tableau.com) to deliver data visualizations in interactive reports. This includes a dashboard with comparative data between each institution and up to two different benchmarks (e.g., one compared to other institutions in the province and the other compared to other colleges only), the institution's results, and an administration summary with the representativeness of the collected data based on the profile of the students invited to participate. All variables in the cohort file and demographic sections are established as filters, and this allows institutional users to examine their data based on their interests. All the dashboards can be exported as PDF, high resolution image, or PowerPoint files to create customized executive summaries of their data that can easily be shared with collaborators and stakeholders at each institution. A case-level dataset of each institution's results is also provided so that institutions can do their own customized analyses. The ability to customize reporting or analyses is meant to support the network of stakeholders who are involved at each institution.

Using the CCWS Data

In 2022, key contact persons from eight institutions in the Canadian Atlantic region and one institution from British Columbia were invited to participate in an interview to explore experiences of deploying the CCWS during the fall of 2020, and to see how institutions were utilizing the collected data. Of the nine institutions invited, six representatives from five institutions participated in the interview. During these interviews, questions were asked to explore barriers and facilitators to deploying the survey, using the data, as well as perceptions of the associated data analyzation tools provided as a part of the survey deliverables.

From these interviews, we learned that the CCWS data was being used at institutions to inform the creation and modification of programs, services, and policies. For example, institutions created health and wellness awareness campaigns after noticing many daily cannabis users at their institution. Another institution used the data to inform initiatives addressing food insecurity on campus. For others, the collected data assisted in the revision of staff member responsibilities after seeing that certain student needs were not being met. Mostly, the CCWS data was used alongside data from other in-house, institutional surveys. For example, institutions with a particular interest in substance and alcohol usage on campus used data collected from the CCWS and CPADS. Participants described the CCWS as another rich data source when considering services and policies, and when communicating with board members, administration, and senior institution staff. The richness of the data and the variety of areas covered in the CCWS also allowed institutions to share the data to various student affairs, and health and wellbeing offices, across their campuses.

Analysing and Using the Collected Data

As discussed, institutions receive their data in the Tableau data visual analytics platform. Tableau provides institutions with the flexibility and autonomy to dive deeper into their data by analysing various questions across different filtered populations and build different visual models. In addition to using Tableau, benchmarking tools were a part of the deliverables available to participating institutions. As a part of this tool, institutions could benchmark their data against other anonymized institutions' data to compare their survey results against other Canadian institutions in a similar deployment window and context. During the interview, we learned that institutions found the benchmarking tool extremely useful and helpful.

However, during the interviews, we learned that the novelty and flexibility of Tableau resulted in challenges to institutions analysing and using the data. As Tableau was a novel way to view and analyse data for many institutions, staff members tasked with analysing the data experienced difficulties navigating the platform. When looking at the process of how data was analysed at institutions, it became apparent that the analysis process varied at institutions depending on the resources available and the key contact person receiving the deliverables. The key contact person deploying the survey at an institution did not necessarily have analytic expertise. Some institutions hired a staff member to conduct data analyses, or the data was passed to internal institutional research staff at larger institutions. For some institutions, hiring another staff member was not financially feasible and in-depth analyses were delayed or not possible. This became a barrier for some institutions when working with the data. Taking note of this challenge, the CCWS team has been working to provide institutions with seminars, tutorial videos, and a frequently asked questions resource to assist institutions in using Tableau. Responding to additional feedback provided from institutions, the CCWS team is planning to provide more traditional summary reports that can be printed and shared.

In 2020, the CCWS was deployed at several campuses in Canada during the height of physical restrictions in response to the COVID-19 pandemic. For many post-secondary institution campuses, this also meant the implementation of online classes and social distancing measures. During the deployment of this survey, some institutions observed lower response rates than usual. It was speculated that the reason for this decline in responses had to do with the increased amount of time students spent looking at screens and monitors. Moreover, the stress from the pandemic resulted in a lower capacity for students to feel motivated to take a health and wellbeing survey. Thus, screen and survey fatigue presented itself as an additional barrier for institutions to collect more robust data.

During the interview, some institutions questioned the value of their data due to the deployment of the CCWS during the second wave of the COVID-19 pandemic. To these institutions, it was perceived that the pandemic represented such an unusual time for students that interpretation of the data was challenging. For others, being able to have a current picture of their students' perceived mental and physical wellbeing during the COVID-19 restrictions allowed for a better understanding of the needs of their student body and the services that were required.

As the CCWS continues to be deployed at campuses each year, ongoing evaluations will track the uptake of the CCWS and continue to monitor how CCWS data informs institutional planning and initiatives. Early evaluation highlights the challenges for some institutions in "actioning" the data, which is moderated by institutional capacity to support data analysis and knowledge exchange within an institution. Notably, a key reason for using the Tableau platform was the perceived ease with which staff without extensive analytic expertise would be able to navigate the data and conduct custom analyses. This has not yet been translated into practice. Addressing this barrier continues to be a focus of the CCWS team.

Challenges and Opportunities

Dealing with Complexity

A systems approach to health promotion on post-secondary campuses must recognize the complexity inherent in the system. This complexity can be seen as the context where numerous interacting elements (i.e., people, entities, actions) in a system make it hard to see, describe, and assess what is happening in the whole. The CCWS is currently a student-level measure of health and wellbeing and is not able to capture changes in the system as a whole because of changes in programs and policies, for example. The CCWS is best seen as one, but not the only, source of information that post-secondary stakeholders can collect in piecing together a more coherent understanding of health promotion on campuses. This may include consultive "town halls" with students and other stakeholders, assessment of administrative data, and interviews and focus groups with potential change agents.

A related challenge with a systems approach is recognizing the number of actors in the system that could use and act on data collected by the CCWS. In our experience, it is not always clear what happens with the CCWS data, with whom it is shared, and whether it gets in the hands of stakeholders who can act on it. This is a focus of current evaluation efforts to understand more about the barriers and facilitators of implementing lessons learnt from the CCWS data.

One aspiration in developing the CCWS was using collected data as a resource and stimulus for action in knowledge exchange fora. Can the data be used to bring Canadian institutions together to discuss trends in the data, to share best practice in response to issues of concern, or to collaboratively identify policy and practice solutions for the future? A systems approach to health promotion necessitates multiple communities of interest working together in a coordinated manner (Norman, 2009). Developing partnerships with organizations with a vested interest in health and wellbeing such as the Canadian Association of College and University Student Services (www.cacuss.ca) and the Best Practices in Canadian Higher Ed: Making a positive impact on student mental health (www.bp-net.ca) will be essential in establishing such a national dialogue.

Our perspective is that the student-level CCWS would be strengthened through linkage to institutional data. Identifying the institutional-level programs and policies that are differentially associated with mental health and physical health risk behaviours at the student level may provide clearer insights for informing the future dissemination of successful practices to other institutions. This could save precious limited prevention resources. Linking interventions with individual-level behaviour over time would strengthen the potential to evaluate natural experiments that occur within institutions, and this would substantially add to our systems-level understanding of what interventions work, for which students, and in which contexts (Faulkner et al., 2019). Future work will consider approaches to capturing information at institutional levels regarding programs, policies, and resources associated with well-being among students.

Sourcing Data

It is commonly acknowledged that response rates to health surveys have been declining in recent decades and in many countries (Czajka & Beyler, 2016; Tolonen et al., 2006). For example, response rates for the NCHA and CCWS appear similar at approximately 18–20 per cent (Faulkner et al., 2020; Linden et al., 2021). A range of plausible explanations for this have been proposed including greater time pressures, the increasing number of surveys in circulation, survey fatigue, and privacy concerns (Galea & Tracy, 2007). This non-response has the clear potential to bias the results if the non-response is systematically related to the outcomes of interest. For example, syntheses of previous work highlight that males, younger ages, lower socio-economic positions, and poorer health and health behaviours such as heavier alcohol intake are associated with non-response (Lallukka et al., 2020). A number of strategies have been reported to increase response rates in Internet surveys including providing incentives, pre-notifying individuals, the use of reminders, and employing more personable questionnaires (Edwards et al., 2009). The CCWS experience consistently finds a greater response rate with at least three reminders and the use of incentives (Faulkner et al., 2020). An important role for institutions is socializing employees and students to the CCWS deployment, and communicating the importance of participation and the steps that will be taken in responding to the collected data. We have encouraged institutions to consider how the CCWS might be integrated and delivered within common learning platforms like Canvas or Blackboard.

It remains to be seen whether new forms of data collection supersede traditional survey approaches like the CCWS. For example, crowdsourcing has been suggested as one alternative approach to surveillance and monitoring (Ranard et al., 2014). Crowdsourcing can be defined as an "online, distributed problem-solving and production model that leverages the collective intelligence of online communities for specific purposes" (Brabham et al., 2014, p. 179). This approach has much in common with community engagement and assumes that citizens are the experts on local issues and their local environment. Institutions could engage in online crowdsourcing to address specific wellbeing challenges and/or to monitor specific health behaviours. With the ubiquity of mobile phones and their geospatial potential, remote sensors could also be used to track engagement with health services or purchases of food items and beverages. The use of ecological momentary assessment approaches could track wellbeing in real time and over time (e.g., Bedard et al., 2017). While such approaches still carry technological and privacy concerns, they do point to future methods that could complement online surveys like the CCWS.

Conclusion

The CCWS was created based on Canadian stakeholders' interest in developing a "home-grown" mechanism for collecting data on the health and wellbeing of post-secondary students during a distinct life stage of emerging adulthood (Arnett, 2000, 2006). The CCWS now provides one tool for supporting the Okanagan Charter's guiding principle of promoting research, innovation, and evidence-informed action (Okanagan Charter, 2015, p. 9). While there has been promising uptake of the CCWS since its piloting in 2019, its sustainability will rest on the impact institutions perceive its implementation has in supporting their health promotion goals. Developing a common Canadian measurement mechanism embedded within the post-secondary system remains an ambitious vision, but we believe such a mechanism remains integral to supporting the health and wellbeing of young Canadians attending post-secondary institutions (Faulkner et al., 2019).

Acknowledgments

The Rossy Foundation and the University of British Columbia provided direct funding, and the University of British Columbia and the University of Toronto were collaborating partners on the development of the CCWS.

REFERENCES

Arnett, J.J. (2000). Emerging adulthood: A theory of development from the late teens through the twenties. *American Psychologist, 55*(5), 469–80. https://doi.org/10.1037/0003-066X.55.5.469

Arnett, J.J. (2006). Emerging adulthood: Understanding the new way of coming of age. In J.J. Arnett & J.L. Tanner (Eds.), *Emerging adults in America: Coming of age in the 21st century* (pp. 3–19). American Psychological Association. https://doi.org/10.1037/11381-001

Arnett, J.J. (2019). Conceptual foundations of emerging adulthood. In J.L. Murray & J.J. Arnett (Eds.), *Emerging adulthood and higher education: A new student development paradigm* (pp. 11–24). Routledge.

Auerbach, R.P., Mortier, P., Bruffaerts, R., Alonso, J., Benjet, C., Cuijpers, P., Demyttenaere, K., Ebert, D.D., Green, J.G., Hasking, P., Murray, E., Nock, M.K., Pinder-Amaker, S., Sampson, N.A., Stein, D.J., Vilagut, G., Zaslavsky, A.M., & Kessl, R.C. (2018). WHO world mental health surveys international college student project: Prevalence and distribution of mental disorders. *Journal of Abnormal Psychology, 127*(7), 623–38. https://doi.org/10.1037/ABN0000362

Bedard, C., King-Dowling, S., McDonald, M., Dunton, G., Cairney, J., & Kwan, M. (2017). Understanding environmental and contextual influences of physical activity during first-year university: The feasibility of using ecological momentary assessment in the MovingU study. *JMIR Public Health and Surveillance, 3*(2), e32. https://doi.org/10.2196/publichealth.7010

Brabham, D.C., Ribisl, K.M., Kirchner, T.R., & Bernhardt, J.M. (2014). Crowdsourcing applications for public health. *American Journal of Preventive Medicine, 46*(2), 179–87. https://doi.org/10.1016/j.amepre.2013.10.016

Cameron, R., Manske, S., Brown, S., Jolin, M.A., Murnaghan, D., & Lovato, C. (2007). Integrating public health policy, practice, evaluation, surveillance, and research: The School Health Action Planning and Evaluation System. *American Journal of Public Health, 97*, 648–54. https://doi.org/10.2105/AJPH.2005.079665.

Cuijpers, P., Auerbach, R., Benjet, C., Bruffaerts, R., Ebert, D., Karyotaki, E., & Kessler, R.C. (2019). The World Health Organization World Mental Health International College Student initiative: An overview. *International Journal of Psychiatric Research, 28*(2), e1761. https://doi.org/10.1002/mpr.1761

Czajka, J., & Beyler, A. (2016). *Declining response rates in federal surveys: Trends and implications.* Mathematica Policy Research. https://aspe.hhs.gov/sites/default/files/private/pdf/255531/Decliningresponserates.pdf

Edwards, P.J., Roberts, I., Clarke, M.J., Diguiseppi, C., Wentz, R., Kwan, I., Cooper, R., Felix, L.M., & Pratap, S. (2009). Methods to increase response to postal and electronic questionnaires. *Cochrane Database Systematic Review, 8*(3), MR000008. https://doi.org/10.1002/14651858.MR000008.pub4

Faulkner, G., Ramanathan, S., Kwan, M., & CCWS Expert Panel Group. (2019). Developing a coordinated Canadian post-secondary surveillance system: A Delphi survey to identify measurement priorities for the Canadian Campus Wellbeing Survey (CCWS). *BMC Public Health, 19*(1), 935. https://doi.org /10.1186/s12889-019-7255-6

Faulkner, G., Weatherson, K., Joopally, H., & Wunderlich, K. (2020). *Provincial deployment of the Canadian Campus Wellbeing Survey (CCWS) in British Columbia — 2019–20: Final report for the Ministry of Advanced Skills, Education and Training.* www.ccws-becc.ca

Galea, S., & Tracy, M. (2007). Participation rates in epidemiologic studies. *Annals of Epidemiology, 17*(9), 643–53. https://doi.org/10.1016/j.annepidem .2007.03.013

Hochberg, Z.E., & Konner, M. (2020). Emerging adulthood, a pre-adult life-history stage. *Frontiers in Endocrinology, 10*, 918. https://doi.org/10.3389 /fendo.2019.00918

Kwan, M.Y., Arbour-Nicitopoulos, K.P., Duku, E., & Faulkner, G. (2016). Patterns of multiple health risk-behaviours in university students and their association with mental health: Application of latent class analysis. *Health Promotion and Chronic Disease Prevention in Canada, 36*(8), 163–70.https://doi .org/10.24095/hpcdp.36.8.03

Kwan, M.Y.W., & Faulkner, G. (2010). The need for a physical education. *The Psychologist, 23*(2), 116–19. https://www.bps.org.uk/psychologist/need-physical -education

Kwan, M.Y.W., Faulkner, G.E.J., Arbour-Nicitopoulos, K.P., & Cairney, J. (2013). Prevalence of health-risk behaviours among Canadian post-secondary students: Descriptive results from the National College Health Assessment. *BMC Public Health, 13*(1), 548. https://doi.org/10.1186/1471-2458-13-548

Lallukka, T., Pietiläinen, O., Jäppinen, S., Laaksonen, M., Lahti, J., & Rahkonen, O. (2020). Factors associated with health survey response among young employees: A register-based study using online, mailed and telephone interview data collection methods. *BMC Public Health, 30*, 184. https://doi.org/10.1186 /s12889-020-8241-8

Leatherdale, S. T. (2019). Natural experiment methodology for research: A review of how different methods can support real-world research. *International Journal of Social Research Methodology: Theory and Practice, 22*(1), 19–35. https:// doi.org/10.1080/13645579.2018.1488449

Linden, B., Boyes, R., & Stuart, H. (2021). Cross-sectional trend analysis of the NCHA II survey data on Canadian post-secondary student mental health and wellbeing from 2013 to 2019. *BMC Public Health, 21*(1), 590. https://doi.org /10.1186/s12889-021-10622-1

McLafferty, M., Brown, N., McHugh, R., Ward, C., Stevenson, A., McBride, L., Brady, J., Bjourson, A.J., O'Neill, S.M., Walsh, C.P., & Murray, E.K.

(2021). Depression, anxiety and suicidal behaviour among college students: Comparisons pre-COVID-19 and during the pandemic. *Psychiatry Research Communications, 1*(2), 100012. https://doi.org/10.1016/J.PSYCOM.2021.100012

Norman, C. D. (2009). Health promotion as a systems science and practice. *Journal of Evaluation in Clinical Practice, 15*(5), 868–72. https://doi.org /10.1111/j.1365-2753.2009.01273.x

Okanagan Charter: An International Charter for Health Promoting Universities and Colleges. (2015). *Okanagan Charter.* Kelowna, BC: Author. Retrieved from http://internationalhealthycampuses2015.sites.olt.ubc.ca/files /2016/01/Okanagan-Charter-January13v2.pdf

Pedrelli, P., Nyer, M., Yeung, A., Zulauf, C., & Wilens, T. (2015). College students: Mental health problems and treatment considerations. *Academic Psychiatry, 39*(5), 503–11. https://doi.org/10.1007/s40596-014-0205-9

Porter, C.D., McPhee, P.G., Kwan, M.Y., Timmons, B.W., & Brown, D.M. (2023). 24-hour movement guideline adherence and mental health: A cross-sectional study of emerging adults with chronic health conditions and disabilities. *Disability and Health Journal, 16*(3), 101476. https://doi.org/10.1016/j.dhjo.2023.101476

Rahn, R.N., Pruitt, B., & Goodson, P. (2016). Utilization and limitations of the American College Health Association's National College Health Assessment instrument: A systematic review. *Journal of American College Health, 64*(3), 214–37. https://doi.org/10.1080/07448481.2015.1117463

Ranard, B.L., Ha, Y.P., Meisel, Z.F., Asch, D.A., Hill, S.S., Becker, L.B., Seymour, A.K., & Merchant, R.M. (2014). Crowdsourcing – H the masses to advance health and medicine, a systematic review. *Journal of General Internal Medicine, 29*(1), 187–203. https://doi.org/10.1007/s11606-013-2536-8

Ross, R., Chaput, J.-P., Giangregorio, L., Janssen, I., Saunders, T., Kho, M., Poitras, V., Tomasone, J., El-Kotob, R., McLaughlin, E., Duggan, M., Carrier, J., Carson, V., Chastin, SF. M., Latimer-Cheung, A., Chulak-Bozzer, T., Faulkner, G., Flood, S., Gazendam, M.K., … Tremblay, M.S. (2020). Canadian 24-hour movement guidelines for adults aged 18–64 years and adults aged 65 years or older: An integration of physical activity, sedentary behaviour, and sleep. *Applied Physiology, Nutrition, and Metabolism, 45*(10 (Suppl. 2), S57–S102. https://doi.org/10.1139/apnm-2020–0467

Statistics Canada. (2020). Canadian post-secondary enrolments and graduates, 2017/2019. *The Daily.* https://www150.statcan.gc.ca/n1/daily-quotidien /200219/dq200219b-eng.

Sussman, S., & Arnett, J.J. (2014). Emerging adulthood: Developmental period facilitative of the addictions. *Evaluation & the Health Professions, 37*(2), 147–55. https://doi.org/10.1177/0163278714521812

Taber-Thomas, B., & Pérez-Edgar, K. (2015). Emerging adulthood brain development. In *The Oxford Handbook of Emerging Adulthood* (pp. 126–41). Oxford University Press.

Tolonen, H., Helakorpi, S., Talala, K., Helasoja, V., Martelin, T., & Prättälä, R. (2006). 25-year trends and socio-demographic differences in response rates: Finnish adult health behavior survey. *European Journal of Epidemiology*, *21*, 409–15. https://doi.org/10.1007/s10654-006-9019-8.

Vadeboncoeur, C., Townsend, N., & Foster, C. (2015). A meta-analysis of weight gain in first year university students: Is freshman 15 a myth? *BMC Obesity, 2*, 22. https://doi.org/10.1186/s40608-015-0051-7

Weatherson, K.A., Joopally, H., Wunderlich, K., Kwan, M.Y., Tomasone, J.R., & Faulkner, G. (2021). Post-secondary students' adherence to the Canadian 24-Hour Movement Guidelines for Adults: Results from the first deployment of the Canadian Campus Wellbeing Survey (CCWS). *Health Promotion and Chronic Disease Prevention in Canada, 41*(6), 173–81. https://doi.org/10.24095/hpcdp.41.6.01

Wunderlich, K., Faulkner, G., & Fang, M. (2022). *Development of the Canadian Campus Wellbeing Survey (CCWS) for Employees – CCWS Technical Report Series.* www.ccws-becc.ca

4 Supporting Indigenous Peoples' Wellbeing on University Campuses

HEATHER J.A. FOULDS AND LEAH J. FERGUSON

Introduction

The original inhabitants of Turtle Island, the land currently known as Canada and the United States, are collectively referred to as Indigenous Peoples and include multiple distinct and diverse nations of First Nations, Inuit, and Métis Peoples (Garner et al., 2010; Greenwood et al., 2018). Having inhabited this land for more than 24,000 years, more than 1.8 million people in Canada self-identified as Indigenous in 2021 (Bourgeon et al., 2017; Statistics Canada, 2022). While collective terms such as "Indigenous" and "Aboriginal" are often used to refer to Indigenous Peoples, hundreds of Indigenous communities and more than sixty distinct Indigenous languages are included in these broad, general identities in Canada (Crown-Indigenous Relations and Northern Affairs Canada, 2017; Statistics Canada, 2012).

Historic and ongoing colonization has fractured Indigenous Peoples' ways of life, community and family structures, languages, independence, self-governance and governance structures, access to traditional lands, and cultural practices (Canadian Human Rights Commission, 2013; Mitchell et al., 2019; Walters et al., 2002). These and other colonial traumas have led to persistent physical, social, emotional, cultural, and spiritual disruptions that have caused profound health and social disparities across all aspects of wellbeing, distinctly disadvantaging Indigenous Peoples (Mitchell et al., 2019). Key outcomes of colonial trauma that underpin many health disparities are ruptured identity, alienation from family, community, and Nation, and loss of culture (Mitchell et al., 2019).

Many Indigenous Peoples embrace a broad understanding of wellbeing recognizing the interconnectedness, interrelatedness, and balance of all four spheres of humanity: physical, mental, emotional, and spiritual components (Graham & Stamler, 2010; King et al., 2009; Lavallee, 2007). Moreover, wellbeing of Indigenous Peoples cannot be understood outside of interactions and context as wellbeing is dependent on identity, community, environment, and economics and politics (Graham & Stamler, 2010; Johnson et al., 2021; King et al., 2009). Given the power of universities as agents of change, institution-wide initiatives, programs, and supports to promote Indigenous Peoples' wellbeing must consider and incorporate all of these aspects (Graham & Stamler, 2010; Lavallee, 2007).

Self-Situating

The authors of this chapter, Drs. Heather Foulds and Leah Ferguson, are Métis academics and members of Métis Nation-Saskatchewan and Saskatoon Métis Local 126. Heather Foulds grew up in Prince George, British Columbia, and descends from the Métis communities of Bresaylor and Langmeade in Saskatchewan. She completed a BSc in Biochemistry and Molecular Biology at the University of Northern British Columbia, and an MSc in Human Kinetics and a PhD in Experimental Medicine at the University of British Columbia (UBC). Dr. Foulds is currently an associate professor and the Heart & Stroke/CIHR Early Career Indigenous Women's Heart and Brain Health Chair in the College of Kinesiology at the University of Saskatchewan (USask). Dr. Ferguson was born in Humboldt, Saskatchewan, and her Métis ancestry stems from her maternal lineage, with roots in Batoche and Fish Creek, Saskatchewan. She completed all of her post-secondary education at USask, including a BA (Hon) in Arts and Science (psychology), and an MS and PhD in Kinesiology. Dr. Ferguson is currently an associate professor in the College of Kinesiology at USask. The University of Saskatchewan is situated on Treaty 6 territory and Homeland of the Métis.

In this chapter, we will critically discuss concepts and examples that are relevant to supporting Indigenous Peoples' wellbeing on university campuses. Recognizing that experiences, supports, and processes to enable wellbeing of Indigenous Peoples on university campuses vary considerably across institutions, programs, and disciplines, we humbly provide our perspectives on supports, experiences, and processes to enable Indigenous Peoples' wellbeing. This chapter is inherently reflective of our experiences, identities, and cultural backgrounds. Our approach is thus consistent with Métis culture in weaving together physical, mental, emotional, and spiritual elements of wellbeing within identity, community, environment, and economic and political systems.

University Systems to Promote Indigenous Peoples' Wellbeing

Despite comprising 5 per cent of the total population in Canada in 2021, Indigenous Peoples comprise only 1.4 per cent of faculty at Canadian universities, and only 10.9 per cent of Indigenous Peoples (vs. 28.5% of non-Indigenous Canadians) achieve a university degree (Gordon & White, 2014; Statistics Canada, 2020, 2022). Though not widely available, the proportion of Indigenous students at universities varies considerably, from reports of approximately 0.4 per cent at McGill to approximately 3 per cent at the University of Alberta (UofA) and UBC to 14 per cent at USask (McGill, 2022a, 2022b; Mukherjee-Reed & Szeri, 2021; University of Alberta, 2022; University of Saskatchewan, 2022). Indigenous Peoples' under-representation in post-secondary education is directly linked to the ongoing legacy of colonization (Canadian Human Rights Commission, 2013). From 1876 to 1961, enfranchisement laws enacted legislation that status First Nations Peoples[1] would lose their "Indian status" if they attended universities (Laferte, 2021; Vescera, 2018). Following earlier schooling systems in the 1600s with a goal of converting and transforming First Nations community belief systems, federally mandated residential schools operated from 1831 to 1996, and their ongoing legacy negatively affected educational attendance and retention of Indigenous Peoples at universities (Bougie & Senecal, 2010; Gordon & White, 2014; Truth and Reconciliation Commission, 2015). The intergenerational legacy of mistrust that Residential Schools and Eurocentric educational practices have fostered greatly impact Indigenous Peoples' attendance, retention, and completion of post-secondary degrees and education programs (Ottmann, 2017). Supporting Indigenous Peoples' engagement at universities requires weaving together appropriate culturally safe supports, communities, environments, and policies to support

---

1. Status First Nations refers to the specific legal identity of "Status Indian" as deemed by the Government of Canada. In 1876 the Canadian government developed criteria for who would be legally considered an "Indian," and the criteria continue to be outlined in Section 6 of the Indian Act Government of Canada. (2019). *Indian Act (R.S.C., 1985, c. I-5)*. Ottawa: Minister of Justice Retrieved from https://laws-lois.justice.gc.ca/eng/acts/i-5/. There are complex rules governing status, based on descent in one's family and historically privileged male lineage and disproportionately discriminated against First Nations women (Greenwood, M., de Leeuw, S., & Lindsay, N.M., [2018]. *Determinants of Indigenous Peoples' Health, Second Edition: Beyond the Social*. Canadian Scholars. https://books.google.ca/books?id=jblaDwAAQBAJ). Status First Nations are registered under the Indian Act on the Indian Register and are eligible for programs and services offered by federal, provincial, and territorial government agencies.

Indigenous Peoples' holistic wellbeing. The Okanagan Charter calls for health to be embedded in all aspects of campus culture, and for universities to lead health promotion action and collaboration locally and globally (Okanagan Charter, 2015). Achieving health and leading health promotion will require recognition and engagement of the needs of Indigenous Peoples. Supporting health of Indigenous Peoples on campus, locally, and globally requires approaches, policies, and environments that consider Indigenous Peoples' holistic world views and the social, mental, cultural, and physical influences on their health and wellbeing.

Identity

Identity is a core tenant of Indigenous Peoples' wellbeing (Johnson et al., 2021). Indigenous identity includes three central threads: Indigenous ancestry to an Indigenous community of specific lands, membership and acceptance within the said Indigenous community, and continuous existence of the Indigenous community from historical[2] to current times (Larivière, 2015). In addition to attaining Western education focused outcomes, Indigenous Peoples' success at university entails maintaining Indigenous identity and cultural groundings (Pidgeon, 2008). Supporting identity for Indigenous Peoples at university requires at least four actions: 1) supporting accurate and authentic identity, 2) honouring distinct and diverse identities, 3) providing identity safety, and 4) respecting the right of Indigenous Peoples *not* to declare their Indigenous identity.

It is important for all individuals, including students, faculty/staff, and administrators, to understand the diversity and distinctiveness of Indigenous identities. Pan-Indigenous approaches that consider all Indigenous identities as one homogeneous group leads to poorer educational outcomes among Indigenous students (Nguyen et al., 2017). Efforts to support Indigenous Peoples' wellbeing must reflect and consider differing identities and unique needs. Within universities, the need for Indigenous representation on all initiatives related to Indigenous Peoples and Indigenous content (e.g., institutional practices, strategies, committees, and instructional content) creates challenges where the few Indigenous individuals on campus are tasked with representing many diverse Indigenous Peoples. Similarly, Indigenous faculty and instructors are often tasked with teaching Indigenous-related course content, including content and courses that may be far from their own Nation's teachings,

---

2. Prior to effective European control.

understandings, culture, and disciplinary field. Pigeonholing individual Indigenous Peoples as stand-ins for all Indigenous Peoples can create mental and emotional struggles for those individuals and undermine their academic expertise, Indigenous identity, and lived experiences. To fully support Indigenous Peoples' wellbeing in universities, a diverse community of Indigenous Peoples, with complementary identities, cultures, and areas of expertise, is needed to share responsibilities, ensure expectations of Indigenous Peoples are focused on their individual knowledges and expertise, and to sustain community and supportive environments.

In efforts to make universities accessible to more Indigenous Peoples, many institutions have embarked on "Indigenization"[3] strategies (Vescera, 2018). Many Indigenization strategies include targeted hiring and admission seats set aside for Indigenous applicants. A likely unintended consequence of this process is a culture of discrimination and devaluing of Indigenous students and faculty/staff. Many Indigenous students, for instance, are hesitant to acknowledge their Indigenous identity within their student cohorts for fear of being seen as "lesser than" given their "equity seat" admission. Similarly, Indigenous faculty/staff not hired for Indigenous-specific positions may fear identifying as Indigenous, due to concerns of being dismissed as less deserving of their positions by their colleagues. A lack of safety in identifying as Indigenous within universities undermines wellbeing by disconnecting individuals from their own identity, community, and culture. Therefore, creating identity safety is essential to promoting Indigenous Peoples' wellbeing at universities.

The identity of Indigenous Peoples is often perceived as a community-centred existence, where identity is understood as being a member of a specific Indigenous Nation, from specific lands, including connection to community members, the lands, and animals and plants of the Nation's home (King et al., 2009). As described by Maria Campbell, Métis Elder and author, identity as an Indigenous person means knowing the heroes and stories of your People and knowing your community and family (Campbell et al., 2021). This interwoven understanding of identity, community, and land is reflected in the way Indigenous Peoples introduce themselves and ground their relationships in kinship, reflecting deeper dimensions and spiritual connections with their land and culture (Kesler, 2020).

---

3. Indigenization is a transformative movement to expand narrow conceptions of knowledge to include Indigenous perspectives, knowledges, and ways of being.

Universities often see Indigenous identity as a concept outside of universities and beyond their responsibility, yet heavily rely on "Indigenous" individuals for Indigenization strategies. If universities are committed to authentic Indigenization strategies, they have a responsibility to ensure the accurate and authentic identity of the individuals they rely on as Indigenous voices. Targeted hires and admission seats set aside for Indigenous applicants often include scholarships and research funding that have led to incentivizing Indigenous identity (Vescera, 2018). These incentives have led to a wave of "pretendians": individuals falsely claiming Indigenous identity based on, at best, re-indigenization, or at worse, false narratives with no Indigenous ancestry, where pretendians claim Indigenous identity without central identity components of community, history, heroes, and kinship ties (Campbell et al., 2021). Enacting re-indigenization, individuals with a "root Indigenous ancestor" 150-400 years ago claiming Indigenous identity, and "descendians," often through mining archives for Indigenous ancestors, positions Indigenous identity as a resource to be extracted in race shifting (Pedri-Spade, 2022). This Indigenous "re-invention" undermines Indigenous self-determination and sovereignties, and the rights of Indigenous communities to determine individual membership (Pedri-Spade, 2022). The rise of pretendians and descendians causes considerable hardship for Indigenous Peoples: mental and emotional strain, furthering colonial trauma by co-opting, claiming, and undermining Indigenous cultures, stories, narratives, and identities, and significantly detracting from the academic and community work and successes of Indigenous Peoples within universities. As Métis academic Janet Smylie (as cited in Leo, 2021) described, allowing pretendians to claim Indigenous identity undermines the integrity of Indigenous identity and in many ways threatens the existence of Indigenous Nations. Moreover, Sisseton-Wahpeton Oyate First Nation academic Kim TallBear (as cited in Harp, 2022) elaborated that eliminating Indigenous Peoples and replacing us with pretendians is an act of genocide – if recognized "Indigenous Peoples" are not Indigenous, then Indigenous Peoples cease to exist. Though false Indigenous identity is a settler colonial crisis (Pedri-Spade, 2022), in the absence of institutional responsibility, it has become Indigenous Peoples' burden to seek out and address such false claims, and positions Indigenous Peoples as assumed frauds who have to prove their identity. This added responsibility further challenges Indigenous Peoples' wellbeing at universities.

In identifying Indigenous Peoples, universities also need to consider who they acknowledge and recognize as Indigenous communities. Internationally, most commonly recognized Indigenous Peoples include only Indigenous Peoples from First World countries: First Nations, Inuit,

Métis in Canada, American Indian and Alaskan Native in the United States, Maori in New Zealand, Torres Straight and First Nations in Australia, and Saami in northern Europe (UN, 2009). However, Indigenous Peoples include all distinct social and cultural groups sharing collective and continual ancestry and ties to lands and resources with pre-colonial or pre-settler societies, forming non-dominant groups of their society. Indigenous Peoples come from lands within ninety countries worldwide (UN, 2009). Universities need to determine if they will recognize Indigenous Peoples from Canada, from First World countries, or more globally.

Identity Systems of Support

Universities need to have clear policies and guidelines to enable Indigenous Peoples to accurately and authentically identify their Indigeneity, when they feel comfortable doing so. As universities regularly rely on Indigenous faculty/staff and students for contributions to Indigenous initiatives and Indigenization strategies, institutions have a responsibility to ensure these solicited contributions stem from people who *are* Indigenous. At the same time, policing Indigenous Peoples' identities through colonial policies reinforces historical traumas and negatively affects Indigenous Peoples' wellbeing. Creating and maintaining environments where it is safe to identify as Indigenous is paramount to supporting Indigenous wellbeing. Moreover, universities need to consider the diversity of Indigenous identities within their institutions. Systems of support for Indigenous identity within universities should also seek to remove barriers and burdens for Indigenous Peoples. For instance, Indigenous identity mining is a settler colonial crisis that does not and should not fall on the backs of Indigenous Peoples to rectify. As leaders of change, universities have an opportunity to partner with Indigenous Nations and communities to lead creation of local and global action for promotion of safe and healthy environments for identity of Indigenous Peoples (Okanagan Charter Call to Action 2.3) (Okanagan Charter, 2015).

Community

A central aspect of Indigenous identity and holistic wellbeing is community. As a minority population on university campuses, developing community among Indigenous Peoples can provide important supports and avenues for wellbeing (Ottmann, 2017). For many Indigenous Peoples who have faced dispossession from land and culture over generations (Richardson, 2004), universities can be important places to reconnect with identity, language, culture, and the wider community. Supporting initiatives and programs to connect Indigenous Peoples with community both broadly and Nation-specific can serve to connect and reconnect spiritual and holistic aspects of wellbeing. This support of personal development is consistent with Call to Action 1.4 of the Okanagan Charter (2015).

Peer support, a form of engaging community, is an important aspect of Indigenous students' success at universities (Gallop & Bastien, 2016). There are numerous examples of undergraduate academic programs designed specifically for Indigenous students, where a community of Indigenous students naturally forms and Indigenous students may have greater educational success (e.g., Indian Teacher Education Program at USask, Indigenous Nursing Entry Program at Lakehead University) (Gallop & Bastien, 2016). Within undergraduate programs where a critical mass of Indigenous students has been reached, many Indigenous student societies have formed, creating a community of Indigenous students within a program (e.g., Indigenous Business Students' Society at USask, Indigenous Law Students Association at UofA). Indigenous student groups have also formed at larger college or institutional levels across programs, providing greater voice for Indigenous students (e.g., Indigenous Students' Union at USask, Indigenous Students' Association at Western University). While some of these communities incorporate Indigenous students and allies, some communities are limited to Indigenous students. Cross-institutional communities of Indigenous students have also been created within disciplines (e.g., Indigenous Medical Students Association of Canada). For graduate students, the ability to form a community with other Indigenous students can be more challenging and represents an important component of wellbeing at university (Ottmann, 2017). To develop these graduate-level communities, some universities have created institution-wide Indigenous graduate student associations (e.g., Indigenous Graduate Students' Council at USask, Indigenous Graduate Students' Association at UofA) or cross-institution associations (e.g., SAGE – Supporting Aboriginal Graduate Enhancement in British Columbia). The Canadian Institutes of Health Research (CIHR) funded Indigenous Mentorship Networks were also a primary source of community among Indigenous graduate students within each respective network. Expanding beyond communities of students, the CIHR-funded Network Environments for Indigenous Health Research (NEIHR) also provide community for students and researchers. Across diverse programs and enrolment tapestries, different supports and student needs arise in forming community among Indigenous students. Creating and supporting community among Indigenous students is an important initiative to support wellbeing.

Most universities have an Indigenous student centre (e.g., Gordon Oakes Red Bear Student Centre at USask, Indigenous Student Resource Centre at Memorial University), including physical space, where supports and programming for Indigenous students can be housed. Having physical spaces on campus where Indigenous students can be themselves, without the self-editing of being in Euro-Canadian spaces, can provide important opportunities to feel safe and provide mental and emotional relief/support (Johnson et al., 2021). Many Indigenous student centres provide services to Indigenous students such as tutoring, cultural activities, education and information sessions, networking opportunities, and smudging facilities. These services can support emotional wellbeing through social interactions, academic supports, and community building, and should be available and accessible to Indigenous students across disciplines and campus locations. Some centres offer family-based programming where Indigenous students and their children/families can engage in activities together. As Indigenous students are generally older than non-Indigenous students, incorporating family activities can weave together Indigenous students' responsibilities to studies and family, and create opportunities for social engagement while supporting self-efficacy (Ottmann, 2017). Community support is an important mediator for physical activity among Indigenous Peoples on campuses (Ironside et al., 2021), and Indigenous Peoples on campuses may benefit from Indigenous fitness programs (e.g., Fit 4 U at USask; Ferguson & Philipenko, 2016). Various "lunch and learn" sessions are common among many universities (e.g., UBC, Vancouver Island University), where community building among Indigenous Peoples on campus is supported around a meal and information sessions. While supports and programs are generally available through Indigenous student centres, siloing of supports through such centres brings supports only to students active in attending and maintaining communication from Indigenous student centres.

Building community among Indigenous faculty/staff is critical for wellbeing and breaking down the isolation of being an Indigenous person in the academy. Initiatives to develop community among Indigenous faculty/staff require university-level support, and should begin from the point of hire. Some universities have undertaken cluster hires of Indigenous faculty to develop community among new hires. Unlike Indigenous student organizations, formal Indigenous faculty/staff organizations at academic institutions are few and far between (e.g., newly established National Indigenous University Senior Leaders' Association). Without support and connection through universities or unions, it can be challenging for Indigenous Peoples hired into institutions to connect with and create community with other Indigenous Peoples, particularly for "orphaned"

Indigenous faculty/staff who are the only Indigenous employees in their academic unit. University-level supports, such as annual Indigenous faculty/staff gatherings sponsored by the institution or other ad hoc or formalized groups of Indigenous faculty/staff provide meaningful ways for engaging community within institutions. Supporting and improving wellbeing for Indigenous faculty/staff requires opportunities for an Indigenous community on campus to meet and visit[4] without specific agendas or mandates to be fulfilled during meeting times. For many Indigenous faculty/staff, community on campus has formed through Indigenous-specific committees or research teams, which may not be equally accessible across academic units. With small numbers of Indigenous faculty nationwide, discipline-specific community requires cross-institution levels of engagement. As these cross-institution communities are not grounded in a specific university, development of such communities is limited to the few disciplines where conferences have developed (e.g., Native American and Indigenous Studies Association, Mawachihitotaak Métis Studies Symposium, CIHR-funded NEIHRs). Further, awareness and engagement of these conferences depend primarily on word of mouth, pre-existing relationships, and research programs fitting conference mandates. For many Indigenous faculty, discipline-specific communities of Indigenous faculty would be a useful support for their wellbeing but remain out of reach without innovative supports from universities.

In addition to individual accountability, Indigenous Peoples hold a higher standard of collective responsibilities to their Indigenous Nations and communities. This collective responsibility for and subsequent support of communities provide a robust support system for Indigenous students and faculty/staff. At the same time, crises, trauma, and challenges in home communities, often unexpected or unplanned, require collective responsibility and support that can take time from academic studies/work and contribute to increased stress and potential mental health challenges for Indigenous Peoples. Providing mental health supports for Indigenous Peoples at universities requires tailored supports, as the legacy of distrust from historic and ongoing colonialism positions "Western" counselling as not relevant or sympathetic to Indigenous cultures (Robertson et al., 2015). Mental health services that allow Indigenous Peoples to engage in more traditionally based services, including Elders, healers, and spiritual

---

4. Visiting was once embedded in Indigenous Peoples' everyday lives and consists of gathering together for dialogue and deliberation, storytelling, celebration, laughter, and sharing and caring for our relatives. Visiting maintains kinship roles, social relationships, and can positively impact wellness (Flaminio et al., 2020).

leaders from individual home communities, traditional medicine people, and traditional ways of engaging with Western mental health professionals, such as storytelling or other non-linear, holistic ways of discussing challenges, can provide benefits for Indigenous Peoples (Robertson et al., 2015). Engaging and supporting community may be a meaningful way to support mental wellbeing among Indigenous Peoples.

Community Systems of Support

Consistent with Okanagan Charter Call to Action 1.3, universities should generate thriving communities and a culture of wellbeing (Okanagan Charter, 2015). Supporting Okanagan Charter Call to Action 1.5 can also provide additional community systems of support by creating and reorienting campus services to meet the needs of Indigenous Peoples (Okanagan Charter, 2015). By providing opportunities for community, universities promote Indigenous students and faculty/staffs' wellbeing and flourishing. Community for Indigenous Peoples needs to be supported on multiple levels, from connections to home communities, to communities within and across disciplines and communities within Indigenous identities. Opportunities to develop community must recognize and support differing histories and unique cultures across these communities that may require differing initiatives, programs, and policies to appropriately support their wellbeing. Supporting Indigenous Peoples wellbeing at universities requires opportunity for community activities, including physical, cultural, spiritual, and culturally grounded supports.

Environment

Indigenous Peoples want to belong to their families and communities, and also to university spaces (Indspire, 2018). As people living within Western, colonized spaces, Indigenous Peoples walk two worlds, which is physically, mentally, and emotionally exhausting (Johnson et al., 2021). In addition to having safe spaces to be themselves, such as Indigenous student centres, Indigenous Peoples need to feel welcome and comfortable in all spaces throughout the university (Indspire, 2018). Indigenous Peoples need to see themselves, their histories, and their cultures woven throughout all aspects of universities from courses, content, processes, supports, and systems to physical spaces, and experienced and perceived environments (Indspire, 2018). Environments need to be supportive and create an atmosphere where Indigenous Peoples and their cultures are a priority, rather than an accommodation (Indspire, 2018). The atmosphere of the environment around universities greatly influences the ability of Indigenous Peoples to succeed and substantially influences their holistic wellbeing. Okanagan Charter Call to Action 2.1 calls for integration of health, wellbeing, and sustainability across disciplines to develop change, which for Indigenous Peoples requires weaving of supports and a sense of inclusion into all aspects of the university environment (Okanagan Charter, 2015).

Universities need to be environments where Indigenous Peoples feel they belong, are safe and supported, and can "see" themselves (Gallop & Bastien, 2016; Ottmann, 2017). Universities need to have transition supports for Indigenous students moving from primarily Indigenous spaces to the university (Lewington, 2017; Ottmann, 2017). The changes in environment and expectations can create tensions and conflicts, requiring academic, social, and personal-emotional adjustments (Ottmann, 2017). Further, Indigenous students need to see Indigenous faculty/staff mentors whom they feel safe turning to for support and can engage with and relate to (Gallop & Bastien, 2016; Indspire, 2018). For Indigenous students, politics of experiences at universities create significant barriers to participation and attendance. With 79 per cent European-descent faculty and low numbers of Indigenous students, universities can be unsafe places for Indigenous students, where being so under-represented can make universities feel isolating (Laferte, 2021). Supports for Indigenous students, such as educational guidance and advising and supports for wellbeing, need to be present throughout all programs, departments, colleges, and faculties, not just within a dedicated Indigenous student centre. The greatest benefits will be seen when a community of Indigenous Peoples can be built around such supports. Examples include the USask Community of Aboriginal Nursing Program and the Indigenous Student Initiatives Manager in the Faculty of Medicine at the UBC.

The ongoing environment and appetite for reconciliation and Indigenization inevitably mean that Indigenous faculty/staff are repeatedly sought out for every Indigenous-related committee, advisory group, and research project seeking Indigenous input (Vescera, 2018). This "race tax" creates unequal service responsibilities due to under-representation, resulting in two or three times more committee/service work than non-Indigenous faculty (Henry et al., 2017; Vescera, 2018). When combined with an environment that is not supportive of Indigenous Peoples, this leads to systemic burnout of Indigenous faculty (Vescera, 2018). Burnout among Indigenous faculty adds complex challenges for initiatives that seek to increase recruitment and retention of Indigenous graduate students and faculty, as Indigenous undergraduates interacting with emotionally rundown Indigenous faculty are less likely to enter graduate school (Vescera, 2018). Moreover, support is needed for Indigenous faculty who experience high burdens of emotional labour in supporting Indigenous students, faculty, and their own communities, while walking two worlds and dealing with historic colonial barriers as minority faculty in academia (Vescera, 2018).

Education and understanding about Indigenous Peoples should begin with courses and content embedded within all programs and degrees (Indspire, 2018). More importantly, this content must be accurate, respectful, and go beyond simple history to include Indigenous culture, and ways of knowing, being, and doing (Indspire, 2018). When this content is cursory or inaccurate, it creates undue burdens, and mental and emotional strain for Indigenous students who are faced with correcting inaccuracies and misinformation presented by instructors (Indspire, 2018). Similarly, Indigenous students are sometimes called to be the "Indigenous experts" and are asked to share or teach this material to their classmates, or to provide the "Indigenous point of view" (p. 5), creating additional stress and discomfort (Indspire, 2018). Indigenous content within classes should be taught by Indigenous Peoples who can provide authentic Indigenous perspectives (Indspire, 2018).

Universities need to provide an environment of anti-racism and anti-oppression. Indigenous faculty across Canada report hostile work environments, facing daily microaggressions, regular racism, and complacent administration providing only lip service towards change (Henry et al., 2017). Experiences of racism and discrimination significantly influence Indigenous Peoples' wellbeing, from participation in physical activities and sports, to willingness to seek out medical help (Ironside et al., 2021; Johnson et al., 2021). The emotional labour of Indigenous Peoples surviving in colonial spaces, microaggressions, or overt racism and balancing walking in two worlds creates significant mental, physical, and emotional burdens for Indigenous Peoples (Indspire, 2018; Johnson et al., 2021). Indigenous students often face racist and discriminatory criticism from peers including the questioning of their identity because students don't "look Indigenous" or didn't grow up on a reserve, or labelling them as a "free loading Indian" (Maracle, 2014). These experiences of hostile and challenging environments leave Indigenous students facing mental and emotional labour, which are not experienced by non-Indigenous students. Further, asking Indigenous faculty to give guest lectures on Indigenous topics across curriculums and courses minimizes the responsibility of European-descent faculty to make universities more inclusive and welcoming (Henry et al., 2017).

Developing a supportive environment for Indigenous Peoples' wellbeing requires a community of informed, educated, and engaged allies. Authentic allies can contribute to a more welcoming and supporting environment for Indigenous Peoples, and subsequently promote their wellbeing. Awareness and education initiatives can support safe environments and promote development of allies (e.g., Indigenous Education Weeks at the University of Toronto and Wilfrid Laurier University, Indigenous Knowledge Public Lecture Series at the University of Calgary). Importantly, beyond allies, strong accomplices are needed for long-term, sustainable change to make universities safe and supportive environments for Indigenous Peoples (Jones, 2021). Accomplices work in solidarity with Indigenous Peoples to overthrow systems of oppression, institutions, and norms that lead to inequality (Jones, 2021). Accomplices take on personal risks and losses to support Indigenous Peoples, disrupt colonial norms, and further equity agendas, particularly when it may not be safe for Indigenous Peoples to push such actions. Within universities, potential ways to be accomplices for Indigenous Peoples include admitting and investing in Indigenous students from a variety of backgrounds, altering financial models to support community initiatives, establishing enforceable goals with penalties for failure, and seeking out research supports, collaborations, and opportunities with and for Indigenous faculty (Jones, 2021). Further supporting Indigenous Peoples' wellbeing at universities will also require advancing research, teaching, and training across all aspects of weaving Indigenous safety and wellbeing into the fabric of universities, consistent with the Okanagan Charter Call to Action 2.2 (Okanagan Charter, 2015).

Celebration of Indigenous student successes at universities can also support creating and promoting safe environments, including mid-year celebrations (e.g., Indigenous Achievement Week at USask) and graduation celebrations (e.g., Indigenous Scarf Ceremony at McGill University, Indigenous Graduation Celebration at UBC). For Indigenous faculty, experiencing acknowledgement and celebration of their achievements (e.g., Academica.ca Indigenous Top 10) can also support feeling included and welcomed in universities. While these initiatives support awareness and knowledge of Indigenous Peoples' experiences, large-scale shifts in attitudes and mindsets across and beyond universities are needed to support identity safety, unpack perceptions of special treatment for Indigenous Peoples, and create safe environments for Indigenous Peoples.

Creating inclusive and supportive environments for Indigenous Peoples includes incorporation of all aspects of Indigenous cultures, including languages, traditional practices, and teachings. Cultural activities hosted at universities, often connected to Indigenous student centres, are associated with greater cultural integrity, promote community, and support Indigenous student self-esteem, confidence, and capacity (Gallop

& Bastien, 2016). Spiritual/cultural practices often engage multiple dimensions of wellbeing, from traditional dances and physical activities/ games, to smudging, sweats, and other forms of prayer and grounding, which support mental and emotional wellbeing (Gallop & Bastien, 2016). Teachings, knowledge sharing, and intergenerational knowledge transmission provide important opportunities for maintaining and expanding connections with culture, land, and identity (Gallop & Bastien, 2016). Cultural identity supports multiple dimensions of wellbeing, from lowering blood pressure, to enhancing mental resilience and reducing fear of assimilation (Foulds et al., 2016; Gallop & Bastien, 2016). Cultural continuity is an important component of mental wellbeing within Indigenous communities (Chandler & Lalonde, 1998). It is important to remember that cultural activities and practices are specific to individual identities and vary from Nation to Nation. Supporting cultural engagement requires ongoing commitment and investment in cultural events across Indigenous identities, which require the support of Elders, Traditional Knowledge Keepers, or others familiar with cultural activities. The ability to engage in Indigenous practices, protocols, and spirituality, such as smudging, needs to be available in spaces throughout campus locations (Indspire, 2018). Spaces and support for Indigenous Peoples also need to be easily identifiable and accessible to the broader Indigenous community. When Indigenous spaces, practices, supports, and content are limited to single buildings, programs/courses, and advisors, Indigenous Peoples continue to be marginalized, essentially recreating the reserve system on university campuses.

The land is the first teacher; all things come from the land (Styres, 2011). There is an interrelationship between Indigenous identity and place, grounding Indigenous knowledges in the land (Styres, 2011). The opportunity to spend time on the land, in natural environments, is important for mental and emotional wellbeing, and brings forth land as a spiritual dynamic (Styres, 2011). Many Indigenous Peoples need time in natural environments to recharge, particularly when embedded in Western, colonial environments such as living in cities and working or studying at universities. Further, land where Indigenous Peoples can practice traditional harvesting/gardening and practice learning on the land (e.g., Indigenous Teaching Garden at the University of the Fraser Valley, gardens at the Ontario Tech University) can provide additional opportunities for traditional subsistence and time on the land. Access to traditional subsistence methods supports Indigenous Peoples' wellbeing, incorporating aspects of cultural and spiritual health with healthy foods. It is important for universities to have natural environment spaces that are easily accessible from campus locations, where Indigenous Peoples can access spiritual land-based connections to reconnect, reclaim, and relate to Indigenous identities and ways of knowing, being, and doing.

Environment Systems of Support

As outlined in the Okanagan Charter Call to Action 1.2, universities should strive to create supportive campus environments (Okanagan Charter, 2015). Creating supportive environments for Indigenous Peoples on campus requires changes and supports throughout all levels, systems, spaces, programs, curriculums, and minds on campus. Supportive environments include physical and natural environment spaces, appropriate workloads for Indigenous faculty/staff considering the additional responsibilities, burdens, and requests of Indigenous Peoples, social environments of anti-racism and anti-oppression, and inclusion of Indigenous cultural and traditional practices. Establishing true supportive environments will require mind shifts and cultural shifts among non-Indigenous people at universities and the support of accomplices and allies.

Economics and Politics

For Indigenous students, insufficient funding for education is often a significant barrier in pursuing and attaining post-secondary education (Indspire, 2018). On average, Indigenous students are older than non-Indigenous students attending universities (Ottmann, 2017), and many are also caregivers to children, family, and community members. Consequently, insufficient funding, including the resources needed for and access to childcare, are considerable barriers for many Indigenous students (Indspire, 2018). Though status First Nations students are eligible to receive funding for post-secondary education through the Indigenous Services Canada branch of the federal government, significant gaps in available funds, which have not kept up with inflation, limit available supports, often creating waitlists of individuals within each First Nation requesting funds to attend post-secondary institutions (Timmons & Stoicheff, 2016). Further, this federal funding is not available to non-status First Nations, Métis, or Inuit students. Indigenous students more often have to relocate to attend universities, limiting support networks while attending (Timmons & Stoicheff, 2016). As community is central to many Indigenous Peoples, Indigenous students also often travel to their home communities mid-semester to attend funerals, gatherings, and other ceremonies requiring extra funds for travel, and time away from studies. Economic challenges faced by Indigenous students are intensified because of limited summer employment opportunities, both due to location of home communities and racial legacies of colonialism (Timmons & Stoicheff, 2016). Overall, economic challenges faced by many Indigenous students limit their ability to attend, continue with, and succeed in university.

Supports available to Indigenous students and faculty/staff on campuses are often limited to Eurocentric world views. Medical plans provided for students and faculty/staff are based on Eurocentric definitions of medicine and often overlook culturally appropriate supports from traditional healers, Indigenous counsellors, and ceremonies. Support for Indigenous students and faculty/staff needs to include medical coverage for Indigenous counsellors and healers as part of standard medical plans. While some Indigenous supports are starting to be included at universities (e.g., Indigenous health expenses added as a category in USask's personal spending account), coverage for these traditional healing services available for students are rare. In addition, Indigenous students and faculty/staff often have to take time away from studies or use vacation time to attend cultural ceremonies celebrated outside of universities' Eurocentric calendars where classes and exams are scheduled around Christian holidays, further challenging Indigenous students and faculty/staff's ability to attain wellbeing across holistic health dimensions. Restricted access to traditional healing, cultural ceremonies, and Indigenous counselling further compounds the economic challenges for Indigenous Peoples at universities.

Success in recruiting Indigenous Peoples into universities requires growing from the grassroots. Recruiting Indigenous students to university "often begins in elementary or high school with Indigenous-infused summer camps, campus visits and transition-to-university boot camps" (Lewington, 2017). While many universities are pushing to increase Indigenous faculty numbers, the small pool of Indigenous candidates has led to a "gold rush" of Indigenous PhDs with sufficient publications and funding records to be considered for faculty positions (Vescera, 2018). Though Indigenous candidates are highly sought after, Indigenous PhD graduates are less likely to attain faculty positions (Henry et al., 2017). The competition for limited numbers of Indigenous PhDs regularly leads to hiring of Indigenous graduate students years earlier than their non-Indigenous peers (Vescera, 2018). Early recruitment places many new Indigenous faculty hires in challenging positions, where non-Indigenous peers may have a cynical view that Indigenous faculty are not as worthy, prepared, or successful (Vescera, 2018). Combined with the increased committee work and fewer years of training to prepare for academic positions, these cynical outlooks can become self-fulfilling stereotypes where Indigenous faculty appear less productive ten years into their careers compared to non-Indigenous hires (Vescera, 2018). New Indigenous faculty face challenging burdens weaving together responsibilities of teaching assignments, the increased committee and service requirements compared to non-Indigenous faculty, and beginning their research programs, while also feeling less confident in declining the avalanche of requests they face to provide Indigenous perspectives across a range of initiatives and curriculums across campus. Indigenous faculty who are hired before completion of their PhD face even further burdens in completing their PhD studies, while also undertaking these extraordinary burdens as new Indigenous faculty. Recruiting Indigenous Peoples into universities can only be successful if they are recruited into supportive and safe environments (Lewington, 2017).

As overviewed by Henry et al. (2017), Indigenous faculty face greater barriers in achieving key career markers. For instance, three per cent fewer Indigenous faculty make tenure, and 14 per cent fewer make full professor, at an average of three years later, compared to European-descent faculty. These delays in attaining career progression milestones lead to lower pay overall among Indigenous faculty. These career delays are amplified by less targeted mentoring of Indigenous faculty, while European-descent faculty are often mentored to succeed in their positions and further progression to administration. Within Eurocentric universities, Indigenous knowledges and Indigenous research are often undervalued, creating further challenges for Indigenous faculty seeking tenure and promotion. Overall, though Indigenous faculty publish more articles and attain more tri-council funding than faculty members of European-descent, Indigenous faculty are paid less, creating a system where Indigenous work and skills are less valued in universities. These tapestries of low Indigenous worth contribute to an ongoing challenge in retention of Indigenous faculty.

Many universities are currently undertaking initiatives towards Indigenization (Ottmann, 2017). To be true Indigenization movements, universities need to weave Indigenous values, principles, and modes of organization and behaviour into every fabric of the university, including structures and processes (Ottmann, 2017). These movements require acknowledgement that change is needed, and recognition of the strengths gained through inclusion of Indigenous voices and knowledges. The process of Indigenization on many post-secondary campuses is structured as a top-down approach, with Indigenous faculty positioned to be the voices of Indigenous Peoples on campuses, though few are involved in executive decision-making processes (McKenzie-Jones, 2019). This top-down approach is superficial and tokenistic to Indigenization (Anti-Racism

Network et al., n.d.). Moreover, this approach paradoxically positions Indigenous Peoples at risk for speaking out against detrimental policies (McKenzie-Jones, 2019). Processes of Indigenization need to proceed cautiously, for fear of losing cultural identities and languages, and becoming another instrument of assimilation (Newhouse, 2016). Further, university administrators seeking Indigenization must acknowledge that Indigenization is not bound by the limits of how Western thinking defines it, and must include weaving Indigenous Peoples, knowledges, and cultures into the fabric of the university (Pidgeon, 2016). Supporting authentic and culturally safe processes and structures of Indigenization requires Indigenous faculty/staff and students to lead Indigenization projects and decision-making processes, and universities' acceptance of the legitimacy of Indigenous legal and cultural systems (Anti-Racism Network et al., 2021; McKenzie-Jones, 2019). Successful achievement of this authentic process also requires systems to alleviate Indigenous faculty workloads in other areas to avoid and prevent overburdening oversubscribed Indigenous faculty (McKenzie-Jones, 2019). Achieving meaningful change occurs when administrators are accomplices, and particularly when leadership positions include individuals other than males of European descent (Henry et al., 2017). While Indigenous Peoples are crucial in leading and directing Indigenization processes, care must be taken to maintain wellbeing of the Indigenous Peoples entrusted with these responsibilities.

Indigenization initiatives begin with increasing visibility of Indigenous Peoples, languages, cultures, and voices (Gaudry & Lorenz, 2018). Visible symbols, boasting of new recruits, enrolled students, and welcoming messages, are easy accomplishments of "Indigenous inclusion" to show the progress of Indigenization. However, meaningful changes to the daily experiences and lives of Indigenous Peoples at universities requires more long-term initiatives. "Reconciliation Indigenization" seeks to achieve meaningful change for greater inclusion of Indigenous Peoples and knowledges at universities within the common threads of Indigenous and non-Indigenous ideals (Gaudry & Lorenz, 2018). Conversely, "Decolonial Indigenization" requires untangling threads of universities to weave together a radically transformed university with knowledge systems and values reoriented towards Indigenous cultures, politics, knowledges, and land-based skills (Gaudry & Lorenz, 2018). Universities need to determine their commitment to reweaving the threads to create something radically different. When universities' Indigenization strategies are limited to increasing numbers of Indigenous Peoples on campus, the lack of holistic inclusion of Indigenous knowledges, cultures, and world views leaves Indigenous Peoples experiencing continued retraumatization, breakdown of trust and relationships, and feelings of exclusion. As commitments and words of change continue, Indigenous Peoples expect and rely on authentic and significant change, which has the potential to positively influence their wellbeing.

The leaders who determine the policies and politics at universities need to consider the balance between Indigenous Peoples upon whose lands universities sit, and the diverse identities, cultures, and knowledges of the Indigenous Peoples they employ, teach, and welcome. The recognition of First Nations, Inuit, and Métis Peoples in Canada reflects the differing legal relationships Canada has with Indigenous Peoples, though this generalized terminology undermines the distinctiveness and diversity of individual Indigenous Nations. While universities across Canada undertake similar Indigenization initiatives, these processes, outcomes, and experiences need to be vastly different from one another. Each university sits on lands that hold different meanings, stories, and knowledges to the original inhabitants of these primarily unceded lands. Incorporating Indigenous ways of knowing, being, and doing will require understandings of the unique places and spaces where each specific university is located. While land acknowledgements reflect the specific lands upon which universities sit, many reconciliation efforts, such as targeted hiring, rarely consider the Peoples with whom Canada or universities specifically are trying to reconcile. Moreover, standard overarching approaches to support Indigenous Peoples' wellness while at university do not consider the varying needs, experiences, and expertise of diverse Indigenous Peoples. University leaders who support the wellbeing of Indigenous Peoples need to consider the diversity of Indigenous Nations, their histories, cultures, and experiences.

Economic and Political Systems of Support

Enacting safe and supportive policies and initiatives (Okanagan Charter Call to Action 1.1) to further enable Indigenous Peoples' wellbeing at universities require substantial change (Okanagan Charter, 2015). Weaving Indigenous ways of knowing, being, and doing into the fabrics of universities needs to include appropriate health care and wellbeing supports, appropriate holidays and ceremonial leaves, and accommodations of time to support the multiple responsibilities held by Indigenous Peoples. Financial supports for Indigenous students need to recognize Indigenous Peoples' increased responsibilities to family and community, childcare needs, and the increased and competing workload demands faced by Indigenous Peoples. Valuing contributions, experiences, and expertise of Indigenous Peoples at universities requires changes to Eurocentric standards, qualifications, eligibilities, interpretations of academic outputs, and rigid colonial policies. Universities need to consider the spectrum of educational systems, from preschool through grade school and to the multiple levels of university education to weave supports throughout all levels. Authentic Indigenization processes will need to go beyond the increased visibility prioritized by most universities to deconstruct universities at the very core and enable the weaving together of Indigenous ways of knowing, being, and doing throughout all aspects of universities.

Weaving Together

Given the many injustices and challenges for Indigenous Peoples within universities that gravely impact their wellbeing, how do we move forward? As a starting place, we highlight the potential utility of an equity indicators framework for universities to begin locating themselves on a spectrum from completely colonial dominant to more equitable and culturally safe. The Anti-Racism Network et al. (2021) developed their equity indicators framework, which evaluates key criteria of an organization's structures, policies, and programs. The framework is rooted in anti-racist methodology whereby rubrics are used to evaluate performance on accountability, budget, human resources, leadership and decision-making (i.e., power), location, partnerships, pay, programs and services, professional development and training, strategic planning, and revenue resources. The result is a visual representation of the extent to which an organization is culturally safe, anti-racist, and anti-oppressive. Utilizing an equity indicator framework may support initial steps towards organizational changes that support Indigenous Peoples' wellbeing, consistent with Okanagan Charter Call to Action 1.1, to embed health in all campus policies. It is imperative that such frameworks be used cautiously and intentionally as a starting place, so as to not perpetuate checklist approaches that superficially support Indigenous Peoples' wellbeing. Engaging in transparent evaluation to identify meaningful action towards structural changes is a step towards becoming a health and wellbeing promoting campus, as called upon in the Okanagan Charter.

Supporting Indigenous Peoples' wellbeing requires careful, critical, and deliberate change throughout every fabric of universities. Indigenous Peoples at universities are under-represented, oversubscribed, and undervalued. Maintaining and retaining Indigenous Peoples at universities will require universities to be safe spaces, supportive of Indigenous Peoples' holistic wellbeing, where meaningful and substantial change towards decolonized Indigenization is realized and forthcoming. Health promoting universities that want to transform the health of our societies, strengthen communities, and contribute to wellbeing demand anti-colonial approaches that bring attention to, and take action against, power structures that assert oppression. As researchers, we encourage the weaving of anti-colonial approaches (Hart et al., 2017) to confront colonial processes, be deeply committed to Indigenous values, centre relationships, affirm Indigenous knowledges, and generate positive change for Indigenous Peoples, as defined by them, thus fostering Indigenous self-determination, self-governance, and sovereignty throughout the fabric of universities. Supporting and promoting Indigenous Peoples' wellbeing needs to consider the diversity of Indigenous Nations, the specific Indigenous Peoples upon whose lands universities sit, and with whom universities are specifically intending to reconcile. Supporting Indigenous Peoples' wellbeing will require unravelling current institutional structures, policies, and mindsets, to fully integrate strands of Indigenous identities, communities, environments, economics, and politics within the existence of universities. Universities that do so will become leaders in health promotion action.

REFERENCES

Anti-Racism Network, Sasakamoose-Kuffner, B., Rosenberg, R., Fitzsimmons, S., Drozd, H., Brophy, C., Walling, E., Battiste, A., & Heimlick, M. (2021). *Equity indicators framework*. https://cooperation.ca/wp-content/uploads/2021/01/20210119-Antiracism-Framework-3.0.pdf

Bougie, E., & Senecal, S. (2010). *School success and the intergenerational effect of residential schooling*. University of Western Ontario. Retrieved from https://ir.lib.uwo.ca/aprci/88

Bourgeon, L., Burke, A., & Higham, T. (2017). Earliest human presence in North America dated to the last glacial maximum: New radiocarbon dates from Bluefish Caves, Canada. *PLoS One, 12*(1), e0169486. https://doi.org/10.1371/journal.pone.0169486

Campbell, M., Belcourt, T., & Lavallee, L. (2021). *Metis identity*, Faculty of Community Services at Ryerson University. https://www.youtube.com/watch?v=KxyJ0b97TIE

Canadian Human Rights Commission. (2013). *Report on equality rights of Aboriginal People*. Government of Canada. Retrieved from http://publications.gc.ca/site/eng/9.697656/publication.html

Chandler, MJ., & Lalonde, C. (1998). Cultural continuity as a hedge against suicide in Canada's First Nations. *Transcultural Psychiatry, 35*(2), 191–219. https://doi.org/10.1177/136346159803500202

Crown-Indigenous Relations and Northern Affairs Canada. (2017). *Indigenous peoples and communities*. Government of Canada. Retrieved from www.rcaanc-cirnac.gc.ca/eng/1100100013785/1529102490303

Ferguson, L., & Philipenko, N. (2016). "I would love to blast some pow music and just dance": First Nations students' experiences of physical activity on a university campus. *Qualitative Research in Sport, Exercise, and Health, 8,* 180–93. https://doi.org/10.1080/2159676X.2015.1099563

Flaminio, A.C., Gaudet, J.C., & Dorian, L.M. (2020). Métis women gathering: Visiting together and voicing wellness for ourselves. *AlterNative: An International Journal of Indigenous Peoples, 16*(1), 55–63. https://doi.org/10.1177/1177180120903499

Foulds, H.J., Bredin, S.S., & Warburton, D.E. (2016). The vascular health status of a population of adult Canadian Indigenous peoples from British Columbia. *J Hum Hypertens, 30*(4), 278–84. https://doi.org/10.1038/jhh.2015.51

Gallop, C.J., & Bastien, N. (2016). Supporting success: Aboriginal students in higher education. *Canadian Journal of Higher Education, 46,* 206–24. https://doi.org/10.47678/cjhe.v46i2.184772

Garner, R., Carriere, G., & Sanmartin, C. (2010). The health of First Nations living off-reserve, Inuit, and Métis adults in Canada: The impact of socio-economic status on inequalities in health. *Health Research Working Paper Series.* Catalogue no 82-622-X(004). https://www150.statcan.gc.ca/n1/en/pub/82-622-x/82-622-x2010004-eng.pdf?st=raytlS9g

Gaudry, A., & Lorenz, D. (2018). Indigenization as inclusion, reconciliation, and decolonization: Navigating the different visions for indigenizing the Canadian academy. *AlterNative, 14*(3), 218–27. https://doi.org/10.1177/1177180118785382

Gordon, C.E., & White, J.P. (2014). Indigenous educational attainment in Canada. *The International Indigenous Policy Journal, 5*(3), 6. https://doi.org/10.18584/iipj.2014.5.3.6

Government of Canada. (2019). *Indian Act (R.S.C., 1985, c. I-5).* Minister of Justice. Retrieved from https://laws-lois.justice.gc.ca/eng/acts/i-5/

Graham, H., & Stamler, L.L. (2010). Contemporary perceptions of health from an Indigenous (Plains Cree) perspective. *International Journal of Indigenous Health, 6*(1), 6–17. https://doi.org/10.18357/ijih61201012341

Greenwood, M., de Leeuw, S., & Lindsay, N.M. (2018). *Determinants of Indigenous peoples' health, Second edition: Beyond the social.* Canadian Scholars. https://books.google.ca/books?id=jblaDwAAQBAJ

Harp, R. (2022, 26 October). The unravelling story of Mary-Ellen Turpel-Lafond. *MEDIA INDIGENA : Indigenous current affairs* (ep 304). https://podcasts.google.com/feed/aHR0cHM6Ly9tZWRpYWluZGlnZW5hLmxpYnN5bi5jb20vcnNz/episode/YmU0OTMwZDMtOGQyZS00ZTM3LThkNWItZTFiYzRiM2NmODIw

Hart, M.A., Straka, S., & Rowe, G. (2017). Working across contexts: Practical considerations of doing Indigenist/anti-colonial research. *Qualitative Inquiry, 23*(5), 332–42. https://doi.org/10.1177/1077800416659084

Henry, F., Dua, E., James, C.E., Kobayashi, A., Li, P., Ramos, H., & Smith, M.S. (2017). *The equity myth: Racialization and Indigeneity at Canadian universities.* UBC Press. https://books.google.ca/books?id=0lcnDwAAQBAJ

Indspire. (2018). *Post-secondary experience of Indigenous students following the Truth and Reconciliation Commission.* Indspire. Retrieved from https://indspire.ca /about/reports/

Ironside, A., Ferguson, L.J., Katapally, T.R., Hedayat, L.M., Johnson, S.R., & Foulds, H.J.A. (2021). Social determinants associated with physical activity among Indigenous adults at the University of Saskatchewan. *Applied Physiology, Nutrition & Metabolism, 46*(10), 1159–69. https://doi.org/10.1139 /apnm-2020-0781

Johnson, S., LaFleur, J., Moore, S., Ferguson, L., McInnes, A., & Foulds, H.J.A. (2021). "It's exhausting to always be self-editing": The importance of culture and social support in the health of Métis Peoples. *Journal of Exercise, Movement, and Sport, 52*(1).

Jones, J.C. (2021). We need accomplices, not allies in the fight for an equitable geoscience. *AGU Advances, 2*(3), e2021AV000482. https://doi.org/https:// doi.org/10.1029/2021AV000482

Kesler, L. (2020). *Aboriginal identity & terminology.* First Nations Studies Program. Retrieved 1 February 2022 from https://indigenousfoundations.arts.ubc. ca/aboriginal_identity__terminology/#:~:text=When%20introducing%20 themselves%2C%20people%20may,of%20their%20community%20or%20nation

King, M., Smith, A., & Gracey, M. (2009). Indigenous health part 2: The underlying causes of the health gap. *Lancet, 374*(9683), 76–85. https://doi .org/10.1016/S0140-6736(09)60827-8

Kuokkanen, R. (2007). *Reshaping the university: Responsibility, Indigenous epistemes, and the logic of the gift.* UBC Press.

Laferte, B. (2021). Indigenous students deal with greater barriers while attending school. *Martlet.* https://www.martlet.ca/uvic-indigenous-students-barriers/

Larivière, P. (2015). *Métis identity in Canada.* Carleton University.

Lavallee, L. F. (2007). Physical activity and healing through the medicine wheel. *Journal of Indigenous Wellbeing Te Mauri – Pimatisiwin,, 5*(1), 127–53.

Leo, G. (2021). *Indigenous or pretender?* Canadian Broadcasting Company (CBC). https://www.cbc.ca/newsinteractives/features/carrie-bourassa-indigenous

Lewington, J. (2017, 5 Dec. 5). Supporting Indigenous students on campus: Finding the best approach. *Macleans.* https://www.macleans.ca/education /truth-and-education/

Maracle, A. (2014, 17 September). Barriers to education remain for Indigenous students. *The Queen's Journal.* https://www.queensjournal.ca/story/2014-09-17 /opinions/barriers-education-remain-indigenous-students/

McGill. (2022a). *Fall 2020.* McGill. Retrieved 25 May 2022 from https://www .mcgill.ca/es/registration-statistics/fall-2020

McGill. (2022b). *Frequently Asked Questions (FAQs).* McGill. Retrieved 25 May 2022 from https://www.mcgill.ca/fph/prospective-students/frequently -asked-questions-faqs

McKenzie-Jones, P. (2019). What does "We are all treaty people" mean, and who speaks up for Indigenous students on campus? *The Conversation Canada.* https://theconversation.com/what-does-we-are-all-treaty-people-mean-and -who-speaks-for-indigenous-students-on-campus-119060

Mitchell, T., Arseneau, C., & Thomas, D. (2019). Colonial trauma: Complex, continuous, collective, cumulative and compounding effects on the health of Indigenous peoples in Canada and beyond. *International Journal of Indigenous Health, 14*(2), 74–94. https://doi.org/10.32799/ijih.v14i2.32251

Mukherjee-Reed, A., & Szeri, A. (2021). *University of British Columbia Annual Enrolment Report 2020/21.* Vancouver, B.C.: University of British Columbia Retrieved from https://senate.ubc.ca/sites/senate.ubc.ca/files/downloads /UBC-Enrolment-Report-2020-21_0.pdf

Newhouse, D. (2016). The meaning of Indigenization in our universities. *Canadian Association of University Teachers Bulletin, 63.* https://bulletin-archives.caut.ca /bulletin/articles/2016/06/the-meaning-of-indigenization-in-our-universities

Nguyen, B.M.D., Alcantar, C.M., Curammeng, E.R., Hernandez, E., Kim, V., Paredes, A.D., Freeman, R., Ngyuen, MH., & Teranishi, R. T. (2017). *The racial heterogeneity project: Implications for educational research, practice and policy.* ACT Centre for Equity in Learning

Okanagan Charter: An International Charter for Health Promoting Universities and Colleges. (2015). *Okanagan Charter.* Kelowna, BC: Author. Retrieved from http://internationalhealthycampuses2015.sites.olt.ubc.ca/files/2016/01 /Okanagan-Charter-January13v2.pdf

Ottmann, J. (2017). Canada's Indigenous Peoples' access to post-secondary education: The spirit of the 'new buffalo.' In J. Frawley, S. Larkin, & J.A. Smith (Eds.), *Indigenous pathways, transitions and participation in higher education,* (pp. 95–118). Springer Open.

Pedri-Spade, C. (2022). We are facing a settler colonial crisis, not an Indigenous identity crisis. *The Conversation Canada* (26 January 2022). https:// theconversation.com/we-are-facing-a-settler-colonial-crisis-not-an-indigenous -identity-crisis-175136

Pidgeon, M. (2008). *It takes more than good intentions: Institutional accountability and responsibility to Indigenous higher education.* University of British Columbia. https://open.library.ubc.ca/collections/24/items/1.0066636

Pidgeon, M. (2016). More than a checklist: Meaningful Indigenous inclusion in higher education. *Social Inclusion, 4*(1), 77–91. https://doi.org/10.17645 /si.v4i1.436

Richardson, C.L. (2004). *Becoming Metis: The relationship between the sense of Metis self and cultural stories* University of Victoria]. https://dspace.library.uvic.ca /bitstream/handle/1828/655/richardson_2004.pdf;sequence=1

Robertson, L.H., Holleran, K., & Samuels, M. (2015). Tailoring university counselling services to Aboriginal and international students: Lessons from native and international student centers at a Canadian university. *Canadian Journal of Higher Education, 45*(1), 122–35. https://doi.org/10.47678/cjhe.v45i1.184262

Statistics Canada. (2012). *Aboriginal languages in Canada 2011.* Statistics Canada

Statistics Canada. (2020). Survey of post-secondary faculty and researchers, 2019. *The Daily, 11-004-X* (22 September 2020). https://www150.statcan.gc.ca/n1/daily-quotidien/200922/dq200922a-eng.htm

Statistics Canada. (2022). Indigenous population continues to grow and is much younger than the non-Indigenous population, although the pace of growth has slowed. *The Daily, 11-001-X* (21 September 2022), 1–22. https://www150.statcan.gc.ca/n1/daily-quotidien/220921/dq220921a-eng.pdf

Styres, S. (2011). Land as first teacher: A philosophical journeying. *Reflective Practice, 12*(6), 717–31. https://doi.org/10.1080/14623943.2011.601083

Timmons, V., & Stoicheff, P. (2016). *Post-secondary education in Canada: A response to the Truth and Reconciliation Commission of Canada.* University of Regina and University of Saskatchewan. Retrieved from https://www.schoolofpublicpolicy.sk.ca/documents/research/policy-briefs/PolicyBrief-Post%20Secondary%20Education%20in%20Canada.pdf

Truth and Reconciliation Commission. (2015). *Honouring the truth, reconciling for the future: Summary of the final report of the Truth and Reconciliation Commission of Canada.* Truth and Reconciliation Commission of Canada. Retrieved from http://trc.ca/assets/pdf/Honouring_the_Truth_Reconciling_for_the_Future_July_23_2015.pdf

United Nations (UN). (2009). *State of the World's Indigenous Peoples.* United Nations. Retrieved from http://www.un.org/esa/socdev/unpfii/documents/SOWIP/en/SOWIP_web.pdf

University of Alberta. (2022). *Aboriginal students.* University of Alberta. Retrieved May 25 from https://www.ualberta.ca/strategic-plan/overview/student-demographics/aboriginal-students.html

University of Saskatchewan. (2022). *USask Indigenous community.* University of Saskatchewan. Retrieved 25 May from https://leadership.usask.ca/priorities/indigenous/#:~:text=14%25,of%20any%20university%20in%20Canada.

Vescera, Z. (2018, 1 Aug.). 'The Gold Rush': Canadian universities' rush to hire Indigenous faculty is taking an aggressive turn. *The Ubyssey.*

Walters, K.L., Simoni, J.M., & Evans-Campbell, T. (2002). Substance use among American Indians and Alaska Natives: Incorporating culture in an "Indigenist" stress-coping paradigm. *Public Health Rep, 117*(Suppl), S104–S117.

5 Promoting Equity, Diversity, and Inclusion (EDI) through Strategic Planning

MAHA KUMARAN AND SURESH KALAGNANAM

Equity, Diversity, and Inclusion (EDI) and Related Concepts

It is important to note that the language of equity, diversity, and inclusion (EDI) has evolved over the years. The Government of Canada (2024) defines equity as "the removal of systematic barriers"; diversity as "the variety of unique dimensions, identities, qualities, and characteristics individuals possess along with other identify factors"; and inclusion as "the practice of ensuring that all individuals are valued and respected for their contributions and are supported equitably in a culturally safe environment" (para What is EDI). The United Nations has seventeen sustainable development goals (SDGs) of which eight could be directly tied to EDI (UN, n.d.). Lately, EDI, social justice, belonging, and accessibility have gained global emphasis.

In the context of higher educational institutions (HEIs), the push for EDI has been in the making for the past forty years and has gained momentum over the last decade (Cardillo, 1993; Employment Equity Act, 1995; Government of Canada, 2022; Milano, 2019; Universities Canada, 2022). EDI initiatives are rooted in the Athena Swan initiative (Wolbring & Lillywhite, 2021) and initially focused on gender equity in higher education and research. Since then, there have been joint initiatives to bring attention to other dimensions of diversity in HEIs (Wolbring & Lillywhite, 2021).

There are several reasons why EDI is now acknowledged as important in HEIs. First, HEIs are a vital component of society because their main purpose is to educate the current and next generation of individuals who will carry their learning and experiences as they move forward and transform societies through their various activities. Second, research-based HEIs also have the potential to transform societies via their discoveries and other research. According to the Dimensions Charter (2022), engaging in EDI strengthens "the research community, the quality, relevance and impact of research, and the opportunities for the full pool of potential participants" (para 2). Third, as the HEI caters to multiple stakeholder groups, understanding EDI can enable balancing potentially diverse stakeholder needs. In summary, "[h]igher education plays a central role in all aspects of the development of individuals, communities, societies and cultures – locally and globally" (Okanagan Charter, 2015, p. 6) and therefore needs to be intentional about EDI in strategic planning processes.

While EDI's importance is acknowledged in HEIs, it is not always as clarified, implemented, or executed as originally intended in strategic plans (Kouritzin et al., 2021). To begin with, there is a lack of definition of EDI-related concepts in HEI strategic plans. Lane (2000) indicated that it is easier to "arrive at a common understanding of efficiency's meaning than the concept of equity, which is also crucial for public sector governance" (p. 23). Therefore, the focus of EDI in strategic plans might shift towards how EDI can be efficient in sustaining the institution. If strategic plans (SP) mention the inclusion of historically marginalized groups, there is no framework for how this inclusion would be implemented, executed, and evaluated. Kouritzin et al. (2021) assessed their institutions' strategic plan for various keywords and their recurring patterns and concluded that EDI mentions were to "just add minorities and stir" (p. 242). Their study concluded that universities are "ill-prepared and ill-equipped to place under-represented populations and equity-seeking groups front and center" (Kouritzin et al., 2021, p. 252). Several scholars have suggested that large organizations, such as universities, that do not align themselves with the changes in their external environments or the needs of their various stakeholders will face extinction (Dowling & Pfeffer, 1975; Schuman, 1995; Warhurst, 2005). For EDI work to go beyond tokenism and representation, the SP process might benefit from clear directions on where, why, and how EDI strategies are implemented. For example, if the focus is on faculty recruitment, the plan could concentrate on recruitment and all retention-related activities such as research support, promotion, mentorship, leadership roles, and so on, with each year of the plan dedicated to a specific effort. If the focus is on students and employees with disabilities, then support systems such as space redesigning and other accommodations might be priorities.

EDI-Aligned Concepts

There are numerous EDI-aligned concepts, but in the context of strategic planning in higher education, three that surface as important are wellbeing, belonging, and flourishing. Figure 5.1 shows how all three concepts are interconnected and connected to EDI.

Figure 5.1. Interconnectedness of EDI and aligned concepts

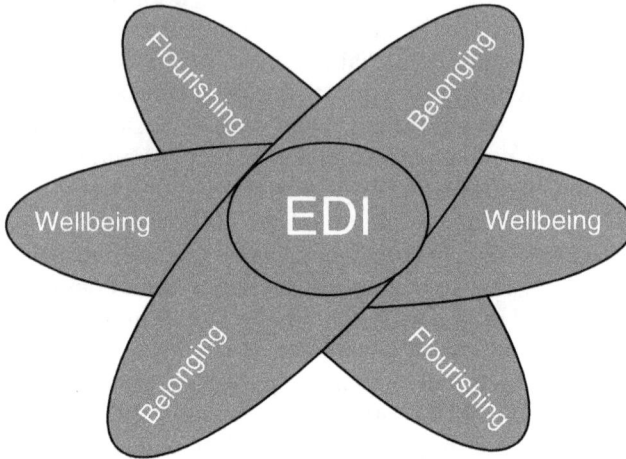

Wellbeing

There are many facets to wellbeing (Amaya et al., 2019; Church, 2023; Holzer et al., 2021; Iordache-Platis, 2020; Minnotte & Pederson, 2023, Peterson et al., 2022). Wellbeing involves physical, psychological, mental, emotional, and spiritual wellbeing. Strategic planning in HEI has typically focused on student wellness and students' mental and physical health. Since the focus of the strategic plan is to compete, it leads to recruiting and retaining students from all over the world, and their success is an important metric to evaluate the success of the institution. However, students' success depends on the wellbeing of all employees in higher education.

International charters such as the Okanagan Charter (2015) recommend a holistic approach to the "wellbeing of people, places, and the planet" (p. 4) by engaging in cross-sector partnerships and "use holistic settings and systems as the foci for enquiry and intervention, effectively drawing attention to the opportunities to create conditions for health in higher education" (Okanagan Charter, 2015, p. 9). This holistic approach also stretches beyond individual health and includes interconnected health determinants such as working spaces. According to a recent report from the College and University Professional Association for Human Resources (2020), more than one-third of American institutions did not have a holistic wellness program. In Canada, there is a community of practice among a group of Canadian universities and colleges that participate in workplace wellness (Canadian Post-secondary Community of Practice for Workplace Wellness, n.d.).

Wellbeing may be very focused or broad. For example, the University of Saskatchewan's wellness focuses on three major elements: a healthy mind, a healthy body, and a healthy life (University of Saskatchewan, n.d.). The University of British Columbia has an even broader approach and focuses on six priority areas of collaborative leadership, mental health resilience, food and nutrition, social connection, built and natural environments, and physical activity for the university community (University of British Columbia, n.d.).

An important driver of wellbeing is inclusion. Bashford (2022) emphasized that "when people feel more included at work, that when their opinions are being sought actively, and they're being respected, valued and included in decision making, that can have a positive effect on their wellbeing at work" (para 2, Inclusion is the birthplace of wellbeing). Within the Canadian HEI context, the University of Toronto is one example where EDI information is integrated into the wellness page (University of Toronto, n.d.). Wellness plans should be guided through an EDI lens for all employees, units, departments, and colleges.

Belonging

Belonging could be the other side of the coin of inclusion. While the institution could provide the necessary inclusive environment, belonging is a sense that comes from the individual. This sense of belonging, although subjective, can only happen if there are efforts towards meaningful integration rather than assimilation. Belonging connects to wellbeing where an individual gains "acceptance, attention and support from members of the group as well as provide[ing] the same attention to other members" (Cherry, 2021, para 2). Belonging is about having a voice, being heard, participating equitably at decision-making tables, and being able to contribute and demand. It suggests "mutual power, access, and opportunity among all groups and individuals within a shared container" (Othering & Belonging Institute, n.d., para 3). Although there are no scales to measure belonging, creating a holistic wellbeing environment could create opportunities and motivations for belonging (Allen et al., 2021)

Flourishing

Flourishing is a multifaceted concept. In simple terms, it is a high level of subjective wellbeing, often complemented by measurable indicators (Hone et al., 2014). In the context of EDI, it is important for all individuals regardless of their status or identities to flourish. Minority faculty flourish with support from their academic communities (Wright-Mair & Marine, 2021). Faculty's positive relationships with students help the latter flourish in academia. All employees flourish "when they experience a sense of belonging and purpose" (Cherkowski & Walker, 2018, p. ii) and for them to find belonging and purpose, they need to be included.

Strategic Planning in Higher Education Institutions

With its origins in a meeting of university planners in 1959 at the Massachusetts Institute of Technology and later Keller's (1983; as cited by Temple, 2018) publication on the topic, SP is often a linear process that generally includes an analysis of the institution's strengths, weaknesses, opportunities, and threats (SWOT). This planning is a complex, formal, and deliberate effort to identify any gaps and help establish future goals for the institution, particularly to stay competitive and sustainable (Temple, 2018; Tromp & Ruben, 2010; William, 2019). Moran (1985) defined strategic planning as a management innovation that provides unity and direction and connects the institution to its environment. Since SP includes many things from analysis to setting directions through goals, it is often a catchall phrase. As a corporate document, the strategic plan commodifies academic practices in pursuit of status, profits, and public image compliance (Kouritzin et al., 2020, 2021). Two significant influences that have shaped strategic planning in HEIs are the concepts of new public management (NPM) and managerial culture.

New Public Management

NPM is a neo-liberal, entrepreneurial, and managerial concept touted as a tool to resolve operational problems in higher education (Carvalho, 2020). NPM is a private-sector concept applied to public services such as publicly funded HEIs and is loaded with arguments and questions about its efficiency for functioning in HEIs, particularly for equity purposes (Lane, 2000). Globalization and fierce competition have propelled many public-sector organizations to focus on competing and therefore move away from socially responsible activities such as equity. This is captured by Fusco and Ricci (2019), who stated that "it is necessary to stress that the public sector has since the 90s been pushed towards focusing on economic and financial targets and responsibilities, on efficiency rather than on effectiveness and – above all – equity" (p. 22), which is referred to in a social sustainability perspective.

Managerial Culture

Based on the Scottish, British, and German higher education models and coming from a Catholic tradition, managerial culture is about administrators controlling all processes for "cost containment, feasibility, and specifiable outcomes" (Bergquist & Pawlak, 2008, p. 45). It is also about leadership, governance and structure, succession planning, decision-making, and people development.

The early models of colleges and universities in North America aimed to serve the underserved, assimilate immigrants into mainstream society, and promote upward social mobility. Immigrants were diverse in terms of their Eastern European and European identities (e.g., French-speaking Catholics). Training and learning in colleges meant a guaranteed place in society. The trend of immigrant students or international students coming to Western universities to improve their educational qualifications and be employed in English-speaking or socio-economically, politically, and religiously stable nations continues today. However, the make-up of immigrant and international students has moved away from Eastern European populations to students from Asia and African countries (Crossman et al., 2021).

As institutions moved away from the Catholic focus towards becoming secular and multipurpose, there was a focus on centralizing managerial efforts, and the state legislature provided the funds, thus forcing the need for strategic and budget planning processes. Outcomes needed to be quantified and tangible to justify the funding from the government. Overall, efficiency, competent administration, effective management of people and resources, and the need to function like an organization rather than an educational institution were pushing HEIs towards adopting managerial cultures. In managerial cultures, students are also expected to be competent. All stakeholders work in a hierarchical structure, have specific roles and expected outcomes, pay attention to generating funds, have detailed meetings and discussions, and plan the future. However, with a focus on high efficiency, the true embedding of EDI in all processes has fallen by the wayside.

Revisioning Strategic Planning

Having a strategy is necessary for HEIs to compete and differentiate themselves from other institutions (William, 2019). A strategic plan allows institutions, as a collective, to make proactive choices, prioritize their needs, and respond to changes and challenges that are sometimes beyond the control of the institution (Mensah, 2020). While budget issues, technology, and political landscape are more commonly addressed in strategic plans, recent challenges of surviving a pandemic and its associated technological and budgetary concerns, and the need to respond to a heightened awareness of social justice (Universities Canada, 2022), especially for racial and ethnic minorities, and the recommendations from the Truth and Reconciliation Report (Government of Canada, 2015) to have inclusive curricula through the integration of Indigenous knowledges, pedagogies, additional funding and programs have meant focusing on inclusion and equity in designing and mobilizing strategic plans.

Strategic planning is not only complex, but also challenging due to multiple factors such as the globalization of education, the steady rise of international students, the need for technological creativity, changes in the political environment, and shrinking budget support. More recently there have been calls for HEIs to plan for a future that is broader and inclusive in its "ethnocentric, ideological and technocratic understanding of knowledge futures" (Mbembe, 2016, p. 41), which requires upskilling and ongoing training for current and future employees, curriculum changes with epistemic diversity for faculty and students, and hiring the right people to institute such inclusive changes. With all these demands and expectations, a comprehensive strategic plan must also consider the needs and demands of multiple stakeholders.

Who Are the Multiple Stakeholders?

There are internal and external stakeholders in HEIs. As mentioned previously, significant internal stakeholders at HEIs are students, staff, faculty, and unions; and the external stakeholders are accrediting bodies, funding agencies, local community organizations, or the community at large. Although planning is well intended, with multiple stakeholders and the need to fulfil their expectations, services and implementation often become large-scale and standardized. Due to multiple forces and their impacts (e.g., COVID-19, calls for social justice in higher education), such standardization could mean that stakeholders and their institutions are not well equipped to handle non-standard issues that become part of the system of related problems or the so-called wicked problems "that are complex, unpredictable, open-ended, or intractable" (Head & Alford, 2015, p. 712). Planners need to remember that standard measures cannot "comprehend the experiences of diverse citizens who are supposed to be helped by these interventions and the values underlying their needs and desires" (Head & Alford, 2015, p. 713). Therefore, strategic planning processes need to go beyond the standard approaches.

Decision-makers need to consider what a strategic plan means for each of the stakeholder groups and how their needs and/or perspectives can be included. If EDI initiatives relevant to communities are fragmented, add-ons, or stand-alone actions, there is a danger of weakening the strategic plan. Including these communities at various stages of designing the plan from its initial to completion stages will thwart such danger and also bring in perspectives directly from those who would either be living the plan or contributing as stakeholders. The next few paragraphs will capture some of the stakeholders in higher education.

Community

A major stakeholder for publicly funded institutions is their local and immediate communities. Partnerships between HEIs and their communities are named the "third mission," and this commitment is highlighted in HEIs' "mission statements and strategic plans" (Plummer et al., 2021). The first two missions are teaching and research. In Canada, one of the most important local communities is Indigenous communities. Decades of hegemonic practices and dominant social structures in HEIs have led to the exclusion of Indigenous voices in curriculum, practices, and decision-making positions. The Truth and Reconciliation Report (Government of Canada, 2015) has resulted in Calls to Action with ninety-four recommendations that prompted actions at HEIs to Indigenize and decolonize all their work. It is only more recently that Canadian HEIs are intentional in their Indigenization efforts including creating positions of power for Indigenous colleagues. There are calls for dehomogenizing Indigenous communities, including Indigenist research principles, building an inclusive curriculum and culturally appropriate pedagogies, and Indigenizing teaching, learning, and knowledge practices in higher education (Hogarth, 2017; Sammel et al., 2020).

One of the ways to be inclusive is to invite community Elders and gatekeepers to not only engage in the planning process but also to participate in actively shaping the strategic framework and the implementation of goals. One illustration of such inclusion is the four "deep-rooted principles that were gifted to the University of Saskatchewan ... through a rigorous Indigenous-led community consultation process" (Carter et al., 2022, p. 163); these lie at the heart of the university's plan (University of Saskatchewan, n.d.).

Students

Students are typically the largest stakeholder group in an HEI, and their experiences within the HEI can have a lasting impact on their future. It is important to hear their voices as their needs change based on their changing demographics. Since HEI landscapes are competing on a global scale, international students are major stakeholders. International students are not only exploring diverse opportunities, but they are also looking for added value for their money (Degtjarjova et al., 2018). Marginalized students' expectations drive curriculum changes and education quality (Forsyth et al., 2020; Friesen & Hermann, 2018). Indigenous students are driven by barriers related to "access, relocation, transportation, family responsibilities, health, employment, and financial needs" (Brunette-Debassige, 2021), all of which might interrupt their student life. LGBTQ students have unique challenges that can be taxing both in their social and student lives. All minority students face marginalization issues due to their gender, race, sexuality, and language issues, which need to be considered during strategic planning. There should be questions during the process about whether the needs of these marginalized students are met in terms of facilities, research support, health, housing, access to open textbooks, inclusive curriculum, inclusive safe spaces, and so on. There should be campus-wide discussions with various student stakeholders to understand, design, and implement new strategies that incorporate international and intercultural dimensions (Andrade, 2017; Tiessen & Grantham, 2017; Xiao, 2018).

Faculty and Staff

Faculty, staff, and the supportive structures they uphold are also important stakeholders and entities in higher education. One example of a support structure is the unions (addressed later). Faculty and staff are responsible for planning, supporting, and mobilizing the quality of education, the equipment and materials needed to ensure quality and inclusive education, and the desired results of such a process (Degtjarjova et al., 2018). They are involved in many aspects of students' lives from finding and recruiting them to the university, seeing them through graduation, and even securing their careers through letters of recommendation, transcriptions, and networking. Since a successful strategic plan would depend on "broad-based support and participation by organizational constituents" (Welsh et al., 2005, p. 21) it would be wise to enable and empower this group of stakeholders through a strategic plan. From an EDI perspective, some questions to ask and address during the strategic planning process with this group of stakeholders could be their general concerns on representation and inclusion, whether existing systems and structures are inspiring or impediments and if so how, and how the institution could help advance a sense of belonging particularly for marginalized staff and faculty.

Unions

Leaders need to work in tandem with structures such as unions to "use those structures as ladders, bridges, staircases for building better worlds" (Darbinski, 2019, p. 56). Most Canadian public universities are unionized, and it is not uncommon to find multiple unions represented in these HEIs. As unions are a key liaison between members of the union and the university's central administration team, it only makes sense that the different student bodies and employee unions become active participants in any university's EDI journey through the strategic plan. Two important aspects of employee unions are to (1) work *collaboratively and harmoniously* with other units across the university to enable the development of the three elements of the EDI triangle (introduced later in the chapter) and (2) introduce flexibility in collective agreements or contracts to enable progress.

In summary, in today's "pluriversities," which are open to epistemic diversity and "radical refounding" of how HEIs function, the planning processes are more challenging and complex and include multiple concepts including EDI (Mbembe, 2016, p. 37). Consequently, how EDI is understood, operationalized, and woven through the fabric of a university can significantly impact the community, students, staff, faculty, and potentially other stakeholders (Wolbring & Lillywhite, 2021).

The EDI Journey of HEIs

How can an organization instill EDI within the DNA of every member? EDI is *not* a typical management intervention or program that is finite in terms of its definition, scope, and measurable outcomes; neither can it be implemented within a certain time period. Implementing EDI is a longitudinal journey. Undertaking an EDI journey involves setting EDI goals, laying the foundation for an EDI structure and culture, and investing time and energy in designing policies or procedures. The authors have captured some of their thoughts in a visual EDI triangle (see figure 5.2).

EDI Triangle

The purpose of EDI is to move an organization forward in a socially sustainable manner. This is possible by conceptualizing EDI in three mutually reinforcing ways – a goal, a foundation, and a set of policies/procedures. Such a three-pronged approach, enabled by other necessary mechanisms, will help individuals and the collective make decisions, and take actions to improve organizational wellbeing. The elements of this triangle are discussed briefly in figure 5.2.

Figure 5.2. The equity, diversity, and inclusion (EDI) triangle

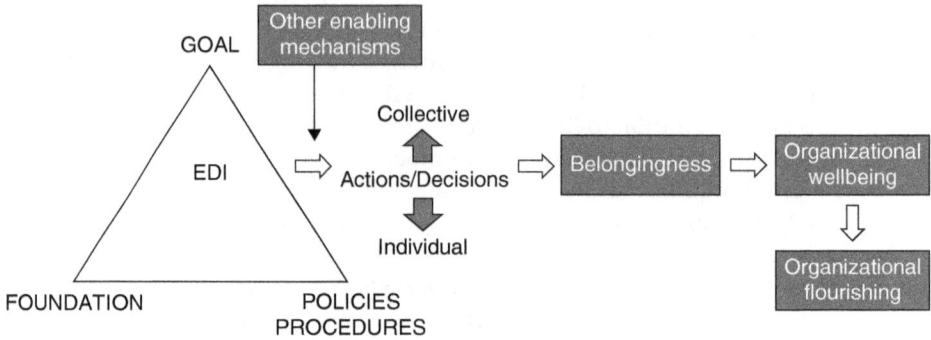

Goal

The first element, "EDI as a goal," pertains to developing a common understanding of EDI within the context of the organization and avoiding the potential of conflicts. A common understanding enables effective implementation. One critical reason for conceptualizing EDI as a goal is that it will allow the organization to formally articulate, emphasize, and reinforce its importance on an ongoing basis.

Foundation

It is common knowledge that any structure is only as strong as its foundation. Within the context of an organization – a collective of individuals – a foundation consists of a set of values or principles (Mishra & Kalagnanam, 2022) that underlie EDI and will form the bedrock of strong institutional values thereby guiding the organization to continuously progress towards the desired goal of organizational wellbeing. According to Hawley (1993, 1995), this set of principles makes up an organization's inner law and serves as the lens – the EDI lens in this instance – which can be used to develop policies and procedures and govern planning and decision-making.

The depth and breadth of a foundation are equally important to ensure that the structure is sustainable over the long term. Additionally, within the context of a collective, continuous reinforcement of these principles is also essential. Questioning the principles or values that form a strong "EDI foundation," removing biases and systemic barriers through the lens of privilege, and providing equal opportunity to every organizational member requires all individuals to recognize, understand, and practice a set of what we call the basic human values of acceptance, adaptability, compassion, openness, respect, and understanding. This list is by no means exhaustive. Moreover, these values may not be mutually exclusive. Finally, it is not essential to think about which value drives which other value. A potentially important outcome of understanding and practising these values is that doing so should lead individuals towards understanding the importance of EDI and taking the responsibility to transform for the sake of their organization's wellbeing.

Policies/Procedures

The foundation of a physical structure should be able to withstand turbulence. The foundation enables an organization to develop/refine its policies and procedures that provide guidance and the tools for employees to take the right actions to achieve the organization's objectives (Hawkins, 2005). However, the most important question from an EDI perspective is 'what are the desirable objectives of any organization when looking through the EDI lens?' Can it be anything other than organizational wellbeing? Raising this question underscores the criticality of organizational wellbeing as a driver of the organization's ability to achieve desired outcomes.

It is common knowledge that policies are often written in broad terms and provide guidance, whereas procedures are relatively more specific thereby providing step-by-step directions. Large organizations typically develop multiple policies to address the scope and scale of their operations, spread, and reach. Instilling EDI within the DNA of an organization requires that policies and procedures be developed using an "EDI lens" so that the EDI foundation is at the forefront of policy development. Does this mean developing a new EDI policy or revising existing policies? The answer is "both." Developing a specific EDI policy allows the organization to formally address the goal element of the EDI triangle, and timely revisions to other policies allow the foundation element of the triangle to be formally incorporated into policies and procedures to guide actions. The University of Saskatchewan has an EDI policy, and other policies were revised (or are currently under revision) (University of Saskatchewan, 2020).

There are three points to consider when developing/refining policies and procedures and avoid creating any new perceived or real inequities. First, policy/procedure development is a continuous, organic, and iterative process to align with internal and external environments. Second, reviewing policies/procedures through an EDI lens requires that they are not revised with an ideal student, staff, or faculty in mind. This is especially important if we accept that the desirable goal of EDI is to enable organizational members, via equitable and unbiased access to opportunities and resources, to enhance their wellbeing, experience a greater sense of belongingness, and realize their full potential for flourishing. Finally, and perhaps most importantly, whose voice is not represented is a critical question to answer considering the stakeholder mix in HEIs. The "gatekeeper" of this process is a critical individual and must be carefully identified.

Enabling Mechanisms

Constructing the EDI triangle is a critical step in guiding the decisions. However, this may not be possible without the existence of other mechanisms that enable such decisions. These enabling mechanisms may include individuals (especially those in decision-making roles), leadership, stakeholders (e.g., unions, student bodies, external bodies), and management control systems (e.g., resource allocation and performance measurement/management).

Individuals

Every organization, small or large, is a collective of individuals who engage in actions that contribute towards achieving the organization's mission and vision. Therefore, how an individual understands, internalizes, and practises EDI is a critical enabling mechanism. An important step is to learn from experts about issues such as unconscious bias, discrimination, and privilege. Qualities underlying the understanding, internalization, and practice of EDI, such as acceptance, adaptability, compassion, openness, respect, and understanding, may already be part of the value systems of individuals, "but really it is up to each individual to prioritize certain qualities and nurture them using a variety of familiar tools and techniques … It could also mean remembering the moral stories that our grandparents read or narrated to us" (Mishra & Kalagnanam, 2022, p. 119). A key outcome of such practices is that they enable the individual, especially one in a position of authority, to develop mutual respect for a fellow human being regardless of the other person's capabilities, status, or role in the organization.

Leadership

The importance of leadership in influencing organizational members is a known fact (Abernethy et al., 2010; Schein, 1992). Both Burns (1978) and Yukl (2013) suggest that regardless of the type(s) of the leadership style adopted, the relationship between leaders and their followers needs to appeal "to the followers' value systems, is respectful, inspirational, and transformational rather than transactional" (Mishra & Kalagnanam, 2022, p. 124). The leader is responsible for articulating and communicating organizational values and role modelling (Klassen et al., 2019; Mishra & Kalagnanam, 2022) and for shaping an organization's culture. However, this is never easy in the context of a large organization like a university, which typically has leaders dispersed at different levels and requires regular communication to ensure that individual goals are aligned with the goals of the institution.

Management Control System

A management control system (MCS) includes a variety of mutually reinforcing elements that hold the collective together and steer the organization in the right direction. It enables senior management to influence employees' behaviour, thereby guiding them towards achieving the organization's vision and mission. MCS includes belief systems that focus on organizational purpose and values (Simons, 1994); boundary systems that communicate the specific risks to be avoided (Simons, 1994); cultural controls that contribute towards defining the organization's norms (Malmi & Brown, 2008); personnel controls that enable employees to perform the desired tasks satisfactorily on their own (Merchant & Van der Stede, 2017); and administrative controls that outline accountability and reporting structures (Malmi & Brown, 2008). Recruitment and training, budgeting/resource allocation, performance management, and communication are some of the critical MCS elements discussed below.

Recruitment and Training

An important aspect of recruiting is the representation of diversity and inclusion among different ranks and positions to develop the desired work or organizational culture. Such representation should not be tokenistic. Sivakumar and Rao (2010) suggested focusing on selecting appropriate personnel, rewarding ethical behaviour, and having checks on unethical behaviour in addition to training members in the values of the organization. When members cultivate values, they will promote ethical behaviour and practices. Recruitment of members who adhere to values and promote ethical behaviour should be conducted through an EDI lens. As mentioned by Klassen et al. (2019), training is an important part of an organization's ethos.

Budgeting/Resource Allocation

As noted by Lew (2011), "budgeting is not just a collection of numbers but an expression of our values and aspirations" (p. WK9). However, budgets alone do not achieve strategic alignment. Planning is important. As Fairbairn (2017) noted, an institution's statements and plans need to align with resource allocation; he went further to suggest that the plan and budget be integrated. Kavanagh and Kowalski (2021) suggest that within the context of EDI, "it's important to understand the concept for budgeting: why it matters, how it might realistically be applied, and practical concerns and challenges" (p. 19). Similarly, Sharp (2003) highlights the importance of equity by suggesting that equity should be added as a fourth "e" in addition to the economy, efficiency, and effectiveness in performance-based budgeting. As clarified by Frenz and Vega (2010), it is important to align resources with needs (vertical equity) while ensuring equal access for equal needs (horizontal equity). The simple message here is that talking about EDI and even the creation of policy documents is meaningless unless significant resources are allocated to enable such transformational change.

Performance Management

The relevant questions regarding performance management "include what to measure ... how frequently to measure ... what to recognize ... and how to recognize" (Mishra & Kalagnanam, 2022, pp. 127–8). While some of the above questions may be more relevant to non-academic personnel in a university, they can be adapted to assess all employees' EDI journey (Klassen et al., 2019).

The idea here is that looking at performance measurement through an EDI lens will require a careful assessment of existing performance measurement systems. Within the context of standards for the tenure and promotion of faculty, a reassessment may necessitate thinking about diversity in the domains of research and teaching, being inclusive of a variety of research agendas, pedagogy, and methods, and providing the resources to avoid horizontal and vertical inequities (Frenz & Vega, 2010). At an institutional level, one way to measure performance is to examine the extent to which systemic barriers that can potentially lead to the presence of inequities are removed to promote organizational wellbeing. Within the context of early childhood and development interventions, Marra and Espinosa (2020) found the existence of five types of barriers that affected effective coverage. These include availability, accessibility, acceptability, contact, and effective coverage; identifying relevant

bottlenecks within an EDI-HEI context and specifically tailoring reme-
diations to individual universities may be a step in the right direction.

Communication

How an organization communicates important issues to its stakeholders
can influence their attitude towards these issues. Recognizing diversity
as an asset rather than as an obstacle (Canadian Centre for Diversity and
Inclusion, 2022) can significantly enhance its value within the minds of
stakeholders. Three other elements pertaining to communication are
(1) frequency of communication, (2) mode of communication, and (3)
who should communicate. Although there is no right answer to these
questions, it is important to note that the objective of communication
is to bring EDI to the mainstream so that it is "front and centre"! Two
examples include explicitly recognizing the importance of EDI in the
mission statement and on the front page of all course outlines.

EDI applies to all stakeholders, so they feel accepted, visible, supported,
and mentored at their institutions (Spafford et al., 2006). Stressing the
importance of EDI goals, strengthening the foundation, developing and
revising policies and procedures, enabling the various mechanisms, and
emphasizing clarity in communicating the importance and need for EDI
throughout the SP process will lead to individual belongingness, organizational wellbeing, and organizational flourishing.

Discussion and Conclusion

Strategic planning is a complex process. It could easily become a complex program of having to untangle many other issues to have a successful strategic plan. Despite this possibility, having EDI strategies integrated
into the strategic plan is important. Strategic plans in HEIs may benefit
from co-creating and designing an equity framework that becomes the
foundation of the SP and emphasizes how people engage with the plan in
their everyday work. Davis and Mendez (2022) suggest an R4P framework
in the context of COVID-19 vaccines, and some of these ideas could be
meaningfully and intentionally included while planning strategically. The
four Rs are to remove negative structures, attitudes, and practices; attempt
to repair by acknowledging the past; remediate by addressing exposures
and offering protection; and restructure by addressing all inequities. The
"P" in R4P stands for providing services centred on cultural and economic
sensitivities that currently disadvantage marginalized communities.

Embarking on any journey requires that the traveller periodically assess
their progress. The equity indicators framework (EIF), collaboratively

developed by the Anti-Racism Network, can serve as a guide for such an assessment (Kuffner et al., 2020). The EIF rubric enables the assessment of structures, policies, and programs using equity indicators along the following dimensions: (1) accountability, (2) budget, (3) human resources, (4) leadership and decision-making, (5) partnerships, (6) pay, (7) professional development and training, and (8) revenue sources. A starting point for any institution is to use this framework to conduct a study to perform a gap analysis and repeat it periodically (once every three or five years) to assess progress.

Recognizing the diversity in capabilities, knowledge, and expertise through equitable and inclusive plans, policies, and procedures, and harnessing this diverse knowledge base are critical in knowledge-based organizations (Sheehan et al., 2005). Practising EDI contributes to increasing belongingness (Cherry, 2021; Othering & Belonging Institute, n.d.). An individual who "belongs'" will likely feel a sense of self-worth and become an active contributor to achieving the organization's objectives. As Wolbring and Lillywhite (2021) stated in the context of students with disabilities, all their needs from housing, feeling safe and secure, interpersonal relationships, self-esteem, and their educational progress should be addressed. The authors believe that EDI-founded strategic planning will empower stakeholders in HEIs including their wellbeing, how they are labelled, and whether they feel like they belong, and can flourish.

REFERENCES

Abernethy, M.A., Bouwens, J., & Van Lent, L. (2010). Leadership and control system design. *Management Accounting Research, 21*(1), 2–16. https://doi.org/10.1016/j.mar.2009.10.002

Allen, K., Kern, M.L., Rozek, C.S., McInerney, D.M., & Slavich, G.M. (2021). Belonging: A review of conceptual issues, an integrative framework, and directions for future research. *Australian Journal of Psychology, 73*(1), 87–102. https://doi.org/10.1080/00049530.2021.1883409.

Amaya, M., Donegan, T., Conner, D., Edwards, J., Gipson, C. (2019). Create a culture of wellness: A call to action for higher education, igniting change in academic institutions. *Building Healthy Academic Communities Journal, 3*(2). https://doi.org/10.18061/bhac.v3i2.7117

Andrade, M. (2017). Institutional policies and practices for admitting, assessing, and tracking international students. *Journal of International Students, 7*(1), I–VI. https://doi.org/10.32674/jis.v7i1.241

Bashford, S. (2022). Ocado group case study: How do you ensure alignment between health and wellbeing and diversity and inclusion? https://makeadifference

.media/culture/ocado-group-case-study-how-do-you-ensure-alignment-between
-health-and-wellbeing-and-diversity-and-inclusion/

Bergquist, W.H., & Pawlak, K. (2008). *Engaging the six cultures of the academy.*
Josey-Bass.

Brunette-Debassige, C. (2021). *The trickiness of settler colonialism: Indigenous
women administrators' experiences of policy in Canadian universities.* [Doctoral
dissertation, University of Western Ontario]. Electronic Thesis and
Dissertation Repository, Western Libraries. https://ir.lib.uwo.ca/etd/7702/

Burns, J. (1978). *Leadership.* Harper and Row.

Canadian Centre for Diversity and Inclusion (2022). *Who we are.* https://ccdi.ca/

Canadian post-secondary community of practice for workplace wellness. (n.d.).
https://hr.ok.ubc.ca/health-wellbeing-2/cop/

Cardillo, B. (1993). Defining and measuring employment equity. *Perspectives on
labour and income* (Statistics Canada, Catalogue 75-001) *5*, 43–56.

Carter, D., Jaisee, T., Nickel, L., & Kalagnanam, S. (2022). Principles-based
budgeting: Resources for revisioning academic planning. *Engaged Scholar
Journal, 8*(2): 163–74. https://doi.org/10.15402/esj.v8i2.70786

Carvalho, T. (2020). New public management and social justice in higher
education. In J. McArthur & P. Ashwin (Eds.), *Locating social justice in higher
education research* (pp. 38–52). Bloomsbury Academic.

Cherkowski, S., & Walker, K. (Eds.). (2018). *Perspectives on flourishing in schools.*
Lexington Books.

Cherry, K. (2021, 5 March). *What is the sense of belonging?* Verywellmind. https://
www.verywellmind.com/what-is-the-need-to-belong-2795393

Church, E. (2023, 15 June). *Clinical leaders warn of financial and human cost of
racism.* Nursing Times. https://www.nursingtimes.net/news/workforce
/clinical-leaders-warn-of-financial-and-human-cost-of-racism-15-06-2023/

College and University Professional Association for Human Resources. (2020).
https://www.cupahr.org/blog/a-comprehensive-look-into-the-wellbeing
-of-higher-ed-employees/

Crossman, E., Choi, Y., & Hou, F. (2021). *International students as a source of
labour supply: The growing number of international students and their changing
sociodemographic characteristics.* Statistics Canada. https://www150.statcan.gc.ca
/n1/pub/36-28-0001/2021007/article/00005-eng.htm

Darbinski, E. (2019). What is critical about critical librarianship? *Art Libraries
Journal, 44*(2), 49–57. https://doi.org/10.1017/alj.2019.3

Davis, A., & Mendez, D. (2022). Applications of an equity framework in
COVID-19 vaccine trial and distribution planning. *Health Equity, 6*(1), 55–8.
https://doi.org/10.1089/heq.2021.0122

Degtjarjova, I., Lapina, I., & Freidenfelds, D. (2018). Student as stakeholder:
"Voice of customer" in higher education quality development. *Marketing and
Management of Innovations, 2*, 388–98. https://doi.org/10.21272/mmi.2018.2-30

Dimensions Charter. (2022, 4 April). *Equity, diversity, and inclusion.* Government of Canada. https://www.nserc-crsng.gc.ca/InterAgency-Interorganismes /EDI-EDI/Dimensions-Charter_Dimensions-Charte_eng.asp

Dowling, J., & Pfeffer, J. (1975). Organizational legitimacy: Social values and organizational behavior. *Pacific Sociological Review, 18*(1), 122–36. https://doi .org/10.2307/1388226

Employment Equity Act (S.C. 1995, c. 44).]Retrieved from the Justice Laws website: https://laws-lois.justice.gc.ca/eng/acts/E-5.401/index.html

Fairbairn, B. (2017). No-brainer or brain-twister? Linking planning and budgeting. *Planning for Higher Education Journal, 45N3,* 31–40.

Forsyth, C., Short, S., Gilroy, J., Tennant, M., & Irving, M. (2020). An Indigenous cultural competence model for dentistry education. *British Dental Journal, 228*(9), 719–25. https://doi.org/10.1038/s41415-020-1480-3

Frenz, P., & Vega, J. (2010). Universal health coverage with equity: What we know, don't know, and need to know. Background paper for the First Global Symposium on Health Systems Research, Montreux, Switzerland, November 16–19.

Friesen, M.R., & Hermann, R. (2018). Indigenous knowledge, perspectives, and design principles in the engineering curriculum. *Proceedings Canadian Engineering Education Association Conference.* https://ojs.library.queensu.ca /index.php/PCEEA/issue/archive

Fusco, F., & Ricci, P. (2019). What is the stock of the situation? A bibliometric analysis on social and environmental accounting research in public sector. *The International Journal of Public Sector Management, 32*(1), 21–41. http://doi .org/10.1108/IJPSM-05-2017-0134

Government of Canada. (2015). *Truth and Reconciliation Commission of Canada: Calls to action.* https://www2.gov.bc.ca/gov/content/governments/indigenous-people /new-relationship/truth-and-reconciliation-commission-calls-to-action

Government of Canada. (2022). *Equity, diversity, and inclusion: Tri-agency EDI action plan 2018–2025.* https://www.nserc-crsng.gc.ca/InterAgency-Interorganismes /EDI-EDI/Action-Plan_Plan-dAction_eng.asp

Government of Canada. (2024, 10 October). *Best practices in equity, diversity and inclusion in research.* https://www.sshrc-crsh.gc.ca/funding-financement/nfrf -fnfr/edi-eng.aspx#2

Hawkins, D. (2005). *Introduction to the Management Control Process.* Harvard Business School Press.

Hawley, J. (1993). *Reawakening the spirit in work: The power of dharmic management* Berrett-Koehler Publishers.

Hawley, J. (1995). Dharmic management: A concept-based paper on inner truth at work. *Journal of Human Values, 1*(2), 239–48. https://doi.org/10.1177 /097168589500100207

Head, B.W., & Alford, J. (2015). Wicked problems: Implications for public policy management. *Administration & Society, 47*(6), 711–739. https://doi.org/10.1177/0095399713481601

Hogarth, M. (2017). The power of words: Bias and assumptions in the Aboriginal and Torres Strait Islander Education Plan. *The Australian Journal of Indigenous Education, 46*(1), 44–53. https://doi.org/10.1017/jie.2016.29

Holzer, J., Lftenegger, M., Korlat, S., Pelikan, E., Salmela-Aro, K., Speil, C., and Schober, B. (2021). Higher education in times of COVID-19: University students' basic need satisfaction, self-regulated learning, and wellbeing. *AERA Open, 7.* https://doi.org/10.1177/23328584211003164

Hone, L.C., Jarden A., Schofield, G.M., & Duncan, S. (2014). Measuring flourishing: The impact of operational definitions on the prevalence of high levels of wellbeing. *International Journal of Wellbeing, 4*(1), 62–90. https://doi.org/10.5502/ijw.v4i1.4

Iordache-Platis, M. (2020). Strategy for wellbeing in universities: A Romanian higher education approach. *Sustainability, 12*(8243). https://doi.org/10.3390/su12198243

Kavanagh, S., & Kowalski, J. (2021). The basics of equity in budgeting. *Government Finance Review,* 18–27 February. https://www.gfoa.org/materials/gfr-equity-in-budgeting-2-21

Klassen, M., Kalagnanam, S., & Vasal, V. (2019). Managing values and financial accountability: The case of a large NGO. *International Journal of Indian Culture and Business Management, 19*(1), 103–27. https://doi.org/10.1504/IJICBM.2019.101195

Kouritzin, S.G., Nakagawa, S., Kolomic, E., & Ellis, T.F. (2020). Academic identities and institutional aims: Critical discourse analysis of neoliberal keywords on U15 University Websites. *International Research in Higher Education, 5*(3), 8–25. https://doi.org/10.5430/irhe.v5n3p8

Kouritzin, S.G., Nakagawa, S., Kolomic, E., & Ellis, T.F. (2021) Neoliberal sleight of hand in a university strategic plan: Weaponized sustainability, strategic absences, and magic time. *Alberta Journal of Educational Research, 62*(2), 236–55. https://doi.org/10.55016/ojs/ajer.v67i2.70164

Kuffner, S.B., Rosenberg, R., Fitzsimmons, S., Drozd, H., Brophy, C., Walling, E., Battiste, A., & Heimlick, M. (2020). Equity Indicators Framework. Anti-Racism Network.

Lane, J.E. (2000). *New public management: An introduction.* Routledge. https://doi.org/10.4324/9780203467329

Lew, J. (2011, 6 Feb.). The easy cuts are behind us. *New York Times* (WK9). http://cyber.usask.ca/login?url=https://www.proquest.com/historical-newspapers/easy-cuts-are-behind-us/docview/1645421048/se-2

Malmi, T., & Brown, D. (2008). Management control systems as a package – Opportunities, challenges, and research directions. *Management Accounting Research, 19*(4), 287–301. https://doi.org/10.1016/j.mar.2008.09.003

Marra, K., & Espinosa, I. (2020). Bottlenecks and barriers to effective coverage of early childhood health and development interventions in Guatemala: A scoping review. *Pan American Journal of Public Health, 44*, E105. https://doi.org/10.26633/RPSP.2020.105

Mbembe, J.A. (2016). Decolonizing the university: New directions. *Arts and Humanities in Higher Education, 15*(1), 29–45. https://doi.org/10.1177/1474022215618513

Mensah, J. (2020). Improving quality management in higher education institutions in developing countries through strategic planning. *Asian Journal of Contemporary Education, AESS Publications, 4*(1), 9–25. https://doi.org/10.18488/journal.137.2020.419.25

Merchant, K.A., & Van der Stede, W A. (2017). *Management control systems: Performance measurement, evaluation, and incentives* (4th ed.). Prentice-Hall.

Milano, B. (2019, 17 October). *Faculty diversity in business schools: 25 years in the making.* AACSB. https://www.aacsb.edu/insights/articles/2019/10/faculty-diversity-in-business-schools-25-years-in-the-making

Minnotte, K.L., & Pedersen, D. (2023). Sexual harassment, sexual harassment climate, and the wellbeing of STEM faculty members. *Innovative Higher Education, 48*, 601–18. https://doi.org/10.1007/s10755-023-09645-w

Mishra, P., & Kalagnanam, S. (2022). *Managing by Dharma: Eternal principles for sustaining profitability.* Palgrave Macmillan.

Moran, B.B. (1985). Strategic planning in higher education: Stratagems for survival in the 80s. *College & Research Libraries News, 46*(6), 288–92. https://doi.org/10.5860/crln.46.6.288

Okanagan Charter: An International Charter for Health Promoting Universities and Colleges. (2015). *Okanagan Charter.* Kelowna, BC: Author. Retrieved from http://internationalhealthycampuses2015.sites.olt.ubc.ca/files/2016/01/Okanagan-Charter-January13v2.pdf

Othering & Belonging Institute. (n.d.). *Our story.* https://belonging.berkeley.edu/our-story

Peterson, D., Krieger, N., Lee, R., & Lawrence, J. (2022, 21 March). *The high cost of racism: Inequality, the economy, and public health.* Harvard T.H. Chan School of Public Health. https://www.hsph.harvard.edu/event/the-high-cost-of-racism-inequality-the-economy-and-public-health/

Plummer, R., Witkowski, S., Smits, A., & Dale, G. (2021). The issue of performance in higher education institution – Community partnerships: A Canadian perspective. *Journal of Higher Education Policy and Management, 43*(5), 537–56. https://doi.org/10.1080/1360080X.2020.1858386

Sammel, A., Whatman, S., & Blue, L. (Eds.). (2020). *Indigenizing education: Discussion and case studies from Australia and Canada*. Springer. https://doi.org/10.1007/978-981-15-4835-2

Schein, E. H. (1992). *Organizational culture and leadership*. Josey-Bass.

Schuman, M. C. (1995). Managing legitimacy: Strategic and institutional approaches. *Academy of Management Review, 20*(3), 571–610. https://doi.org/10.2307/258788

Sharp, R. (2003). *Budgeting for equity: Gender budget initiatives within a framework of performance oriented budgeting. United Nations development fund for women*. UNIFEM. https://www.unwomen.org/sites/default/files/Headquarters/Media/Publications/UNIFEM/BudgetingForEquity1stHalf.pdf

Sheehan, N., Vaidyanathan, G., & Kalagnanam, S. (2005). Value creation logics and the choice of management control systems. *Qualitative Research in Accounting and Management, 2*(1), 1–28. https://doi.org/10.1108/11766090510635361

Simons, R. (1994). How new top managers use control systems as levers of strategic renewal. *Strategic Management Journal, 15*(3), 169–89. https://doi.org/10.1002/smj.4250150301

Sivakumar, N., & Rao, U. (2010). An integrated framework for values-based management – Eternal guidelines from Indian ethos. *International Journal of Indian Culture and Business Management, 3*(5), 503–524. https://doi.org/10.1504/IJICBM.2010.034385

Spafford, M. M., Nygaard, V. L., Gregor, F., & Boyd, M. A. (2006). Navigating the different spaces: Experiences of inclusion and isolation among racially minoritized faculty in Canada. *Canadian Journal of Higher Education, 36*(1), 01–27. https://doi.org/10.47678/cjhe.v36i1.183523

Temple P. (2018). Academic strategy: The management revolution in American higher education, by George Keller (1983). *Higher Education Quarterly, 72,* 170–7. https://doi.org/10.1111/hequ.12160/

Tiessen, R., & Grantham, K. (2017, January). *Faculty participation in North-South student mobility*. North-South Research, Universities Canada. Available at https://www.univcan.ca/programs-and-scholarships/north-south-research/

Tromp, S. A., & Ruben, B. D. (2010). *Strategic planning in higher education: A guide for leaders* (2nd ed.). National Association of College and University Business Officers.

United Nations (UN). (n.d.). The 17 goals: Sustainable development. Department of Economic and Social Affairs. https://sdgs.un.org/goals

Universities Canada. (2022, July). Building a race-conscious institution: A guide for university leaders enacting anti-racist organizational change. https://www.univcan.ca/wp-content/uploads/2022/07/UC-2022-Report_Building-a-Race-Conscious-Institution_EN_FINAL.pdf

University of British Columbia. (n.d.). *Wellbeing*. https://wellbeing.ubc.ca/

University of Saskatchewan. (n.d.) *Wellness.* https://wellness.usask.ca/

University of Saskatchewan. (2020). *Equity, diversity, and inclusion policy.* https://policies.usask.ca/policies/equity/equity-diversity-inclusion. php#AuthorizationandApproval

University of Toronto. (n.d.). *Wellness: Support for all dimensions of wellbeing.* https://people.utoronto.ca/culture/wellness/

Warhurst, A. (2005). Future roles of business in society: The expanding boundaries of corporate responsibility and a compelling case for partnership. *Futures, 37,* 151–86. https://doi.org/10.1016/j.futures.2004.03.033

Welsh, J.F., Nunez, W.J., and Petrosko, J. (2005). Faculty and administrative support for strategic planning: A comparison of two and four-year institutions. *Community College Review, 32*(4), 20–39. https://doi.org/10.1177/009155210503200403

William, T.M. (October 2019). Does strategic planning matter? *Academic Medicine, 94*(10). 1408–11. https://doi.org/10.1097/ACM.0000000000002848

Wolbring, G., & Lillywhite, A. (2021). Equity/equality, diversity, and inclusion (EDI) in universities: The case of disabled people. *Societies, 11*(2), 49. https://doi.org/10.3390/soc11020049

Wright-Mair, R., & Marine, S.B. (2021). The impact of relationships on the experiences of racially minoritized LGBTQ+ faculty in higher education. *The Journal of Diversity in Higher Education.* https://psycnet.apa.org/doi/10.1037/dhe0000373

Xiao, J. (2018). Internationalization of higher education: Considerations for adult education. *Alberta Journal of Educational Research, 64*(2), 202–7. https://doi.org/10.55016/ojs/ajer.v64i2.56585

Yukl, G.A. (2013). *Leadership in organizations* (9th ed.). Pearson.

6 The Student Health Imperative: Elevating Student Health as a Prime Directive of Student Affairs

AINSLEY CARRY

Background Context

My career in college administration began in the early 1990s. Then, student services focused on fundamental needs such as career services, leadership development, academic support, and social engagement. Meanwhile, marginalized student populations (e.g., Black, Indigenous, Hispanic, LGBTQ, and students with disabilities) pleaded for greater attention to their unique learning and social needs. Conferences, seminars, and publications emerged to help practitioners think creatively about delivering these services. Meanwhile, student health needs lingered in the shadows, awaiting appropriate attention. For the past thirty years, few things have been more consistent, yet ignored, than students' health and wellness as a determining factor in their success. Although colleges and universities now pay more attention to student health services such as counselling, clinical care, and wellbeing programs, the ethic of care has not yet permeated the thick outer shell of institutional culture and practice. Institutional policies and procedures still resemble the outdated frameworks from which they were conceived. Accreditation agencies and faculty still craft requirements based on ancient guidance. New student programming is still based on 1980s and 1990s models. These approaches continue to disregard diverse student populations and contemporary needs.

This chapter is somewhat different from the others. This chapter does not describe a specific student health dilemma or solution. Instead, in this chapter, the author calls for elevating student health among institutions' top priorities. Just as social and intellectual development was prioritized for the first century of the student affairs profession, student health must take centre stage to begin the next century.

Since the early 1900s, student affairs professionals utilized social science theories to understand young adult behaviour. Vincent Tinto (student development theory), Arthur Chickering (identify development), Lawrence Kohlberg (moral development), and William Perry (intellectual and ethical development) laid a foundation for understanding how college-bound young adults developed. Practitioners leaned on social science and psychological theories to anticipate young adult behaviour and design appropriate programs and services. Student development theories heavily informed residence life, career services, leadership development, new student orientation, and academic advising. Practitioners employed constructs from these theories to design programs and services. For example, Tinto's work heavily influenced student retention initiatives and residential learning communities. However, initiatives grown from Tinto's theories have not adapted to account for cultural nuances now present on many campuses.

As universities became more culturally and intellectually diverse, theoretical frameworks developed in the 1920s and 1930s failed to account for diverse perspectives. Women, students of colour, veterans, international students, and students with disabilities were under-represented in the populations sampled for the original theoretical models. As a result, the effectiveness of these theories in explaining student behaviour and providing guidance withered over time. Later, William E. Cross (People of Colour Racial Identity), Kevin Nadal (Filipino American Identify Development), John W. Berry (Ethnic Minority Identify Development), and Kimberlé Crenshaw (Intersectionality) developed more inclusive models that acknowledged racial identity development.

By the late 1930s, student affairs practitioners sought to define "student affairs" work. Student housing, dining, recreation, and health services consumed more institutional resources. In some cases, institutions made decisions between residence halls and academic buildings. Funds were diverted outside the classroom that once were available for academically focused activities. From its inception until the early twentieth century, American higher education emphasized students' social, moral, and religious development. However, in the early twentieth century, American universities shifted away from students' social development and focused on research-driven priorities. Student affairs practitioners realized the field did not have a unified framework, and the shift to research would erode students' social development. It was time for the student affairs profession to be clarified. The relationship of the work to other parts of the university needed to be defined, and research was required to justify ongoing expenses. Practitioners did "what seemed right" without a common agenda or industry standards. Guideposts for the work were non-existent. In response, the American

Council on Education hosted a two-day meeting in 1937 to develop professional standards. The outcome of the meeting was the *Student Personnel Point of View* (Williamson et al., 1937, 1949) – a framework for how student affairs professionals should think about the work. In 1949, the group updated the original document with new information and came to the following conclusion:

> The concept of education is broadened to include attention to the student's well-rounded development – physically, socially, emotionally, and spiritually – as well as intellectually. The student is considered a responsible participant in his development and not a passive recipient of an imprinted economic, political, or religious doctrine or vocational skill. As a responsible participant in the societal processes of our American democracy, his full and balanced maturity is viewed as a major end goal of education and, as well, a necessary means to the fullest development of his fellow citizens. The realization of this objective – the full maturing of each student – cannot be attained without interest in and integrated efforts toward the development of each and every facet of his personality and potentialities. (p.3)

The *Student Personnel Point of View* defined the student as a holistic being with intellectual and social interests. Shifting towards a research focus, universities were devaluing students' social development. Authors of the *Student Personnel Point of View* stressed that universities should invest in students' intellectual growth (e.g., teaching, research, academic advising, classroom facilities) and social interests (e.g., housing, clubs and organizations, recreation, and mental health). They emphasized that the student is multidimensional and ignoring one dimension diminishes their capacity to excel in others.

More than fifty years after the *Student Personnel Point of View* debuted, the profession was called again to define its role in the academy, specifically, its relationship to the academic mission. What is the value of the outside-the-classroom experience to student learning? As expenses grew for student services and athletic programs, parents, faculty, and taxpayers wanted to understand the relationship between student programs and student learning. In 1996, the American Council of Student Personnel Administrators (ACPA) deliberated for four days. Their work culminated in the release of the *Understanding ACPA's Student Learning Imperative* (Bloland, 1996). The authors examined how "student affairs professionals can intentionally create the conditions that enhance student learning and personal development" (Bloland, 1996). The document refocused student-affairs work for greater alignment with the academic mission. The authors advised student affairs divisions to do the following:

1 Develop a mission statement that compliments the institution's mission statement.
2 Allocate resources to encourage student learning and personal growth.
3 Collaborate with other institutional agents and agencies to promote student learning and personal development.
4 Include staff who are experts on students, their environments, and teaching and learning.
5 Base policies and programs on promising practices from research on student learning.

The *Student Learning Imperative* had widespread appeal; practitioners embraced the core theory of the model – students learn outside the classroom. Although most agreed that student learning occurred both inside and outside the classroom, the challenge was finding a consistent measure for that learning. Learning outcomes in non-classroom settings could not be reliably measured. Assessment tools and techniques were developed but lacked scientific validity and reliability. Program assessment and evaluation science grew during the period, but the *Student Learning Imperative* movement eventually withered. The imperative did solidify an important tenant – students learn outside the classroom, and learning outcomes could be intentionally designed. Outside the classroom, initiatives such as experiential learning, high-impact practices, study abroad, and work-integrated learning expanded from this insight.

Student development theories and frameworks for defining student affairs work have been instrumental to the profession. These tools guided student affairs for a century. Institutions and practitioners tweaked and customized these frameworks and theories to understand the unique needs of students and develop more effective programming. The *Student Personnel Point of View* (1937) and *Understanding ACPA's Student Learning Imperative* (1996) shaped the profession during their era. Practitioners looked towards these models for guidance on prioritizing work and how to best incorporate the principles.

Yet again, the profession has reached another turning point. Like the 1930s and 1990s, a growing gap emerged between what students need and how universities function. That gap is defined by growing expectations that universities support a broader array of public health services. Students, parents, and taxpayers expect universities to provide more public health assistance than they had in the past. Students describe this gap as threatening to their health. Institutional responses that begin with, "When I was in college ..." do not ease students' concerns. The line between student and institutional responsibility for health has been redefined. A new framework is needed to guide the profession. It is time for a student health imperative.

A Public Health Approach

Policymakers and health care providers turn to public health models to reconsider remedies to seemingly unsolvable challenges. Health care frameworks have been used to reimagine environmental challenges (Browne & Rutherford, 2017), child abuse (O'Donnel et al., 2008), tobacco regulation (Deyton et al., 2010), violence prevention (Bloom, 2001), STD and HIV prevention (Aral et al., 2013), gun violence (Hemenway & Miller, 2013), and gambling addiction (Bowden-Jones et al., 2019). The approach uncovers novel perspectives and infuses community problem solving.

For example, scientists have used a public health approach to reimagine environmental disasters such as floods, tornados, mudslides, hurricanes, and earthquakes. These events once occurred every fifty to one hundred years, but now they occur more frequently. Changes in global temperatures – warmer ocean temperatures combined with atmospheric pressure – are contributing to catastrophic weather events. In 2013, the World Health Organization (WHO) employed a public health approach at the Global Conference on Health Promotion in Helsinki. They challenged attendees to evaluate public policies across multiple sectors (e.g., government, transportation, agriculture, education, energy, import/export markets, and travel). These sectors have different responsibilities but shared environmental aspirations. Policymakers used the model to integrate ecological health with transportation, agriculture, and energy policies. The goal was to create multisector policy decisions that improve environmental health. A public health approach to ecological health improves accountability at multiple levels.

The most commonly cited success story in public health applications involves vehicle safety (JAMA, 1999). The National Center for Health Statistics (NCHS) and National Safety Council (NSC) reported, "In 1923, the first year miles driven was estimated, the motor-vehicle death rate was 18.65 deaths for every 100 million miles driven. Since 1923, the mileage death rate has decreased 92% and now stands at 1.46 deaths per 100 million miles driven" (Centers for Disease Control and Prevention, 1999). Charts diagramming the number of vehicle deaths on the Y-axis and year on the X-axis show a peak in the mid-1930s followed by a steady downward decline for the next sixty years. By all measures, a 90 per cent reduction in vehicle mortality (while vehicle miles driven were increased) is a significant achievement. The credit for this precipitous decline is attributed to the prolonged commitment to a public health approach to vehicle safety. In the 1960s, policy advocates, lawmakers, and vehicle manufacturers focused on reducing vehicular deaths by shifting attention from user error (Who caused the accident?) to vehicle safety (What caused the injuries?). Not that user error was no longer a factor, but there was plenty of room for improvement in vehicle safety that had not yet been explored. The paradigm shift invited car manufacturers, policymakers, and health providers into the same conversation and focused on the same problem – vehicle mortality rates. Together, they defined the problem, identified risk and protective factors, developed and tested prevention strategies, and assured widespread adoption of effective programs. Over the next forty years, the public health approach to vehicle safety, accompanied by mandatory vehicle safety improvements (e.g., seat belt requirements, child restraint systems, brake lights, and braking systems), reduced fatal car accidents.

Policymakers at the Centers for Disease Control and Prevention (CDC) adopted Dahlbergand Krug's (2002) four-step description of the public health approach: (1) define and monitor the problem, (2) identify risk and protective factors, (3) develop and test prevention strategies, and (4) assure widespread adoption of effective programs. Health is socially determined, and decision-making in diverse policy areas, often unrelated to health, certainly affects health (Browne & Rutherford, 2017). Public health policy is about the health, safety, and wellbeing of a population. A public health approach describes a shift from individual treatment to population-wide solutions. In other words, rather than a patient-centred care model that emphasizes health education and behaviour change, a community-care model focused on the population would generate better outcomes. Likewise, a public health approach starts with the public. The process draws in various disciplines (e.g., sociology, psychology, economics) and sectors (e.g., education, law, health) to view problems from multiple perspectives and uncover more elegant solutions. Stakeholders must act collaboratively and collectively to implement solutions conceived from shared aspirations.

The public health perspective brings distinct advantages to problem solving. First, solutions tend to address the root causes of problems rather than symptoms. Because the public health approach begins with "defining the problem," solutions are more likely to address the underlying problem rather than peripheral issues. Activities focused on symptoms rather than root causes will prove ineffective over time. For example, efforts that address individual cases of sexual assault, mental health, and racism do not account for the root causes of these offences. Hiring counsellors, building "safe spaces," and launching new programs are like putting Band-Aids atop broken bones. Problem solvers must consider more profound questions and test multiple answers. Second, public health solutions require collective rather than individual action. Meaningful change happens when cross-functional groups/teams take collective action. The most significant social movements in the world (e.g., Civil Rights, climate change, marriage equality, Black Lives Matter, and women's rights) achieved success when people worked together across units, departments, political parties, cultures, and genders. Collective action requires a common agenda, shared measurements, mutually reinforcing activities, continuous communication, and supporting structures.

The Student Health Imperative

Since the early 2010s, a new wave of student activism has emerged on university campuses. Students have demanded universities take more action in response to climate change, racial justice, affordability, sexual assaults, and COVID. In 2022, more than three hundred universities and high schools across the United States experienced on-campus protests targeting sexual violence (Migdon, 2022). Students protested conditions that allowed sexual violence to flourish after several college women reported sexual assaults in the first few weeks of the fall 2022 semester. Protestors demanded more accountability and action from administrators to prevent sexual violence and punish perpetrators. Sexual violence prevention is not a new demand. In 2010, the Obama administration made improving university responses to sexual violence a critical initiative. The administration investigated hundreds of universities and issued new legislation, rules, and procedures binders. Universities scrambled to adjust to the new guidance and made plenty of mistakes. More than a decade later, calls for more comprehensive sexual prevention measures remain. Sexual violence creates trauma and guilt for survivors, leading to anxiety, depression, and poor academic performance. At the same time, incidents of sexual violence have public health consequences (McMahon et al., 2020). Survivors experience lifelong psychological harm, and past survivors are reminded of their victimization. Their extended community – families, friends, classmates, and parents – feels a wave of remorse, anger, and fear when sexual violence goes unaddressed.

However, sexual violence is not the only challenge to which a public health lens can be applied. Racial violence, climate anxiety, food and housing insecurity, anxiety, depression, and alcohol abuse are public health threats. Although universities have responded to these challenges via policy changes, conduct rules, educational programs, staffing changes, and new offices, the solutions remain single-sided. Practitioners work in silos confronting complex, multi-dimensional issues. Because these challenges are multi-dimensional, single-sided solutions often fall short. Because there are strong correlations between alcohol consumption, Greek life, and sexual assault (Jordan-Simmons, 2001), solutions that do not bring these entities together are destined to fail. Therefore, confronting alcohol abuse and sexual assault separately often results in inadequate solutions.

A long list of student challenges has public health implications. Scholars and practitioners have applied public health strategies – (1) define and monitor the problem, (2) identify risk and protective factors, (3) develop and test prevention strategies, and (4) assure widespread adoption of effective programs – to devising solutions to hazing (Archibald & Banks, 2020), alcohol abuse (Krupa et al., 2018), suicide prevention (VanDeusen et al., 2015), racial discrimination (Leath et al., 2019), and drug overdoses (Hill et al., 2020). In addition to solutions residing in public health approaches, these issues have incalculable consequences. For example, the entire campus community suffers when a fraternity pledge dies in an alcohol-fuelled hazing ritual. Students with deep concerns about climate change report increased levels of climate or eco-anxiety (Ojala et al., 2021). Many college students are requesting long-term and acute mental health care, but few universities are equipped to provide critical and long-term care. Food and housing insecurity on campus is a public health concern that has implications for student health, wellness, academic performance, and retention (Payne-Sturges et al., 2018; Zein et al., 2019).

The scale and interrelatedness of these challenges cannot be approached individually or as the responsibility of a single campus department. The problems are not isolated but interrelated, and addressing them in silos is ineffective and inefficient. These challenges are seemingly impossible because universities tackle them independently. These are public health issues and, therefore, must be addressed from a collective impact approach – an approach that considers related issues and leverages the joint action of multiple stakeholders and disciplines.

Without a public health framework, universities are offering Band-Aid for critical injuries. Universities spend millions on mental health services, sexual violence prevention, affordable food and housing, transportation, low-cost childcare, and climate change. Yet, responses to these public health challenges are poorly coordinated. Students, especially new students, will spend at least a semester trying to connect with student health services (e.g., counselling services, disability services, cultural centres, food, and housing assistance). These services are hidden on websites and scattered across campus. Students learn about them for the first time in new student orientation programs during their first week on campus; two weeks later, many will forget the resources they were introduced to during orientation. Universities do a disservice to students when public health services are packaged in a theoretical model that does not make sense to them.

The Okanagan Charter

Universities are not starting from scratch in advancing a public health strategy; much of the work has been done. In 2015, public health experts and higher education practitioners gathered to produce the Okanagan Charter: An International Charter for Health Promoting Universities and Colleges (Okanagan Charter, 2015). The Okanagan Charter was built from the World Health Organization's Ottawa Charter for Health Promotion (1986). For three days, practitioners from forty-five countries gathered in Kelowna, British Columbia, and drafted the Charter. Attendees focused on the unique role of higher education in promoting health and wellbeing. The Charter challenged universities to create healthier campuses and communities by incorporating "health promotion values and principles into their mission, vision, and strategic plans, and model and test approaches for the wider community and society" (p. 5). The Okanagan Charter (2015)placed student health at the centre of student affairs work. Like its predecessors, the Okanagan Charter (2015) defined, prioritized, and organized student affairs work. The Okanagan Charter offered a common language, principles, and framework for collective action. Whereas the *Student Personnel Point of View* (1936, 1949) centred on students as multidimensional beings and the *Student Learning Imperative* (1996) elevated learning as a central function of the student experience, the Okanagan Charter (2015) drew attention to student health as a compelling shared interest.

The Charter prescribed universities to take two actions. First, embed health into all aspects of campus culture across the administration, operations, and academic mandates. This step involved embedding health in all campus policies, creating supportive campus environments, fostering thriving communities and a culture of wellbeing, supporting personal development, and orientating campus services to emphasize student health. Many university policies are outdated and lead to unintended health consequences. In some cases, registration deadlines, housing, dining policies, learning accommodations, academic rules, and degree requirements accelerate poor health outcomes rather than institutional effectiveness.

The Charter also prescribed universities to lead health promotion action and collaboration locally and globally. Doing this involved integrating health, wellbeing, and sustainability in multiple disciplines to develop change agents, advancing research, teaching, and training for health promotion knowledge and action, and leading local and global initiatives for health promotion. Public health extends beyond campus boundaries (e.g., off-campus housing, bars and clubs, and transportation). A comprehensive public health approach considers internal and external environmental factors that impact health and wellbeing. To the degree universities can influence or advocate for health and wellbeing off-campus, they should consider doing so.

A Call to Action

Students sometimes bring or experience trauma on campus. Sexual violence, drug and alcohol abuse, anxiety and depression, racial discrimination, suicidal ideation, and affordability are public health challenges that students experience before and during enrolment. Classifying these challenges as a "rite of passage" or "just part of growing up" will undoubtedly result in these challenges evolving from urgent to crisis. Universities that medicate these issues with short-sighted and reactionary responses will wonder why the problems always seem to re-emerge. Universities must take a public health approach and bring partners and allies on board.

Students must advocate for long-term solutions rather than performative and symbolic actions (e.g., space, staffing, funding); these remedies do not address the root cause of the problem. Students are sometimes manipulated into protesting for increased office space, furniture, and programmatic funding; these actions rarely address systemic public health problems. Most student government administrations are in office for one year; therefore, student leaders are compelled to lobby for short-term rather than long-term solutions. This pressure for fast solutions dampens intelligent, sustainable solutions.

Simply adopting the Charter is not enough. Universities must make structural commitments to prioritize public health. First, institutional leadership's commitment to a health-minded strategy is essential. The president, senior student affairs officer, or provost must prioritize public health as an institutional strategy. Properly elevating public health is not a bottom-up or grassroots initiative but requires institutional leaders at the highest levels. Senior leaders must communicate, in word and deed, their commitment to the community's public health.

Second, public health competence is essential in the model. The designated institutional leader should be a public health leader, knowledgeable about public health strategies, or committed to educating themselves in the discipline. Many universities have Public and Population Health degree programs to lean on for expertise and information. In addition, some universities introduced a Vice President for Student Health role. The role oversees student health care units (e.g., counsellors, physicians, nurses, and health promotions) and collaborates across the institution to implement health-minded changes.

Finally, the organizational structure must pivot to support a public health strategy. Student health is often buried on organizational charts. It may be organized under a revenue-generating division focused on profit margins rather than students. Its position on the organizational chart communicates its level of funding and advocacy. Student health must be elevated by role (i.e., a Vice President for Student Health) and position in the organization.

Universities must centre student and population health. This suggestion is not revolutionary or groundbreaking. Hundreds of universities have adopted the Okanagan Charter and verbally committed to elevating public health. However, few have prioritized the structural commitments that advance health care. Academic policies remain outdated and harmful. Support services remain disconnected from one another. Short-term, performative solutions still dominate headlines. The rising tide of public health challenges (e.g., sexual violence, racial discrimination, drug and alcohol abuse, mental health stigma) requires new thinking, greater collaboration, and committed leadership at the highest levels.

REFERENCES

Aral, S., Fenton, K.A., and Lipshutz, J. (2013). *The new public health and STD/HIV prevention approach: personal, public and health systems.* Springer Sciences+Business Media,

Archibald, J., and Banks, S.A. (2020). The state of fraternity and sorority life in higher education. *Georgia Journal of College Student Affairs, 36*(1), 24–32. https://doi.org/10.20429/gcpa.2020.360103

Bloland, P.A. (1996). *Understanding ACPA's Student Learning Imperative.* Paper presented at the Annual Meeting of the American College Personnel Association. Baltimore, MD., March 6–10.

Bloom, S.L. (2001). *Violence: A public health menace and a public health approach.* Forensic Psychotherapy Monograph Series. Karnac Books.

Bowden-Jones, H., Dickson, C., Dunand, C., and Simon, O. (2019). *Harm reduction for gambling: A public health approach.* Taylor & Francis Group.

Browne, G.R., and Rutherfurd, I.D. (2017). The case for "environment in all policies": Lessons from the "health in all policies" approach in public health. *Environ Health Perspect, 125*, 149–54. https://doi.org/10.1289/EHP294

Centers for Disease Control and Prevention. (2024). *The public health approach to violence prevention.* https://www.cdc.gov/violenceprevention/about/publichealthapproach.html

Centers for Disease Control and Prevention (1999). Motor-vehicle safety: A 20th century public health achievement. *JAMA. 281*(22), 2080–2. https://doi.org/10.1001/jama.281.22.2080

Dahlberg, L.L, and Krug, E.G. (2002). Violence: a global public health problem. In E. Krug, L.L. Dahlberg, J.A. Mercy, A.B. Zwi, R. Lozano (Eds.), *World report on violence and health* (pp. 1–21). World Health Organization.

Deyton, L., Sharfstein, J., and Hamburg, M. (2010, May) Tobacco product regulation – A public health Approach. *The New England Journal of Medicine, 362*(19), 1753–6. https://doi.org/10.1056/NEJMp1004152.

Hemenway, D., and Miller, M. (2013). Public health approach to the prevention of gun violence. *The New England Journal of Medicine, 368*(21), 2033–5. https://doi.org/10.1056/NEJMsb1302631

Hill, L.G., Holleran Steiker, L.K., Mazin, L., & Kinzly, M.L. (2020). Implementation of a collaborative model for opioid overdose prevention on campus. *Journal of American College Health, 68*(3), 223–6. https://doi.org/10.1080/07448481.2018.1549049

Journal of the American Medical Association. (1999). Motor-vehicle safety: A 20th century public health achievement. *JAMA, 281*(22), 2080–2. doi:10.1001/jama.281.22.2080

Jordan-Simmons, K. (2001). Sexual violence on campus: The relationship between sorority membership, fraternity contact, and alcohol consumption. (Order No. 3038246). Available from ProQuest Dissertations & Theses Global.

Krupa, T., Henderson, L., Horgan, S., Dobson, H., Stuart, H., and Stewart, S. (2018). Engaging male post-secondary student leaders to apply a campus cultural and gender lens to reduce alcohol misuse: Lessons learned. *Canadian Journal of Community Mental Health, 37*(3), 116–26. https://doi.org/10.7870/cjcmh-2018-015

Leath, S., Mathews, C., Harrison, A., and Chavous, T. (2019). Racial identity, Racial discrimination, and classroom engagement outcomes among Black girls and boys in predominantly Black and predominantly White school districts. *American Educational Research Journal, 56*(4), 1067 – 1551. https://doi.org/10.3102/0002831218816955

Lucas, G.H., Holleran Steiker, L.K., Mazin, L., and Kinzly, M.L. (2020). Implementation of a collaborative model for opioid overdose prevention on campus. *Journal of American College Health, 68*(3), 223-226. https://doi.org/10.1080/07448481.2018.1549049

McMahon, S., Burnham, J., and Banyard, V.L. (2020). Bystander intervention as a prevention strategy for campus sexual violence: Perceptions of historically minoritized college students. *Prevention Science, 21*, 795–806. https://doi.org/10.1007/s11121-020-01134-2

Migdon, B. (2022, 10 Feb.). Campus protests around sexual assault look different this year. *The Hill.* https://thehill.com/changing-america/respect/equality/593592-campus-protests-around-sexual-assault-look-different-this-year

O'Donnell, M., Scott, D., and Stanley, F. (2008). Child abuse and neglect – Is it time for a public health approach? *Australian and New Zealand Journal of Public Health, 32*(4), 325–330. https://doi.org/10.1111/j.1753-6405.2008.00249.x

Ojala, M., Cunsolo, A., Ogunbode, C.A., and Middleton, J. (2021). Anxiety, worry, and grief in a ime of Enevironmental and climate crisis: A narrative review. *Annual Review of Environment and Resources, 46*, 35–58. https://doi.org/10.1146/annurev-environ-012220-022716

Okanagan Charter: An International Charter for Health Promoting Universities and Colleges. (2015). *Okanagan Charter.* Kelowna, BC: Author. Retrieved from http://internationalhealthycampuses2015.sites.olt.ubc.ca/files/2016/01/Okanagan-Charter-January13v2.pdf

Payne-Sturges, D.C., Tjaden, A., Caldeira, K.M., Vincent, K.B., and Arria, A.M. (2018). Student hunger on campus: Food insecurity among college students and implication for academic institutions. *American Journal of Health Promotion, 32*(2), 349–54. https://doi.org/10.1177/0890117117719620

World Health Organization (WHO). 1986. Ottawa Charter for Health Promotion.

World Health Organization (WHO). (2014). Helsinki statement on health in all policies. In *Proceedings of the 8th Global Conference on Health Promotion.* WHO. https://iris.who.int/bitstream/handle/10665/112636/9789241506908_eng.pdf?sequence=1

VanDeusen, K.M., Lewis Ginebaugh, K.J., and Walcott, D.D. (2015). Campus suicide prevention: Knowledge, facts, and stigma in a college student sample. *Sage Open, 5*(2), https://doi.org/10.1177/2158244015580851

Williamson, E.G., Blaesser, W.W., Bragdon, H.D., Carlson, W.S., Cowley, W.H., Feder, D.D., Fisk, H.G., Kirkpatrick, F.H., Lloyd-Jones, E., McConnell, T.R., Merriam, T.W., and Shank. D.J. (1937, 1949). *The Student Personnel Point of View.* American Council on Education Series, v. 13.

Zein, A.E., Shelnutt, K.P., Colby, S., Vilaro, M.J., Zhou, W., Greene, G., Olfert, M.D., Riggsbee, K., Morrell, J.S., and Mathews, A.E. (2019). Prevalence and correlates of food insecurity among U.S. college students: A multi-institutional study. *BMC Public Health, 19*(1), 660. https://doi.org/10.1186/s12889-019-6943-6

7 Is That Our Responsibility? The Role of Academic Units in Campus Wellbeing

CHAD LONDON AND TANYA FORNERIS

Introduction

The COVID-19 pandemic has heightened the urgency of supporting wellbeing in post-secondary contexts. A recent Canadian study found that 74 per cent of students believed that their university has a responsibility to ensure their wellbeing, but only 47 per cent felt that their institution does well in supporting their wellbeing (Academica Group, 2022). In addition, students are struggling at an unprecedented rate. A 2019 study found that within the previous twelve months, 51.6 per cent of Canadian students felt so depressed that it was difficult for them to function, while 16.4 per cent seriously considered suicide and 2.8 per cent attempted suicide (ACHA, 2019). In addition, an increasing number of students are presenting with mental health disorders as they enrol in post-secondary education (Lattie et al., 2019). Thus, there is a pressing need to address the wellbeing of post-secondary communities.

The parallel wellbeing of faculty and staff impacts work with students and the overall climate of campuses. Academic staff are being challenged as they experience increased fatigue in supporting students while trying to mitigate their own psychological and emotional consequences of the pandemic (Cordaro, 2020). Physical health is also at risk, with recent research having shown that workers are sedentary for an average of 9.5 hours per weekday (Alberta Centre for Active Living, 2019) and linking high rates of sedentary behaviour to higher rates of cardiovascular disease, cancer, and type 2 diabetes (Owen et al., 2010). Thus, there is a clarion call for post-secondary institutions to find better ways to support campus wellbeing, with a promising approach for doing so being a whole systems approach that includes contributions from all stakeholders across the institution.

Post-secondary educational institutions are known for being complex, disconnected organizations, which poses challenges when attempting to advance wellbeing using whole systems approaches that consider all aspects of campuses and the integration of various roles in implementing wellbeing strategies. Improving the health of people on campuses has been seen as the primary responsibility of student services and human resources departments, which tend to operate as silos rather than collaborating to serve students, staff, and faculty in integrated ways (Squires & London, 2022). Research related to campus wellbeing has likewise focused on students' wellness as delivered by student service units on campus, with a secondary (and limited) focus on employees through efforts of human resources and faculty relations offices. An oft-neglected stakeholder group in healthy campus practice and research has been the faculty and staff that comprise academic units (such as discipline-based faculties, schools, and departments).

Even though academic units are directly responsible for delivering academic programming to students and supporting their educational experience, there has been little attention paid to the role of academic units in advancing wellbeing. There is a strong rationale to consider academic impacts on students' wellbeing as studies have revealed that the leading cause of stress in students' lives is academic workload and course difficulty (Academica Group, 2022). Research on stress among faculty members has also highlighted the high workload, in particular the multifaceted demands that are placed upon faculty with little training provided in support of those demands (Owens et al., 2018).

Academic units can affect wellbeing in various ways, such as how they deliver courses and assess learning and how they evaluate faculty performance and enhance cohesion among employees. It is possible for those functions to be delivered through a lens to support wellbeing, but to date, academic units are infrequently encouraged or mandated to do so. Furthermore, academic units are comprised of faculty and staff who have vast expertise across a broad range of wellbeing topics but remain a largely untapped pool of talent when it comes to campus wellbeing. For example, it would be difficult to find a post-secondary institution that did not employ disciplinary subject-matter expertise in wellbeing, with experts commonly found across health disciplines, the social and natural sciences, and the humanities. Faculty and staff in such disciplines are designing and delivering research programs and curricula that have the potential to influence campus wellbeing initiatives, but far too often those research and academic programs are disconnected from the institution's wellness strategy.

With the creation of the Okanagan Charter (2015), many universities and colleges have taken up the Calls to Action to "1) Embed health [defined holistically] into all aspects of campus culture, across the administration, operations and academic mandates, and 2) Lead health promotion action and collaboration locally and globally" (p. 3). A recent study examined how initial signatory institutions are implementing and evaluating their healthy campus initiatives (London & Squires, 2020; Squires & London, 2019), but there has been no apparent attempt to investigate how academic units are contributing to the Okanagan Charter implementation.

In this chapter we present the results of a multi-case study of Canadian university exercise science units (often referred to as "kinesiology," "physical education," or "sport studies") to explore the ways in which they are using the Okanagan Charter as a foundational building block for contributing to a systemic approach to advancing campus wellbeing. The study, which addressed the prominent issue of student, staff, and faculty wellbeing, was the first to examine the implementation of the Okanagan Charter by exercise science units, and one of the first to explore the ability of this pan-Canadian framework to promote student and campus wellbeing.

The Evolution of the Mandates of Exercise Science Units

To understand the role of exercise science units in campus wellbeing, it is helpful to consider how the mandate of the discipline has evolved over time. Out of concern for student health, in the 1920s and 1930s, it was common for universities to require students to complete physical activity courses such as swimming in order to graduate. For example, at that time 97% of American colleges and universities offered physical activity-based courses as part of their general education requirements (Cardinal, 2020). From 1950 to 1980 there was a surge in the number of programs developed to train physical educators (Schultz, 2021), and as those programs grew over time, they began to be organized as independent academic units such as departments and schools. As a result of their expertise, experience, and capacity for providing physical activity courses, many of those units also were responsible for delivering campus-wide non-credit programming such as student intramurals. Faculty members often doubled as coaches of the university's varsity sports teams, and the oversight of varsity sports was also part of the mandate of the academic unit. Universities took a greater interest as external community-serving institutions, and sport and recreation programming for non-university audiences became the norm. The mandates of these academic units often included the delivery of academic programs, research, varsity sports programs, campus recreation, and physical activity programming for the broader community.

Physical education was not only viewed as a subject in elementary and high schools, but it was evolving into a discipline that could share knowledge about physical activity and human movement in broader settings. Academic units were becoming multidisciplinary and included many different sectors that allowed students and researchers alike to explore a wider range of topics under an umbrella of "kinesiology" (Schultz, 2021). Approximately forty years ago the world's first two "kinesiology" units were formed in Canada at the University of Waterloo and Simon Fraser University, and many began changing the names of their academic units from "physical education" to "kinesiology" (Elliott, 2007). From an academic standpoint, the scope of these units expanded, and they began creating programs that considered the role of human movement in health and health care settings that went beyond the traditional focus on school and community recreation settings. Students' demand for exercise science programs skyrocketed as students saw clear pathways from kinesiology to other health professional programs such as physical therapy, medicine, and occupational therapy.

Around the year 2000, there began to be a shift in mandates of these academic units to solely focus on teaching and research. Varsity sports and campus recreation responsibilities were moved into other parts of the institution such as units focusing on the student experience. For example, at the Canadian Council of University Physical Education and Kinesiology Administrators' (CCUPEKA) table, there are fewer members whose academic unit is also responsible for athletics and recreation. There are currently forty exercise science units in Canada, and they take various organizational forms including faculties, colleges, schools, and departments. At the time of writing this chapter, only nine were responsible for athletics and recreation, which is a reduction of approximately 50 per cent from the number responsible in 2000. This shift away from having athletics and recreation tied together with the academic unit has been a result of the field moving away from a focus on physical education to kinesiology in the laboratory (Vertinsky, 2017). One could argue that with the recent focus on knowledge mobilization of research, and experiential learning in academic programs, we are in the midst of a shift to exercise science in the community.

Exercise science units that are responsible for facilitating physical activity for students, faculty, staff, and the broader community, have a direct mandate to enhance campus wellbeing. But that does not mean other units are devoid of the responsibilities outlined in the Okanagan

Charter. In fact, through the delivery of academic programs, research, and community engagement initiatives, all exercise science units have the opportunity to contribute to a health-promoting campus. But are they contributing? And if so, how? And what can other disciplines learn from how exercise science units are advancing campus wellbeing?

To answer those questions, a multi-case study of Canadian exercise science units is described below, with consideration given as to how other academic units beyond exercise science can contribute to wellbeing. The overall purpose of the study was to examine the ways in which exercise science units are advancing wellbeing on Canadian universities' campuses, using the Okanagan Charter as a foundational building block for contributing to a systemic approach to wellbeing. Three specific objectives were proposed: (1) to identify how exercise science units are involved in health-promoting campus initiatives that advance the Okanagan Charter; (2) to examine how exercise science units are developing trans-disciplinary collaborations that promote campus health and wellbeing; and (3) to construct an analysis of similarities and differences in the implementation of healthy campus initiatives across campuses.

Theoretical Framework

Howlett et al. (2009) posited that policy development can be framed as an examination of a series of stages within a policy cycle: 1) Adoption, 2) Formulation, 3) Implementation, and 4) Evaluation. This exploratory study examined the third stage, policy implementation, to identify initiatives that have been enacted and the ways in which they are advanced through collaboration with other disciplines. Several units had implemented strategies that arose from the Charter's Calls to Action, and a small number were developing their own evaluation plans including specific targets and milestones. Analysis of the data led to the identification of clear leaders in both the implementation and evaluation of healthy campus initiatives.

Methods and Data Sources

The researchers employed a qualitative, multi-case study methodology suited for studies embedded in higher education (Jones et al., 2006), whereby a multiple-case study framework across campuses was undertaken in the context of the Okanagan Charter. Data were gathered across two phases after the researchers received approval from the Institutional Research Ethics Board.

The first phase consisted of an online survey designed to meet the first objective, which was to identify how exercise science units are involved in health promoting campus initiatives that advance the Okanagan Charter. The second phase was designed to examine the second objective, which was to further examine how exercise science units are developing trans-disciplinary collaborations that promote campus health and well-being. During this second phase, semi-structured interviews were conducted with academic leaders of units identified as being at the forefront of this work. In both phases, data were analysed to meet the third objective, which was to examine similarities and differences across campuses. Details on each phase are presented below.

Phase 1 Methods

An invitation to complete an online survey was sent to all forty CCUPEKA member representatives (i.e., deans, directors, heads of exercise science units across Canada). Of those, twenty-three consented and participated in the survey with seventeen completing all questions of the survey. More specifically, the survey consisted of thirteen open-ended questions. The first two questions were demographic in nature to seek information about the institution and academic unit. The remaining eleven questions asked representatives to share how their respective units had been involved in healthy campus and/or Okanagan Charter initiatives, barriers they have experienced, perceived opportunities for the unit as well as CCUPEKA at large for advancing the Okanagan Charter, resources allocated to the unit for support, experience with evaluating progress or impact of this work, impact of COVID-19, collaborations happening with units across the campus or in the community as well as the opportunities and/or challenges in developing collaborations.

Phase 2 Methods

From Phase 1, five leaders of academic units seen as being at the forefront of advancing healthy campus initiatives in support of the Okanagan Charter were identified and invited to participate in a semi-structured interview. In this phase, data were collected and analysed using processes proposed by Saldaña (2013) to identify major themes, similarities, and differences. The semi-structured interview guide consisted of six overarching questions with prompts to gain an in-depth understanding, with specific examples, of how these units were able to successfully advance the Okanagan Charter including establishing collaborations with others. Questions also focused on the continued challenges in this work and advice interviewees would offer members of other units in their own efforts to advance the charter. In the results section below, "LU1" to "LU5" are used to identify the five interviewees of leading (L) units (U).

Results

The results are broken down into four main sections that combined the results from both phases. The first section details the most common form of initiatives, which were led by exercise units and were perceived as having a strong impact on advancing the Okanagan Charter. The second section outlines the barriers and/or challenges in this work experienced by exercise science units. The third section focuses on the impact of the COVID-19 pandemic. Finally, the fourth section summarizes the perceptions of those leading exercise science units on what academic units, exercise science, and beyond need to do to continue this important work.

Initiatives Led by Exercise Science Units Perceived as Having an Impact

A consistent theme for units, regardless of whether their mandate included physical activity programming on campus, was the use of curricular initiatives within credit-based courses to integrate practical or hands-on student learning with healthy campus programming. For example, as part of exercise and cardiovascular physiology courses, students were involved in the delivery of cardiac rehabilitation programming for community members. Another example involved having students in various health promotion courses form groups and complete applied projects in partnership with the health and wellbeing service unit on campus to assist with different month-long wellness initiatives on campus for students, staff, and faculty across the academic year. LU4 and LU5 also highlighted the importance of co-curricular contributions to enhance wellbeing, such as those led by their student societies, which provide programs to students, staff, and faculty that are consistent with the health and wellness framework of the broader institution. Extensive volunteering is made possible through the student society and serves as "a complement to their academic courses" (LU5).

Units also indicated how many curricular initiatives have also led to or are expanded into the larger community. As a result, students are provided with "work-integrated learning" opportunities such as community placements or practicums, where they lead community-based programming for extended periods of time over the course of an academic term or year. For example, LU3 described a required practicum for exercise science students that "gets our students doing practical work with health promotion in the community and on campus. Using our campus setting is a perfect environment for them to build the skills … they lead it, they enact it, they develop it, they evaluate it, and it's been meaningful work." Leading units also spoke about approaches to teaching and learning that enhance wellbeing and are infused across their programs. LU5 described the pedagogy of kindness in this way:

> We're actually starting to think about how you design courses with the pedagogy of kindness. Thinking about everything from the amount of content to how assignments are structured. We actually review course outlines and think about how it's built across the curriculum. We've put in reading weeks in the fall term. We've put in reading weeks for graduate courses that didn't exist previously.

Similarly, LU3 described advocating for bringing a focus on wellness into the classroom. This initiative was designed to support faculty in thinking about how the design of their course (e.g., flexible grading), approaches in the classroom, and activities such as movement breaks in the classroom can have a positive impact on student wellbeing.

A number of leading units had also moved beyond curricular initiatives within their own exercise science units to deliver curriculum to students in disciplines beyond exercise science. For example, LU1, LU3, and LU4 described first-year health and wellness courses that are required for exercise science students and are available to students from other programs across campus as an elective. Those courses assist students in the transition to university and "all of the struggles that people might have with eating well, and time management, stress, alcohol abuse, and stuff like that" (LU1). A theme arising from leading units was a desire that those courses be required for all first-year students across all academic units.

Existing Barriers and/or Challenges Experienced in Advancing the Okanagan Charter

While respondents recognized various curricular-related opportunities as strong mechanisms for advancing wellbeing on campus, they also noted barriers to implementing healthy campus initiatives such as a lack of resources from central administrative units. With regards to central support, leaders discussed that challenges arise when little to no resources are allocated to units from central administrative units to support initiatives and also when higher level leaders at the institution are unaware of this work. As one respondent from a leading institution shared, "until just recently, our Provost was not even aware of the Okanagan Charter; however, in conversations that I have had with him, I believe there is an openness and willingness to adopt this charter in the future … in my opinion, too many of these initiatives, and the resources for implementing them, are downloaded to individual Faculties/units, making it difficult to establish any kind of campus-wide support and impact" (LU4). Another perceived barrier was the decreased capacity of faculty members to be able to contribute to initiatives, which LU2 described as "faculty fatigue from being stretched to support an increasingly large number of non-teaching requests." Similarly, LU3 noted the workload challenges of faculty members and capacity to be involved in non-research activities as well as a lack of awareness regarding the relationship between student wellbeing and academic performance.

Many respondents indicated that very little collaboration was occurring across units that were involved in healthy campus work, with reasons being limited time and energy, silos within the university and with community, and gaps between academic and service-oriented units (such as student affairs and human resources). Leaders of exercise science academic units noted the subject-matter expertise that their faculty, staff, and students could bring to improving campus wellbeing, but which is not sufficiently accessed. "It aligns so closely with the mission of our faculty and the content that we actually teach … but I don't think we have an active role right now across the institution" (LU5). LU3 observed that "we should be role modelling and promoting this and it's been done very, very, quietly. That's one thing that I'm quite disappointed in and LU5 added that "I think we have strong commitments, but I actually don't think there is coherence or consistency on what that actually means." However, some of the leading campuses had found ways to structure the governance of healthy campus work in collaborative ways where various stakeholders from within the unit were at key decision-making tables and advocated for enhancing campus wellbeing.

The Impact of the COVID-19 Pandemic

Since data for this research was collected during the global COVID-19 pandemic, institutions were asked what impact the pandemic was having on their healthy campus work. One common theme was the increased awareness of mental health challenges being faced by university communities. For exercise science units, a benefit was also increased awareness of the role of physical activity in enhancing mental health. As a result, many of the institutions reported being able to develop new and inno-vative interventions or programming. For example, with reduced access to in-person recreation and physical activity programs, many institutions pivoted and created a large variety of online wellness programming to support students, staff, and faculty. LU5 shared that the pandemic "got me the resources ... we were doing small things ... but because of COVID it was an emergency and ... we threw resources into it."

However, there were also a number of challenges for exercise science students that resulted from the pandemic. Many of the units responsible for delivering athletics and recreation programs reported having to lay off individuals and close campus physical activity facilities, which severely impacted the ability to implement healthy campus initiatives, including remotely delivered ones. Similarly, a number of units reported major budget cuts during this time that resulted in the halting of a number of initiatives that they had been leading on their respective campuses. Leaders of exercise science units also described going into "emergency only mode" and thus having very limited capacity to start or continue ini-tiatives that would advance the Okanagan Charter during the pandemic.

Lessons Learned and Moving Forward

A number of lessons learned and advice were shared by leaders of ex-ercise science units to others hoping to embark on advancing healthy campus initiatives. First, the leaders advised looking for ways to connect research to healthy campus initiatives in a collaborative manner to de-crease challenges or barriers related to capacity and workload. More spe-cifically, there was a recognition by leading units that tying the research projects of faculty and students with healthy campus initiatives is an ex-cellent way to leverage resources in a win-win approach. LU2 suggested,

> make it feasible so faculty members aren't launching a whole program, tak-ing care of the scheduling, getting all the participants up and running ... we've turned a lot of these programs to research hubs, our community is getting programs that typically aren't offered, at a much-reduced cost and our faculty members are getting in-house research hubs and getting sup-port for that. They don't have to take it on all themselves and keep rein-venting the wheel. It seems to get easier and easier to do because we have kind of the structures and the paperwork and the formatting and we know how to do it.

Second, while a light was shone on wellbeing and new ways of delivering programming during the pandemic, awareness of inequities with regards to access to healthy campus initiatives and opportunities increased. Respondents highlighted the decreased time that was available for physical activity and recreation because of individual circumstances. For example, caregiving responsibilities and remote study or work demands were often factors that limited individuals' ability to access health promotion opportunities. Respondents also mentioned that increased awareness of the Indigenous Lives Matter and Black Lives Matter movements had an impact on the wellbeing of university communities in both negative and positive ways depending on the context. While marginalized groups continued to not have equitable access to resources, there seemed to be a renewed commitment to equity, diversity, and inclusion when it came to healthy campus initiatives as described by respondents. LU5 stated,

> we've also seen with a focus on anti-black racism, oppression, decolonization, that you can't have a healthy culture in an environment where there's discrimination and oppression. Thus, for exercise science units a significant lesson learned was related to health inequities and the work needed to enhance equity and inclusion, particularly in their work to advance wellbeing. It is not enough to be developing and implementing initiatives and/or programming for individuals to enhance their wellness, but there is a need to ensure the contexts in which they operate are inclusive and accessible for all.

There is a need for greater collaboration and integration of resources. LU1 and LU4 noted that the structure of their academic units, which combined exercise science with other health-related units, facilitates interdisciplinary collaboration. In providing advice to units that may be about to embark on healthy campus initiatives, LU2 suggested that they "intentionally reach out to the health and sustainability faculty members to seek out those champions ... bring the best of what we have to offer to the table and maybe then we can create something that will start to shift [the] narrative and create healthy spaces." Leading units seemed to place equal emphasis on external collaboration as they did on working together within their universities. "We probably do better at reaching out to the broader community than we do to our internal community" because of practicum placements, remarked LU4. Ongoing discussions were integral in a health care partnership described by LU2:

> they well know what kinesiology can offer and I think that's how we get connected there ... 2 hospitals ... we offer Think Tanks once a month where you show up ... people are launching usually a very raw idea and the idea is to get the people in the room who maybe have expertise and want to

join that team or provide support or get students involved. A lot of those initiatives now are really starting to get stronger connections especially with kinesiology in the hospital.

The primary barrier to collaboration as identified by leading units was a perceived lack of resources:

> We're talking about global climate change ... decolonizing curriculum, EDI. There is a long list of very important commitments that we need to be making progress towards. And they all do definitely take resources ... I think the biggest question then is what resources are we putting into staff and augmenting our student services office versus resources going directly into faculty members and hiring on of new faculty members. (LU5)

What Can Academic Units Outside of Exercise Science Learn from This Study?

Those from disciplines beyond exercise science might be tempted to think that while healthy campus work might be an opportunity for an exercise science unit because it is a health discipline, their non-health-related disciplines do not have much to offer in promoting health on campus. However, the whole systems approach to health promotion that runs as a theme throughout this book advocates for an approach where all members of a community are collectively responsible for the wellbeing of the community and its members. Two of the particular calls to action outlined in the Okanagan Charter (2015) are relevant to the work of academic units. Those two actions will be used to organize a summary of how the findings of this study can inform what all academic units (including the social sciences and humanities, the natural sciences, and more) can do to contribute to a healthy campus.

Action 1.2 of the Okanagan Charter (2015) calls for the creation of supportive campus environments by using cross-cutting approaches to "embed an understanding and a commitment to health, wellbeing and sustainability across all disciplines and curricula" and seeing the campus as a "living laboratory, identifying opportunities to study and support health and wellbeing, as well as sustainability and resilience in the built, natural, social, economic, cultural, academic, organizational and learning environments" (p. 8). This provides an all-encompassing opportunity for disciplines across the academy to create curricular and non-curricular initiatives to support wellbeing. Academic units can go beyond the individual health behaviours that have typically been addressed by health disciplines such as exercise science, and develop learning opportunities that help students, faculty, and staff understand how the physical (built), social, economic, and cultural environments can be designed to enhance wellbeing. Schools of architecture, design and engineering can offer programming related to wellbeing and the built environment. Programs that inform social and cultural wellbeing (and their determinants) can be a focus of social sciences and humanities units. The economic impacts of wellbeing fall directly in the realm of schools of economics and business. These are but a few obvious examples of how studies within different disciplines can be connected to wellbeing.

One particular way that academic units can use the campus itself as a living laboratory to support health and wellbeing is to develop experiential learning opportunities for students from across various academic units that serve individuals and communities on campus. Participants from exercise science units in our study indicated that they tend to look beyond the campus for experiential learning, which causes them to potentially miss out on opportunities for students that directly benefit others on campus. All academic units could consider community service-learning projects, practicum and co-op placements, and applied research projects where students explore topics related to student, faculty, and staff wellbeing and the impact that different service models, learning environments, resource allocations, and/or policies may have on the advancement of the Okanagan Charter. Conducting those projects in collaboration with other units on campus such as student service and human resource departments can inform future initiatives of those campus-serving units in evidence-based ways.

All academic units can ask themselves how they are enhancing wellbeing with the approaches they are using for teaching and learning. Are they using student-centred approaches and pedagogies of kindness that were described by participants in our study? From the outcomes we intend students to achieve, to the content delivered and how it is assessed, teaching and learning practices influence the learning environment and have been shown to have an impact on student wellbeing (Baik et al., 2017). Students can feel overwhelmed if the courses contain excessive content, when connections between concepts are not clear, or when expectations of assessments are vague and the assessments themselves are mistimed in relation to other demands students are facing within their program (TLARC, 2022). Instructors can support wellbeing by creating inclusive and respectful environments, allowing students some autonomy in assessments while also providing constructive feedback, and delivering course content in ways that allow students to connect with each other and the instructor (UBC, 2022). How they design and deliver their courses also has an effect on faculty wellbeing, which should be taken into consideration.

At the level of the academic unit, leaders can facilitate wellbeing through strategies such as incentivizing and rewarding teaching and learning practices that support wellbeing, encouraging collaborative curricular design to support coherent and balanced demands across courses, and creating policies and processes that support pedagogies of kindness and teaching and learning that support wellbeing (TLARC, 2022).

Call to Action 2.2 of the Okanagan Charter (2015) challenges universities to "contribute to health promoting knowledge production, application, standard setting and evaluation that advance multi-disciplinary and trans-disciplinary research agendas relevant to real world outcomes" (p. 8). With research being one-third of the tripartite mandate of the modern university, it should not be ignored when considering how academic units can support health and wellbeing. Findings from our study highlighted opportunities for researchers to work across disciplinary boundaries to examine health and wellbeing questions, which have been proven to be one of those complex, befuddling problems facing modern-day societies across the globe. Academic leaders should be facilitating research collaborations across and beyond the university, with advancing a healthy campus as one of the real-world problems to address.

Finally, Call to Action 2.3 of the Okanagan Charter (2015) indicates that we need to "build and support inspiring and effective relationships and collaborations on and off campus to develop, harness and mobilize knowledge and action for health promotion locally and globally" (p. 8). The experiences of those leading exercise science units show that functions of university governance provide opportunities for academic units to advance a healthy campus. One way to collaborate is for those leading healthy campus efforts at the institution to invite subject-matter experts that are housed in academic units to broader institution-wide tables when developing wellbeing strategic plans. Participating at the front end of planning can open new possibilities for engagement with academic units. Further, teams tasked with implementing and evaluating those plans should include subject-matter expertise across disciplines. While faculty may see this as an administrative service activity that will take time away from teaching and research responsibilities, as described above there are innovative ways to connect faculty work with healthy campus initiatives in a win-win approach. For example, student services and other staff or roles on campus can engage with research teams to support the implementation of initiatives while researchers use their capacity for evaluation and knowledge-sharing activities. There is no better example of a subject-matter-led contribution to wellbeing evaluation than the development of the Canadian Campus Wellbeing Survey (CCWS; www .ccws-becc.ca), described in chapter 3 of this book.

Resources that are allocated through central units within the university are more likely to support healthy campus initiatives involving academic units when representatives from those units are at decision-making tables. Through collaborations that view health and wellbeing in a whole systems manner, increased resources may be allocated to support institution-wide initiatives with multiple levels of benefits such as those being invested in decolonization and anti-racism. Investments in those initiatives are critical in their own right, yet they are also critical for the wellbeing of students, staff, faculty, and the broader community.

Conclusion

This chapter started by asking whether academic units have a responsibility for campus wellbeing, and if so, what was their role in those efforts? The results of a multi-case study were presented to explore how exercise science units at Canadian universities are contributing to healthy campus initiatives to show that those units can play a critical role. Academic units beyond exercise science share the responsibility of developing and maintaining healthy campuses as does everyone in the university community. Expecting that only student services and human resources departments will be the ones to ensure wellbeing of students, staff, and faculty is a misplaced view and a missed opportunity in many ways.

Reviewing the results of the study presented only provides an introductory look at the role of academic units in advancing wellbeing. Further study is needed to better understand how wellbeing can be embedded across all aspects of post-secondary institutions to address the Okanagan Charter's calls to action, and further consideration is needed of the context of any particular institution. It is clear, though, that all academic disciplines and the units where they reside should be at the institutional tables where discussions are happening about wellbeing on campus. It is through these discussions that innovation and collaboration can be fostered to advance health promotion locally and globally through teaching, research, and experiential learning.

REFERENCES

Academica Group. (2022). *Student wellness and the post-secondary institution.* Academica Forum. Retrieved from https://forum.academica.ca/forum/whos-responsible-for-student-wellness

Alberta Centre for Active Living. (2019). *Alberta survey on physical activity.*
    Retrieved from https://www.ualberta.ca/kinesiology-sport-recreation/media
    -library/research/centres-and-units/centre-for-active-living/alberta-survey-of
    -physical-activity/2019/2019-ab-survey-exec-summary.pdf
American College Health Association (ACHA). (2019). *American College Health
    Association–National College Health Assessment II: Canadian Reference Group Data
    Report Spring 2019.* American College Health Association.
Baik, C., Karcombe, W., Brooker, A., Wyn, J., Allen, L., Brett, M., Field,
    R., & James, R. (2017). *Enhancing student mental wellbeing: A handbook for
    academic educators.* https://melbourne-cshe.unimelb.edu.au/__data/
    assets/pdf_file/0006/2408604/MCSHE-Student-Wellbeing-Handbook
    -FINAL.pdf
Cardinal, B.J. (2020). Promoting physical activity education through general
    education: Looking back and moving forward. *Kinesiology Review, 9*(4),
    287–92. https://doi.org/10.1123/kr.2020-0031
Cordaro, M. (2020). Pouring from an empty cup: The case for compassion
    fatigue in higher education. *Building Healthy Academic Communities Journal,
    4*(2), 17–28. https://doi.org/10.18061/bhac.v4i2.7618
Elliott, D. (2007). Forty years of kinesiology: A Canadian perspective. *Quest,
    59*(1), 154–62. https://doi.org/10.1080/00336297.2007.10483544
Howlett, M., Ramesh, M., & Perl, A. (2009). *Studying public policy: Policy cycles
    & policy subsystems* (3rd ed.). Oxford University Press.
Lattie, E.G., Adkins, E.C., Winquist, N., Stiles-Shields, C., Wafford, Q.E., &
    Graham, A.K. (2019). Digital mental health interventions for depression,
    anxiety, and enhancement of psychological wellbeing among college
    students: Systematic review. *Journal of Medical InternetResearch, 21*(7), e12869.
    https://doi.org/10.2196/12869
London, C.L., & Squires, V. (2020, January). *Adopting the Okanagan Charter:
    Exploring the impact on Canadian campuses.* A paper presented at the NASPA
    (Student Affairs Administrators in Higher Education) Strategies Conference.
    New Orleans, Louisiana.
Okanagan Charter: An International Charter for Health Promoting Universities
    and Colleges. (2015). *Okanagan Charter.* Kelowna, BC: Author. Retrieved
    from http://internationalhealthycampuses2015.sites.olt.ubc.ca/files/2016
    /01/Okanagan-Charter-January13v2.pdf
Owen, N., Healy, G.N., Matthews, C.E., & Dunstan, D.W. (2010). Too much sitting:
    The population health science of sedentary behavior. *Exercise and Sport Sciences
    Reviews, 38*(3), 105–13. https://doi.org/10.1097/JES.0b013e3181e373a2
Owens, J., Kottwitz, C., Tiedt, J., & Ramirez, J. (2018). Strategies to attain faculty
    work-life balance. *Building Healthy Academic Communities Journal, 2*(2), 58–73.
    https://doi.org/10.18061/bhac.v2i2.6544

Saldaña, J. (2013). The coding manual for qualitative researchers (2nd ed.). Sage.

Schultz, J. (2021). A history of kinesiology. In C.A. Oglesby, K. Henige, D.W. McLaughlin, & B. Stillwell, *Foundations of kinesiology* (2nd ed., pp. 41–51). Jones & Bartlett Learning.

Squires, V., & London, C. (2022). The Okanagan Charter: Evolution of health promotion in Canadian higher education. *Canadian Journal of Higher Education, 51*(3), 100–14. https://doi.org/10.47678/cjhe.vi0.189109

Squires, V., & London, C. (2019, June). *Gauging the impact of the Okanagan Charter on the wellbeing of Canadian campuses.* A paper presented at the Canadian Society for the Study of Higher Education Conference. Vancouver, BC. https://csshe-scees.ca/wp-content/uploads/2019/05/2019_csshe_prog _20190528.pdf

Teaching, Learning and Academic Resources Committee (TLARC). (2022, January). *Learning and teaching practices that support student mental health and wellbeing.* University of Saskatchewan University Council.

University of British Columbia (UBC). (2022). *Supporting student wellbeing at UBC.* Retrieved from https://blogs.ubc.ca/teachingandwellbeing/files /2017/05/TLEF-Infographic_Round2_v2.pdf

Vertinsky, P. (2017). A question of the head and the heart: From physical education to kinesiology in the gymnasium and the laboratory. *Kinesiology Review, 6*(2), 140–52. https://doi.org/10.1123/kr.2017-0006

8 Promoting Food Security for Post-secondary Students

SARA KOZICKY, VANESSA CUNNINGHAM, MIN-JUNG KIM,
SAM LABAN, AND PHILIP A. LORING

Introduction

Food insecurity can be defined as inadequate or insecure access to food due to financial constraints (PROOF, n.d.). Evidence from a multitude of studies indicates that approximately 30–40 per cent of post-secondary students in Canada are food insecure (Meal Exchange, 2021). Food insecure students may be worrying about where their next meal will come from, choosing between paying rent or paying for groceries, making all sorts of compromises to their needs, or dropping out of their program because they were too tired and unwell. There are numerous interconnected drivers that put students at risk of experiencing food insecurity, including challenges related to finances, time, access to and availability of cultural foods, social identities, and socio-economic positions. Campuses are not food-secure spaces and as a result, the health, wellbeing, and academic success of students is suffering.

Imagine if campuses were flourishing spaces instead, and what that would look like. Surely food insecurity would not exist. There would not be a single student making any of the impossible decisions we describe above. In a flourishing campus, health, wellbeing, and relationships would be prioritized, and in doing so, students would feel safe in a setting where they were cared for and empowered to fully engage in their studies.

We, the authors, are describing a vision of what we believe campus communities can look and feel like in the future. For campuses across Canada, this is not the reality at present, as food insecurity is indeed prevalent (Ahmadi et al., 2020; Bessey et al., 2020; Blundell et al., 2019; Entz et al., 2017; Frank, 2018; Hamilton et al., 2020; Maynard et al., 2018; Meal Exchange, 2021; Olauson et al., 2018; Power et al., 2021; Reynolds et al., 2018) and mental health issues are a concern (Linden & Stuart, 2020). Post-secondary institutions (PSIs) face numerous complex challenges that negatively affect students' health, wellbeing, and academic success. They are not impervious to historic and ongoing structural oppression that form the basis of economic and social inequities (Wilcox et al., 2021; Willis, 2021). Nor are they to other complex challenges of our time, such as the COVID-19 pandemic, inflation, war, and the climate emergency, all of which exacerbate underlying inequities.

Concerns about the realities of being a student are increasing among students, researchers, and university administrators as is attention directed to health-related problems such as food insecurity. Now, more faculty, staff, and partners outside of campus communities are joining students to elevate these issues and develop innovative solutions. A greater number of students with lived experiences are also sharing their stories, which help us all to better understand food insecurity and inform what actions are needed to address it (Bessey et al., 2020; Cunningham, 2022; Frank, 2018; Henry, 2017; Maynard et al., 2018; Power et al., 2021). Based on existing literature and our personal experiences working in the fields of student food insecurity and health, we argue that comprehensive approaches that are multifaceted, systems-based, and overall united are needed.

We also believe that there is an immense opportunity for PSIs to be leaders, locally, regionally, and globally, in demonstrating to the rest of society that food-secure communities are possible and showcasing the myriad of benefits that come along with them. Fortunately, knowledge, passion, and resources already exist and can be readily garnered to generate meaningful change. But action must happen now.

In this chapter, we aim to 1) build knowledge on food insecurity, providing insight into the nuanced experiences of food insecurity within PSIs; 2) inspire post-secondary leaders to act on food insecurity with urgency; and 3) highlight promising practices and critical perspectives to achieving food-secure campuses, predominantly through the use of a case study on the University of British Columbia. Although we focus on post-secondary institutions in Canada, the content in this chapter is applicable to institutions elsewhere that are interested in addressing food insecurity and issues related to health and wellbeing on their campuses.

To help fulfil these aims, we organize the chapter into three main sections. Section 1 provides general context on the various facets of post-secondary student food insecurity. Here, we include quotes from participants[1] (from various research publications) with lived experiences

---

1   All research participants' names presented in this chapter are pseudonyms and any quotes used have received consent from the appropriate participant.

to exemplify concepts, amplify students' voices, and support our position for a systems approach to address student food insecurity. Next, in Section 2, we provide an overview of the current state of campus responses to addressing student food insecurity in Canada, including existing issues that we have observed in our fields of research and practice, as well as a selection of promising examples from across the country. We start with three shorter examples, including the Sliding Scale Fresh Food Market at the University of Guelph, Loaded Ladle at Dalhousie University, and the Canadian Campus Wellbeing Survey, and then move into a more in-depth exploration of the University of British Columbia's Food Security Initiative. Finally, in Section 3, we provide a list of recommendations for post-secondary institutions' leadership to apply as they work towards creating food-secure campuses.

We, the authors of this chapter, have different experiences with food (in)security work and are situated at different institutions, including the University of British Columbia, Vancouver campus, and the University of Guelph in Ontario. Our roles include a food security project manager, researchers, facilitator, and student-staff. We too continue to learn about student food insecurity, health, and wellbeing, and view this chapter as part of our own learning process, as well as a contribution to the larger journey that we are all on together to create these flourishing campus communities.

Section 1. Building an Understanding of Post-secondary Students' Food Insecurity

We begin this section with a brief introduction to food insecurity, followed by a more detailed overview of post-secondary student food insecurity. This overview includes a series of themes we identified in the literature that can help build an understanding of student food insecurity. These themes include drivers, impacts on health, wellbeing, academics, and coping mechanisms.

Introduction

Food is a basic human right (United Nations General Assembly, 1948), and food security is a social determinant of health and wellbeing. Yet for decades, food insecurity – "the inadequate or insecure access to food due to financial constraints" (PROOF, n.d.) – has remained a pervasive public health problem, one that disproportionately affects certain subgroups of the population, such as individuals who are Indigenous (Batal et al., 2021; Tarasuk et al., 2019), racialized (Dhunna & Tarasuk, 2021;

Odoms-Young & Bruce, 2018; Tarasuk & Mitchell, 2020b), disabled (Coleman-Jensen, 2020), and single parents, especially single mothers (Tarasuk & Mitchell, 2020b). Food insecurity is a symptom of structural inequities and has a myriad of negative impacts on all dimensions of health and wellbeing (Dhunna & Tarasuk, 2021; Odoms-Young & Bruce, 2018). Research has found that food-insecure adults are more likely to experience a multitude of chronic health conditions and diseases, such as cancer, diabetes, asthma, and high blood pressure (Coleman-Jensen et al., 2019; Leung et al., 2020; Vozoris & Tarasuk, 2003), psychological distress (Davison et al., 2015; Hamelin et al., 2002; Jessiman-Perreault & McIntyre, 2017; Muldoon et al., 2013), and premature death (Men et al., 2020).

Food insecurity, as a societal problem, has important implications for those concerned with justice. It denies individuals of a human right and necessity, alienates them from their culture, environment, and relationships, and prevents them from choosing how to participate in society. How can we create and sustain healthy, thriving communities that are equitable and just when even a single person is faced with the realities of food insecurity?

In Canada, many people experience food insecurity. In 2017–18, prior to the COVID-19 pandemic, results from the Household Food Security Survey Module (HFSSM)[2] found that 12.7 per cent of all Canadian households were food insecure (Tarasuk & Mitchell, 2020b). The prevalence of food insecurity varies across Canada, with some of the highest rates occurring among Black households (28.9%); Indigenous households (28.2%); female lone-parent households (33.1%); and in Nunavut (57%) (Tarasuk & Mitchell, 2020b). This confirms the increased vulnerability that certain groups face.

Post-secondary Student Food Insecurity

Students have also been identified as another subgroup of the population that is more vulnerable to food insecurity. There are more than two million post-secondary students in Canada (Statistics Canada, 2020a), many of whom pursue higher education to support their knowledge

2 In Canada, household food insecurity is measured using the Household Food Security Survey Module (HFSSM) – a validated measurement tool – through Statistics Canada. From 2004 to 2018, the HFSSM was administered through the Canadian Community Health Survey (CCHS); however, it is now incorporated in the Canadian Income Survey, a component of Canada's Poverty Reduction Strategy (Caron & Plunkett-Latimer, 2022).

interests and career goals as well as increase their chances of upward social mobility. Education, like food, is a social determinant of health and a key component of upward social mobility (Shankar et al., 2013). It also helps to protect against food insecurity, as evidence indicates that households with higher levels of education are more likely to be food secure (Tarasuk & Mitchell, 2020b). However, in the last decade, studies from campuses across Canada have consistently reported that 30–40 per cent of students experience some level of food insecurity (Blundell et al., 2019; Entz et al., 2017; Farahbakhsh et al., 2017; Meal Exchange, 2021; Olauson et al., 2018; Reynolds et al., 2018; Silverthorn, 2016). Every person has their own experiences with food insecurity, which can range from worrying about accessing adequate food, feeling embarrassed, declining social events, and skipping meals (Choubak et al., 2020; Henry, 2017; Maynard et al., 2018). For example, Basir, a participant from a study conducted by Cunningham (2022, p. 86), shared some of the thoughts he had while experiencing food insecurity:

> The thoughts in my mind were all sad, sometimes leading to regret, and in some cases depression. I was always turning to myself and asking, why do I have to eat the same food? Why do I have to make something that I don't like? Why does this rice taste different from what I had before [back home]? And why are these vegetables so expensive that I can buy only once a month, or not even once a month?

With the emergence of these high prevalence rates and increased knowledge of students' lived experiences, more students, researchers, and health practitioners are raising alarm out of concern for the number of food-insecure students, and how it negatively affects their health, wellbeing, and academic success.

Drivers of Post-secondary Student Food Insecurity

There are various drivers of student food insecurity. Some are unique to students, including specific financial and time challenges as well as damaging narratives about the student experience that normalize food insecurity and stunt the responses to it. There are also other drivers that are relevant, but not unique, to students, including the availability of and access to culturally preferred foods (Hattangadi et al., 2019), social identities (Cunningham, 2022), and socio-economic positions (Willis, 2019). These drivers do not exist in isolation from each other; they are interconnected, and often students experience more than one of them at the same time.

Starving Student Narrative

Unfortunately, the starving student narrative, a belief that normalizes students' lack of access to sufficient, quality food while attending post-secondary school, is prevalent within and outside of institutions (Maynard et al., 2018). Being a starving student is framed as a typical post-secondary experience, a "rite of passage," but in doing so, it obscures the harmful realities of food insecurity (Crutchfield et al., 2020). Furthermore, normalizing student food insecurity means that students are less likely to recognize their experience and act accordingly, either in requesting help, voicing concerns, or demanding action. Campuses and society are also more likely to minimize the negative impacts and not take action. Another participant, Roxanne, in the same study by Cunningham (2022, p. 109) explained how she did not identify with being food insecure and instead felt like a broke student:

> I think it's sometimes hard to tell that you're food insecure because you're really just broke, that's what it comes down to. It's not so much that you can't afford food, it's like you can't afford anything, so it doesn't really strike you ... you don't identify with that phrase [food insecurity] when it comes up cause you just feel like a broke student.

Alongside this narrative, students also contend with financial and time-related burdens.

Financial

The financial challenges that students face are multifaceted. Tuition is a unique cost that only students face, and it can be a substantial financial burden, especially since students also still have to pay for other typical living expenses, such as housing and food, which have risen dramatically with record-breaking inflation in 2022 (Statistics Canada, 2022). With less flexible income, these types of price increases can be particularly hard on students. Not all students can afford these costs on their own, nor do they necessarily have parents who can pay for them (Cunningham, 2022). Some students in this position rely on various forms of financial aid, such as scholarships, bursaries, and loans, whereas others cannot because of eligibility requirements that they do not meet (Meal Exchange, 2021). For example, in the same study conducted by Cunningham (2022, p. 96), one of the participants, Nicole, shared that the loan payments she received from the Ontario Student Assistance Program (OSAP) were lower because of the fact that she also received income assistance from the Ontario Disability Support Program (ODSP):

My income is Ontario Disability Support Program; I get the bare minimum and unfortunately it's not enough because none of the students are in town. They're all in other provinces, other towns [living with their parents because of COVID]. There are no shared housing rentals, which has led me to have to rent a one-bedroom with nobody else. So my entire ODSP goes towards rent, which just leaves whatever OSAP is able to provide, which is not a lot. Because of being on ODSP, they give enough to cover tuition, books, and that's about it. Maybe an extra couple hundred dollars on top of that, but there's not much.

Even with both sources of funding, Nicole still did not have sufficient income to buy the food that she needed. Although she was not entirely ineligible for the Ontario student loan program, the eligibility requirements limit the funding she received and thereby contributed to the food insecurity she experienced.

Relying on loans is far from ideal for numerous reasons. The loan payments that students receive can be lower than expected, delayed, and received in lump sums at the beginning of the semester, all of which make it difficult for students to manage their finances (Bessey et al., 2020; Maynard et al., 2018). Studies have found that students who rely on loans are more likely to experience food insecurity (Frank, 2018). Furthermore, having a loan means taking on debt, which is associated with stress and negative health outcomes (Richardson et al., 2013). In addition to financial aid, it is also common for students to work one, or even multiple, jobs on top of their coursework. However, studies have found that, like relying on loans, students who work are more likely to experience food insecurity (Frank, 2018; Hughes et al., 2011). Even with these various sources of revenue in place, the amount of money students receive may still not be enough, as stagnated funding and wages do not match the true costs of being a student (Patton-López et al., 2014). In a study by Power et al. (2021), one of the Indigenous student participants, James, shared that the funding support he received from the federal government for Indigenous students and from his band amounted to $1000 per month. Because he paid $750 per month for rent at the graduate student residence, he only had $250 per month for all his other expenses, such as food, cell-phone bill, and transportation.

For international students, these financial support mechanisms are not always an option. Depending on the conditions of their study permit, international students may be ineligible for financial aid and/or prohibited from working completely, or limited in the hours they are allowed to work (Government of Canada, 2022). These limitations are an issue, especially considering that international students typically pay four times the amount domestic students pay for tuition (Statistics Canada, 2020b). High costs for education with limited financial support options put these students in a precarious situation.

Time

Time-related challenges have also been identified as barriers to food security (Garcia et al., 2010; Hattangadi et al., 2019; Zigmont et al., 2021).
It is well known and accepted that obtaining a post-secondary education
involves learning in a fast-paced environment with a large workload and
competing deadlines from classes, labs, tutorials, exams, and research.
In addition to academic responsibilities, working additional part-time
or full-time jobs out of financial necessity, commuting (e.g., to and from
campus), and fulfilling additional commitments leave students with minimal time, as well as energy to spend on food and health (Hattangadi et
al., 2019). It is not simply a matter of lacking cooking skills or interest
that prevent students from spending time on food, but rather the fact
that they are forced into time- and energy-scarce situations that leave
them without choice. In addition to (but not separate from) increasing
barriers to food security, a lack of time, finances, and the broader academic work culture can cause implications in other areas of health as
well. For example, anxiety and stress as well as loneliness and isolation
from the inability to participate socially in the campus community are all
possible outcomes (Meza et al., 2019).

Social Identities and Socio-Economic Positions

The financial and time-related challenges that elevate students' risk of
food insecurity are not experienced by all students. Research indicates
that students who embody certain social identities (e.g., Indigenous, racialized, women, LGBTQ2S+, and disabled) are more likely to experience food insecurity (Hamilton et al., 2020; Haskett et al., 2020; Maroto
et al., 2015; Payne-Sturges et al., 2018; Willis, 2021) and correspondingly
negative effects to their health and wellbeing. Students who embody
multiple of these social identities experience an even greater risk of food
insecurity (Hamilton et al., 2020). Other social identities that are also at
elevated risk include international students (Sherry et al., 2010), graduate students (Coffino et al., 2021), first-generation students (Camelo &
Elliot, 2019), students who are first-generation Canadians (Power et al.,
2021), and students who have children (Lee et al., 2020).

Most of these social identities are ones that are marginalized, stigmatized,
and disadvantaged by structural systems of oppression and discrimination
that produce inequities (e.g., racism, sexism, heterosexism, ableism).
These structural systems can determine the socio-economic classes
that students are in and therefore influence how accessible a post-secondary education is to them (Canadian Federation of Students, 2018).

They can also exacerbate the financial and time-related challenges for students who are able to attend post-secondary school. As such, the challenges and risks of being a student are experienced differently depending on the social identities that students have. Historically, students with these social identities were under-represented in universities. Encouragingly, this is changing as campus communities are now made up of diverse individuals. This shift has the potential to support the transition to a more just and resilient campus community, but only if post-secondary institutions understand the connections between food insecurity, social identities, and larger structural systems, and work to ensure their health-promoting approaches align with students' diverse needs.

Consequences of Food Insecurity to Health, Wellbeing, and Academics

Health and wellbeing. Food insecurity is extremely stressful and stigmatized, just like other basic needs insecurities, and therefore negatively affects all dimensions of health and wellbeing (e.g., physical, social, psychological). As this section outlines, students experiencing food insecurity may face numerous uncertainties around food access, not have access to culturally important foods, alter their food consumption – such as eating low-quality foods, reducing portion sizes, or skipping meals entirely – decline opportunities to socialize with friends in order to save money, and work more hours at a job (in addition to the hours spent on their studies) to help pay for their expenses. As a result, health can be impacted in a myriad of ways, including an onset of new health conditions as well as exacerbating those that pre-exist.

Typically, food-insecure students report their overall health to be poor (Hughes et al., 2011; Knol et al., 2017). While food insecurity can produce physical sensations of hunger, it also manifests in the mind and body in a multitude of ways (Chilton & Booth, 2007). Physically, students can experience nutritional deficiencies (Wattick et al., 2018), fluctuations in weight, fatigue (Bessey et al., 2020; Frank, 2018), and disrupted sleep (Crutchfield et al., 2020; Hagedorn et al., 2021).

The stressors associated with food insecurity, such as the uncertainties around food access, can also take a serious toll on students' mental health. Numerous studies have reported that food-insecure students experience persistent worry, anxiety, depression, loneliness, anger, jealousy, and low self-worth (Bruening et al., 2016; Farahbakhsh et al., 2017; Hagedorn et al., 2021; Meza et al., 2019; Power et al., 2021; Stebleton et al., 2020). It has also been documented how the stigma around food insecurity (Crutchfield et al., 2020) and food bank use causes shame and isolation (Pineau et al., 2021). For example, Myra, an international PhD student-parent, shared that she did not have money or time for leisure, like participating in activities with her lab. Out of necessity, she focused her attention on her work and family, and over time her lab colleagues stopped inviting her, stopped talking to her so that they would not disturb her. "Definitely I feel alone sometimes," said Myra.

The isolation, loneliness, and exclusion Myra experienced are indeed related to food insecurity, and many other food-insecure students have similar experiences. However, other factors such as race (and racism), cultural differences, and a lack of understanding of the unique challenges international students can face (e.g., language barriers, limited access to cultural foods, and those related to finances) could also contribute (Hanbazaza et al., 2021; Heng, 2017; Sherry et al., 2010).

Academics. Like health, students' academic performance can also decline. Difficulty concentrating because of fatigue and physical hunger (Hanbazaza et al., 2021; Meza et al., 2019), dropping classes (Frank, 2018), lower attendance and Grade Point Average (GPA) (Martinez et al., 2020; Patton-López et al., 2014), and degree completion have all been associated with food insecurity (Weaver et al., 2020). For example, Karen, a participant in a study conducted by Bessey et al. (2020), shared that sometimes she was so fatigued that she skipped class. She also dropped one of her classes so that she could have more money for food.

Coping Mechanisms. As we have outlined thus far, food insecurity is linked to numerous implications to all dimensions of health, wellbeing, and academics. As a result, students rely on many different coping mechanisms to avoid, manage, and mitigate food insecurity (Brescia & Cuite, 2019). Often students use multiple mechanisms simultaneously – these are dynamic, as they can change depending on students' circumstances and personal contexts. Coping mechanisms can temporarily alleviate the effects of food insecurity, but they are not long-term solutions that eliminate the root causes (e.g., financial precarity, lack of time, structural systems of oppression). Food banks are a strong example of this: research on student food insecurity indicates that although food banks may provide emergency relief to some food-insecure students who use this resource,[3] they do not move these students into financially stable positions where they can reliably access sufficient foods that meet their

---

3 Research on household and student food insecurity shows that food-insecure individuals do not use food banks because they are physically inaccessible and users can feel stigmatized and ashamed, therefore choosing other coping mechanisms instead, like relying on support from friends or family members (Frank, 2018; Olauson et al., 2017; Tarasuk et al., 2020a).

needs (Farahbakhsh et al., 2017). Nor do they always ensure that students get the nutrients they need from the foods that food banks provide (Farahbakhsh et al., 2017). As such, students can remain food insecure, even though they use the food bank as a coping mechanism.

Coping mechanisms can also cause harm in different ways, even if they superficially appear to help students with food insecurity. Research has documented that students engage in behaviours like restricted eating (e.g., smaller portion sizes and eating less frequently), drinking fluids in place of food, eating low-quality foods, and skipping meals entirely (Beam, 2020; Bessey et al., 2020; Cunningham, 2022). Students may also decline invitations to social events and attend those that offer free food, rely on strict budgeting, make trade-offs between food and other fixed costs (e.g., tuition, rent, transportation, medication), and focus on coursework instead of food to help cope with food insecurity (Henry, 2017; Smith et al., 2020). For example, Roxanne, a participant from a study by Cunningham (2022, p.107), who was a domestic master's student, made all her meals from scratch because it was the only way she could afford to eat. When she was evicted from her apartment on short notice, she suddenly did not have time to spend preparing food. Searching for a new place to live during an affordable housing shortage while continuing to work on her studies was incredibly stressful and time consuming: "If I have a really busy or stressful week, like last week when my landlord told me I had to move and I was trying to manage school and finding a new place I just didn't have time for cooking, so I went an entire week just eating raw vegetables basically and I actually lost four pounds and it was not good."

Summary

The research we present in this section highlights some of the facets of food insecurity, including the multitude of drivers, impacts, and coping mechanisms. Importantly, we demonstrate that post-secondary student food insecurity is a complex, nuanced, and multifaceted phenomenon that infiltrates all aspects of students' lives. Our position is that to effectively address food insecurity, it is essential to understand these characteristics and develop intervention strategies that are founded on them. We argue that health-promoting approaches informed by the Okanagan Charter's Key Principles for Action – which are already in use for similar issues, like mental health – can be a way to do so.

Knowledge of student food insecurity has expanded over the years, and we now have a better understanding of what kinds of approaches are needed. There is an opportunity to shift away from traditional status quo approaches to addressing food insecurity, which usually operate in isolation from other areas of health, offer short-term relief, and do not address the root causes of food insecurity. In the next section, we outline key issues in these traditional approaches and explore examples from institutions that are addressing these issues in various ways.

Section 2. State of Affairs of Campus Responses to Student Food Insecurity

In this section we discuss status quo approaches to promoting student food security. These are the primary approaches used in post-secondary institutions that tend to focus on short-term relief from food insecurity led by student organizations, in addition to the role of PSIs in supporting student finances. We describe some of the key issues with these approaches, but also explore promising actions across Canada, including those at the Universities of Guelph and Dalhousie. The bulk of this section discusses an in-depth case study of the University of British Columbia's (UBC's) Food Security Initiative (FSI), which takes on a health-promoting university approach informed by the Okanagan Charter to promote food security, aiming to address issues in the current status quo approaches. In addition to the information presented in Section 1, this section will be used to inform a series of recommendations for Post-secondary Institutions (PSI) leadership to promote food security in Section 3.

Status Quo Approaches to Promote Food Security

Although responses to food insecurity are evolving, they continue to primarily be student-led and focused on short-term, emergency food provision (e.g., food banks or pantries) (Glaros et al., 2021). Predominantly, the student community has led programming and advocacy to promote food security on post-secondary campuses (Clarke et al., 2019). The majority of campus food banks and pantries, which provide emergency food and sometimes other supplies (e.g., toiletries), are run by student organizations or student unions. Some campuses also have student-led community cafes, which provide lower cost meals, emphasize community, and advocate for sustainable food systems. Students have also relied on various platforms to raise concern about food insecurity and affordability challenges to PSI leadership, including student unions, PSI boards, media articles in student-led newspapers (e.g., Hunger Gap series at UBC by Nguyen, 2018), and mobilization through grassroots food organizations.

However, students have not been entirely alone in their push for food-secure campus communities. Meal Exchange, a former pan-Canadian non-profit, was instrumental in supporting and empowering students to increase access to quality food for thirty years (Meal Exchange, 2022). They believed in student power, campus collaborations, and post-secondary institution leadership to create resilient, just, and sustainable food systems (Meal Exchange, 2022). A notable contribution from Meal Exchange was a study conducted in 2016 that assessed the prevalence of food insecurity on five Canadian campuses (Silverthorn, 2016). The study was influential as it provided quantitative food-insecurity prevalence data that confirmed concerns brought forward by students for years.

PSIs also have a traditional role of supporting student finances – including assistance in creating a financial plan, navigating scholarships, bursaries, and loans, and managing emergency financial needs. They also play a role in providing health and wellbeing support, including student medical clinics, counselling services, and health education.

Despite student leadership and support from community partners and post-secondary institutions, the consistently high prevalence rates of student food insecurity across Canada indicate that the approaches being used to address the problem are not sufficient. To best determine how to move forward on addressing food insecurity, there is great value in first identifying issues with the status quo.

Issues with Status Quo Approaches to Promote Food Security

Despite years of effort to reduce the prevalence of food insecurity within higher education, the problem still persists, which signals a need for a different approach informed by the Okanagan Charter. Based on our fields of practice and the existing area of scholarship on post-secondary student food security, we've generated the following list of current issues within the status quo approaches by PSIs to promote food security:

Initiatives are student funded and run, and overall poorly resourced
– Such initiatives aimed at addressing food insecurity in PSIs are typically funded and run by students. For example, funding for campus food banks is primarily sourced from student fees. Individuals, such as faculty and staff, who try to support students are often working "off the side of their desks."

Food banks as a solution are problematic – This is so because they do not address root causes and have many barriers to access (including stigma).

Approaches remain siloed and lack cohesion – Responses to food insecurity are often a patchwork within campuses and are not woven all together in a whole campus strategy. Results from the Student Food Insecurity Campus Readiness Assessment found that coordination around student food insecurity as a whole campus and the volume and diversity of activities was low for nearly half (thirteen out of twenty-two) of participating Canadian campuses (Glaros et al., 2021).

Lack of a holistic and intersectional approach – This lack limits understanding of food insecurity in a holistic way including the determinants (e.g., race, gender, sexual orientation) and interconnected areas (e.g., climate, equity, decolonization).

Limited understanding of lived experiences – Food insecurity is a complex phenomenon, nuanced and unique to each person, and shaped by context and the intersection of identities. Understanding this as a starting point is essential to developing strategies, yet it appears that not all PSIs are aware of this.

Roles and responsibilities to address food insecurity between government, PSIs, and students are unclear – This absence of clarity leads to confusion or lack of initiative taken by PSIs to address the complex problem despite significant academic and health and wellbeing impacts.

Missing validated food insecurity measurement tool specific to post-secondary students and no plan for regular measurement across Canada – The standard tool used to measure food insecurity (i.e., HFSSM) in the Canadian Campus Wellbeing Survey is not validated specifically for the student population (only the general population). Currently, it appears that there is no long-term plan for measuring food insecurity in PSIs across Canada, nor for monitoring regional differences and changes over time, including the impact of interventions.

At present, a number of significant issues exist within the current status quo PSIs' approach to addressing food insecurity. By identifying key issues in the current PSIs' approach there is a clear opportunity to take a different approach – a health promoting university approach informed by the Okanagan Charter. There are a number of PSIs working on encouraging efforts to challenge the status quo, which we can learn from when identifying recommendations for PSIs approaches.

Encouraging Student Food Security Approaches Across Canada

Here, we highlight a selection of promising examples addressing some of the issues identified above, including a sliding scale produce market at the University of Guelph, the Loaded Ladle at Dalhousie

University, the Canadian Campus Wellbeing Survey, and an extended case study from UBC's Food Security Initiative. Specifically, UBC's case study demonstrates the most significant efforts attempting to address issues within current PSI approaches to promote food security (Glaros et al., 2021) informed by the Okanagan Charter and a health promotion approach.

Sliding Scale Campus Fresh Food Market, University of Guelph, Ontario

This on-campus food market at the University of Guelph aims to increase physical and financial access to affordable fresh produce. It is a collaborative initiative led by peer helpers from the Feeding Nine Billion Lab and supported by other campus partners including the Community Engaged Scholarship Institute's Guelph Lab, Arrell Food Institute, Sustainability Office, and Hospitality Services as well as a local, off-campus community partner called the SEED. The market sells fresh produce using a sliding scale model – the upper end is similar to retail value and the lower end is 30–50 per cent below – allowing customers to decide what they want to pay. Findings from an evaluation study of the market conducted in spring 2022 indicate that it has numerous benefits. For example, the market increased access to nutritious foods for students because of its convenient location and more affordable prices, and it also helped to build social connections in the campus community (Duncan et al., 2022). The sliding scale market is an example of a promising practice as it is a partnership of university, community, and students to promote food access for all in more dignified ways beyond food banks and pantries.

Loaded Ladle, Dalhousie University, Nova Scotia

The Loaded Ladle is a collaborative non-profit organization that provides "accessible, sustainable, locally sourced free food on the Dalhousie University campus" (Loaded Ladle, 2022). It is led by a diverse and non-hierarchical team of students, volunteers, and staff, and a board of directors. This team runs a variety of programs and workshops including a free lunch program as well as other community programs, such as the Garden Bed Project, Solidarity Servings, and Community Cook-Alongs. It also self-publishes free, accessible content, such as recipes, a community digital cookbook, and newsletters. These activities provide educational and actionable community capacity building opportunities related to food security, food sovereignty, and food justice. The Loaded

Ladle is a promising example of a holistic, community-based approach to promote food security that also provides opportunities to be involved in advocacy for systems change.

Canadian Campus Wellbeing Survey

The Canadian Campus Wellbeing Survey (CCWS) is a tool designed to assess population-level health and wellbeing metrics, including food insecurity, for Canadian post-secondary institutions (Faulkner, 2019). In 2019, it was piloted in a small selection of campuses, followed by implementation at universities throughout British Columbia in 2020. As of 2021, more than fifty campuses have participated in the CCWS. Having CCWS is essential to using the "best" tool to measure food insecurity and other dimensions of health and wellbeing (vs proxy measures) as well as monitor the progress of interventions over time and across Canada within comparable PSIs. These data can support greater understanding of who is most impacted by food insecurity, and thereby help develop targeted interventions. Additionally, the survey is intended for the whole campus community, including faculty and staff, and provides further opportunity to support the health and wellbeing of the whole community.

The University of British Columbia Case Study – An Okanagan Charter–Informed Approach to Food Security

The purpose of this case study is to share UBC's Food Security Initiative (FSI) story, including how it started, key milestones to date, and factors contributing to successes and challenges. These learnings along with other information presented in the chapter will be synthesized into recommendations for all PSIs looking to promote food security (section 3). UBC is one of many partners actively engaged in capacity building across Canada and has identified along with others (including those in the examples above) the need for more united, strategic, and holistic approaches to promote food security and address issues within the current status quo approaches. Currently, the work of UBC's FSI can offer other PSIs key learnings and reflections from their approach, informed by the Okanagan Charter and academic literature on food security, as they are recognized as leaders across Canada. It is also important to note that although food security is the main issue FSI is attempting to address, the approach can be adapted to other complex issues such as mental health. The information shared within the case study was collected through a series of interviews with FSI members.

How It Started – UBC's Food Security Initiative Story

The University of British Columbia (UBC) is a public research university in British Columbia with two campuses totalling over 71,000 students in Vancouver and Kelowna. UBC is also committed to community wellbeing and was one of the first universities in the world to adopt the Okanagan Charter in 2016 (UBC Wellbeing, n.d.b). Led by a community of students, faculty, staff, and stakeholders, UBC is home to a promising network of food-security resources, research, and advocacy. Students have long known food insecurity was a concern at UBC, despite not having institutionally collected prevalence data. For many years they have led diverse programs and services, including a food bank and cafes providing access to affordable food and food literacy education. The institution has also dedicated efforts to address student food insecurity, such as through the UBC Social Ecological Economic Development Studies (SEEDS) Sustainability Program (SEEDS Sustainability Program, n.d.) and VOICES Participatory Research (Campus Health, n.d.), which applied knowledge from research projects to further understand and alleviate students' food insecurity on campus. As these cross-campus initiatives grew individually, it became clear that collaborative, community-led solutions were needed to address the complex issue of campus-based food insecurity instead of tackling the issues individually.

In recent years, various activities and events took place that were important to UBC's journey to creating a food-secure campus:

- The UBC Wellbeing Strategic Framework (UBC Wellbeing, n.d.c) identified food security as a priority with a target to reduce food insecurity prevalence by 2025.
- The Undergraduate Experience Survey (UES) data based on the Household Food Security Survey Module (HFSSM) showed 37 per cent of students at UBC Vancouver and 42 per cent at UBC Okanagan reported low to very low food security, which confirmed what students and some faculty and staff already suspected (Carry et al., 2019).
- The Food Insecurity Action Team (FIAT) was formed to develop a collaborative, multi-disciplinary, and systems-based approach to addressing food insecurity at UBC.
- The FIAT proposal was accepted by the UBC Executive and Board of Governors and included two years of funding for staff capacity and food security projects.

The Food Security Initiative launched in 2020, with the mission to serve as an interdisciplinary and multi-stakeholder platform for students, academics, and practitioners to collaborate in promoting food-security solutions through cross-campus, regional, and national collaboration and inclusive, student- and faculty-led research opportunities. FSI aims to create scalable solutions to further policy, advocacy work, and practices as part of efforts to transform food and social systems through four priority goals (UBC Wellbeing, n.d.a):

1 Deepen understanding of food security within the higher education context.
2 Alleviate immediate pressures of campus-related food insecurity through dignified solutions.
3 Address longer-term campus community food security and affordability.
4 Foster knowledge exchange and advocacy efforts to promote food security within UBC and beyond.

FSI has a dynamic and systems-wide governance structure that includes a "core" team of student workers and representatives, staff and faculty partners that meet monthly to provide oversight, expertise, and decision-making capabilities to the initiative. A project manager supports planning, facilitation, implementation, and evaluation for the initiative including projects. Additional advisors (including those with lived food insecurity experiences) support the FSI on an as-needed basis.

Key Milestones

Since its formation in January 2020, FSI has reached many milestones worth celebrating, including formalizing a governance structure, expanding engagements with key stakeholders and partners within the university and beyond, and beginning long-term work to support systems-wide transformative change. The FSI has two milestones to achieve the 2025 target: establishing community food hubs and supporting (as appropriate) the creation of UBC's affordability plan.

UBC's Transition from Food Banks to Food Hubs

Food hubs are accessible spaces that promote community food security, social connection, and access to food, and financial and wellbeing resources. They support students with food skills development, provide spaces for social connection and cultural celebrations, provide opportunities for student leadership and action, and more. Food hubs are increasingly seen as sustainable, high-impact, community-based approaches as they facilitate capacity building, self-sufficiency, and advocacy efforts for systems change rather than a reliance on emergency food support (Booth et al., 2018). Food hubs are commonly becoming part of the conversation in PSIs including UBC, acknowledging that food banks and pantries are inadequately addressing food insecurity.

UBC's Food Hub model (see figure 8.1) is adapted from the United Way of British Columbia's Hub and Spoke model (United Way British Columbia, n.d.), where a central hub provides a coordination role for existing food and wellbeing assets, or partners known as spokes. The central hub space at UBC provides services like a student-led at-cost grocery store, food, financial and wellbeing programming, and community meeting and advocacy space. The central hub also aims to improve awareness and access to other existing food assets on campus (spokes), including student-led affordable cafes, the student wellness centre, and community-based satellite or mini hubs.

The Food Hub (including a low-cost grocery store) was piloted for nine weeks in the spring of 2022 in tandem with student-led community-based participatory action research to determine the UBC community's vision for a food hub. The pilot and community engagement were initiated to inform future iterations of the Food Hub, including an expanded relaunching of the Food Hub (including Market) in fall 2022.

UBC's Affordability Plan

Affordability challenges continue to be pressing issues brought forward to UBC's leadership by students. As a result of student advocacy and leadership engagement, UBC has recently taken a step forward in articulating institutional roles and responsibilities by developing an affordability plan (Carry et al., 2022), outlining recommendations to address affordability challenges including food security and housing, financial aid, and engagement and advocacy with the provincial government. The plan will be further developed and implemented over time and is an important step and recognition of income-based determinants of food insecurity.

In advancing UBC's Food Hub and affordability plan, the FSI has reflected on facilitators of successes, challenges, and recommendations for other PSIs across the country.

Facilitators of Success

In a reflective dialogue, FSI Core members outlined the various success factors that have led FSI to where it is today: supportive institutional

Figure 8.1. UBC's Hub and Spoke food model

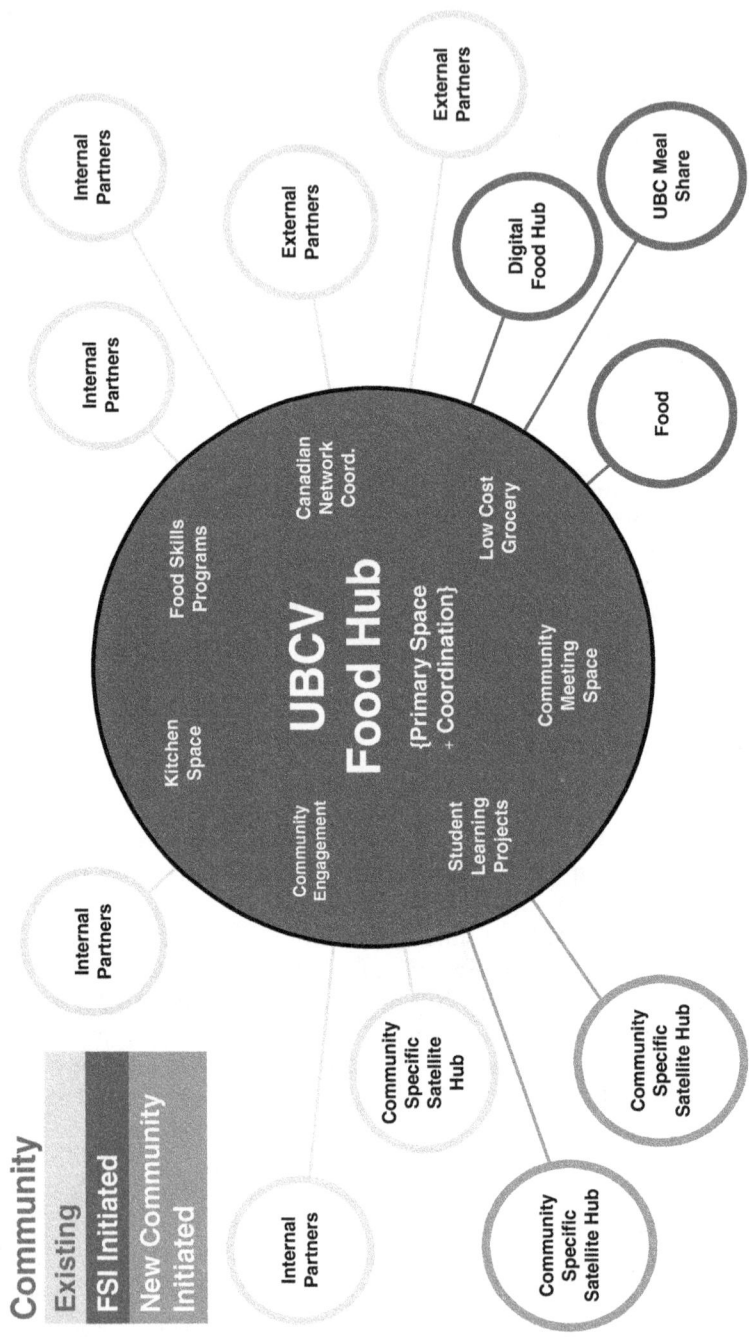

Community

Existing

FSI Initiated

New Community Initiated

Internal Partners

Internal Partners

External Partners

External Partners

Digital Food Hub

UBC Meal Share

Food

UBCV Food Hub

{Primary Space + Coordination}

Kitchen Space

Food Skills Programs

Canadian Network Coord.

Low Cost Grocery

Community Meeting Space

Community Engagement

Student Learning Projects

Internal Partners

Community Specific Satellite Hub

Community Specific Satellite Hub

Internal Partners

Community Specific Satellite Hub

mandate; evidence-informed approach; cohesive whole campus strategy; community-based approach; addressing the food security continuum from immediate relief to systems change; holistic multi-solving approach; capacity to support the initiative.

Supportive Institutional Mandate

An important first step in establishing the FSI and securing high-level leadership support was to align the "why" behind prioritizing campus-based food security and the call to action with a greater mandate – the Okanagan Charter and UBC's Wellbeing Strategic Framework. The Okanagan Charter has been a powerful guiding mandate to shape and identify FSI's mission as a campus-based initiative to alleviate food insecurity and advocate for the health and wellbeing of students. Guided by the calls to action in the Okanagan Charter, UBC's Wellbeing Strategic Framework outlines UBC's collective approach to embedding wellbeing into organizational plans, policies, practices, and decision-making, with one of its targets to reduce food insecurity for UBC community members by 2025.

Evidence-Informed Approach

Taking an evidence-informed approach grounded in student-led research, institution-specific food insecurity prevalence data and evaluation has enabled many successes for the FSI.

The formation of the initiative was called for by student-led research, which also continues to shape projects including conducting a Health Equity Impact Assessment on the Meal Share program (Chan et al., 2021) and informing the emerging governance structure of the Food Hub (Fazal et al., 2022). Student feedback through compensated surveys and focus groups have been an essential component of implementing and adapting successful new pilot programs (UBC's Meal Share program, the food hub market pilot) as they are happening, being responsive to community needs. An evidence-informed approach utilizing institution-specific food insecurity prevalence data has also been especially useful when garnering support from institutional stakeholders, such as the UBC's Board of Governors, to support the initiative with dedicated resources and funds. An FSI staff partner confirmed that the student research was critically important. They noted that "The outcomes of student-led research was a huge driver in bringing attention to campus food security with university administration and resulting in funding."

Cohesive Whole Campus Strategy

A success that is foundational to FSIs is having a whole campus strategy involving various units and partners, including student leaders, that develop a common agenda and strategic plan for action. Campus-based food insecurity is a complex challenge, and employing a "collective impact" approach (Collective Impact Forum, 2022) has been helpful to tackle such a complex issue with many people involved, including with the implementation of the food hub. An FSI staff partner confirmed that the student research was critically important. They noted that "Partnering to create change is key, including involving those at many levels of influence, 'power,' and leadership. It's really helpful to have the capacity to support the work, create a strategy with a vision, mission, goals and target for creating change."

Community-Based Approach

While operating under an institutional mandate, FSI's community-based approach has been a key factor in successful outcomes. Prioritizing community-based practice in this way has given many community members the opportunity to be part of the change-making process, including the voices of people who are directly impacted and hold the lived experience with food insecurity. Having an established group, such as FSI Core, shows the effectiveness of a cohesive, dedicated team bringing together community members to prioritize work and facilitate change. Relationship building, communication, and collaboration have been the grounding principles of successful community engagement for FSI. An FSI student worker confirmed that the student research was critically important. They noted that "It is really helpful to have both institutional partners and students around the table for things to work and feel legitimate. When it's just students, oftentimes it doesn't feel like a project will be able to get to the scale that you want, and if it's just UBC institutional partners without students, it's missing the input and perspective of actual students on campus."

Addressing the Food Security Continuum from Immediate Relief to Systems Change

The FSI's actions were intentionally planned to support a continuum of action from immediate food relief to systems change because no singular action will "solve" food insecurity given the complexity of the issues, and addressing the root causes of food insecurity may be slow to see results. For these reasons, FSI has found success utilizing an adapted food-security continuum (Northern Health, 2022) (see figure 8.2), which categorizes actions

Figure 8.2. UBC's Adapted Food Security continuum (FSI's strategy)

Food Security Continuum

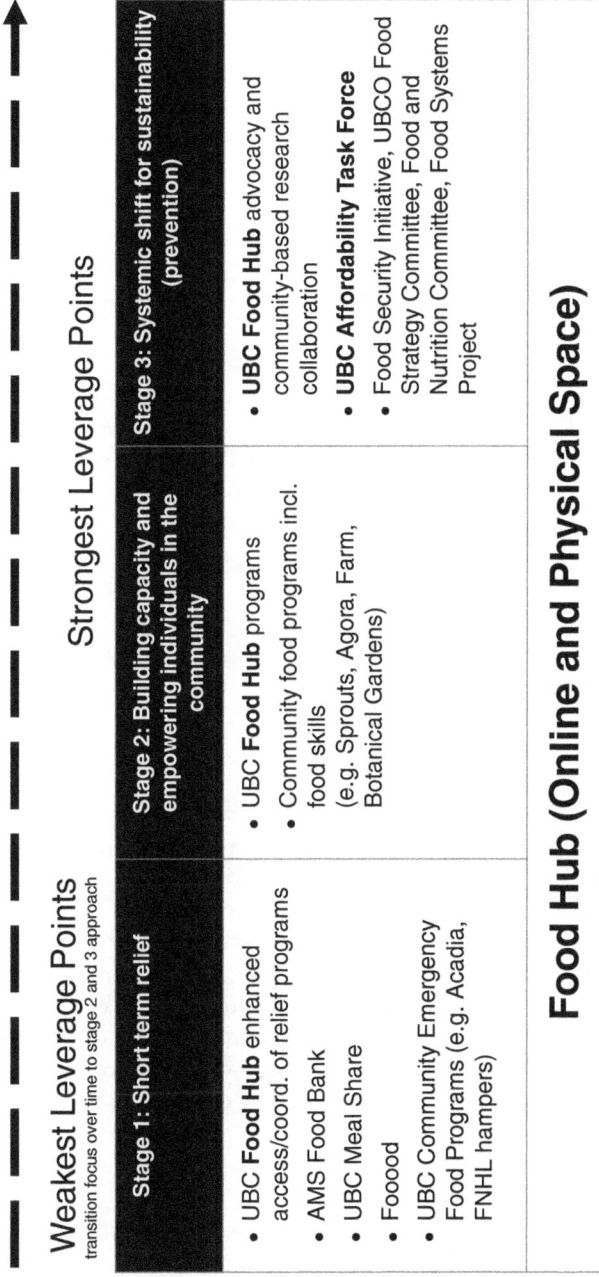

Weakest Leverage Points ————————————— Strongest Leverage Points

transition focus over time to stage 2 and 3 approach

Stage 1: Short term relief	Stage 2: Building capacity and empowering individuals in the community	Stage 3: Systemic shift for sustainability (prevention)
• UBC **Food Hub** enhanced access/coord. of relief programs • AMS Food Bank • UBC Meal Share • Fooood • UBC Community Emergency Food Programs (e.g. Acadia, FNHL hampers)	• UBC **Food Hub** programs • Community food programs incl. food skills (e.g. Sprouts, Agora, Farm, Botanical Gardens)	• **UBC Food Hub** advocacy and community-based research collaboration • **UBC Affordability Task Force** • Food Security Initiative, UBCO Food Strategy Committee, Food and Nutrition Committee, Food Systems Project
Food Hub (Online and Physical Space)		

along a spectrum: from stage 1 weaker, short-term relief interventions (e.g. dignified and lower barrier food access programs) to stage 3 stronger more preventative actions (e.g. addressing root causes of affordability issues including systemic racism). Stages 2 and 3 are stronger leverage points of action that FSI wants to focus more efforts and resources on because they support systems-level changes that prevent food insecurity and promote community food security as opposed to perpetuating a system of emergency food provisions like food banks. UBC has recently made great progress in working towards a systems shift through its two milestones – piloting implementation of a food hub and exploring further issues of affordability.

Holistic Multi-Solving Approach

UBC's FSI has intentionally viewed food security in a holistic, collaborative, and comprehensive way guided by the "multi-solving" approach described as the "process of building solutions to multiple problems into a single act" (Multisolving Institute, 2022). FSI's multi-solving flower (see figure 8.3) demonstrates co-benefits of a holistic approach to promoting food security and UBC's strategic plan connections. UBC's multi-solving framing of food security has facilitated the planning of more fruitful strategies that have multiple co-benefits, including the food hub market pilot where at-cost groceries were sold, providing lower cost access to food on campus. The market also intentionally provided only plant-based protein options, advancing UBC's sustainability, climate, and nutrition goals.

Capacity to Support the Initiative

As one FSI staff partner remarks on capacity, "Never underestimate the importance of good capacity to facilitate the change process. It's not an overnight thing – it takes a lot of time." FSI has added capacity through a project manager, facilitator, and dot connector for relationship building and maintenance with the many people who are doing work within the initiative. Such a role has been essential in managing the various engagement and evaluation processes embedded in FSI's ongoing projects, through which community members come together to brainstorm and lead change on campus. In order for FSI to sustain progress, it has been essential to have a continued staff capacity to support the initiative.

Challenges

Along with successes, FSI has also encountered its fair share of challenges, which include resourcing barriers, breaking down silos on campus, and

Figure 8.3. UBC's co-beneficial "multi-solving" flower approach to promoting food security

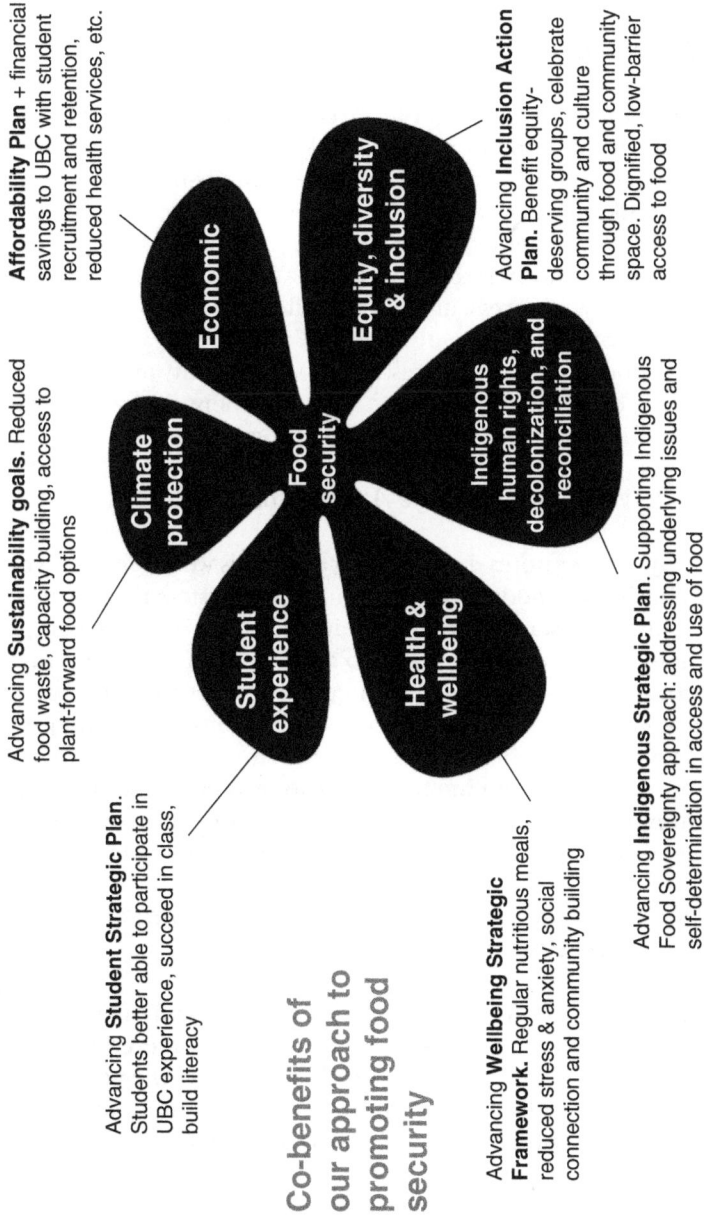

Advancing **Sustainability goals.** Reduced food waste, capacity building, access to plant-forward food options

Affordability Plan + financial savings to UBC with student recruitment and retention, reduced health services, etc.

Advancing **Inclusion Action Plan.** Benefit equity-deserving groups, celebrate community and culture through food and community space. Dignified, low-barrier access to food

Economic

Equity, diversity & inclusion

Climate protection

Food security

Indigenous human rights, decolonization, and reconciliation

Student experience

Health & wellbeing

Advancing **Student Strategic Plan.** Students better able to participate in UBC experience, succeed in class, build literacy

Co-benefits of our approach to promoting food security

Advancing **Wellbeing Strategic Framework.** Regular nutritious meals, reduced stress & anxiety, social connection and community building

Advancing **Indigenous Strategic Plan.** Supporting Indigenous Food Sovereignty approach: addressing underlying issues and self-determination in access and use of food facing rising demand for emergency food services while needing to establish multipronged approaches. In this section, FSI reflects on the ways in which they are continually navigating barriers to further progress in campus-based food-security work.

Resourcing and Long-Term Commitment

Ensuring resources for a longer-term commitment has been a major source of uncertainty for the initiative. Though FSI was able to make steps in having the university acknowledge campus-based food security as a priority and offer commitment to fund various project expenses, the recent COVID-19 pandemic has resulted in uncertain funding from the university. Time is another constraint – it is important to identify a few key priorities, show progress, and launch pilots. This type of progress requires a long-term funding commitment. The university is navigating its roles and responsibilities in addressing food insecurity and affordability and balancing other funding needs, and it is evident that this may be an ongoing tension as key projects and plans progress.

Breaking Down Silos to Engage All Stakeholders

One FSI staff partner notes that, "Having done this work for many years at UBC, the challenge of getting the whole university system to prioritize well-being, as similar to sustainability and equity issues, has been breaking down silos." It has been an ongoing effort to address prominent silos in food-security work on campus. The challenge that comes with such an inter-disciplinary, cross-campus team is dispersing responsibility amongst units while engaging many different groups. Therefore, in developing a community approach to promoting food security, it is essential to have established committees that hold ownership and accountability and have those involved dedicate their capacity for involvement including leading action.

Addressing the Food-Security Continuum from Immediate Relief to Systems Change

Taking an approach across the food-security continuum of balancing immediate food relief and systems change can be considered a success of FSI but it also is an ongoing challenge with the onset of the pandemic and rising inflation. Considering the significant needs of students right now, it can be challenging for some to understand or agree with allocating a higher percentage of limited funding and resources on more preventative actions that take longer to see results. Despite this, UBC would then just continue to rely on unsustainable, undignified food-access supports versus better understanding and addressing the underlying multifaceted determinants of food insecurity. FSI continues to operate with this tension while also seeking opportunities for additional financial support for dignified food-access efforts until they are no longer needed. An FSI staff partner remarks that "It is not acceptable that food insecurity has become a norm – especially not in a privileged space where people should be supported and set up for success to support the broader community."

Section 3. Recommendations to Advance the Current State of Affairs in Promoting Food Security in Higher Education

In recent years, universities have been taking notice of the impacts that food insecurity has on students' wellbeing and academics, and are looking to do more. This interest has increased particularly since the onset of the pandemic, which illuminated the precarity involved with being a student as well as the pervasiveness of systemic inequities and the ways in which these systems create layers of vulnerability for certain people and not others. Challenges clearly exist, but we have reason to be optimistic. There is evidence that individuals within PSIs care, working in various roles and capacities to address the issue within their PSIs. Although student initiatives have been operating with limited institutional support for many years, evidence from our case studies and other initiatives that focus on food and health suggest that this has recently begun to change with PSIs taking on some levels of responsibility. Additionally, through the examples presented, it appears that PSIs recognize that food banks as a solution to food insecurity are problematic and more proactive action is needed.

In UBC's case study, we explored the history and progress of the FSI. UBC's story stands out among Canadian institutions because of the promising work under way to advance food security as a whole campus utilizing a health promotion approach informed by the Okanagan Charter. UBC is developing innovative projects and programs to meet its food-security targets, like the Food Hub and Affordability Plan, and using approaches that are holistic, collaborative, community based, and multipronged to do so. This is built on and informed by decades of student leadership when students tackled these issues predominantly all on their own (Clarke et al., 2019). Things are beginning to change at UBC though, and now the institution is taking on its own leadership role by supporting the FSI. This signals that UBC, as a post-secondary institution, is recognizing the responsibility it has in creating a food-secure campus, and demonstrating its willingness to uphold its commitment to the Okanagan Charter.

Still, just like other PSIs in Canada, UBC has more work to do. The institution has not addressed all the issues we outlined in Section 2 or within the FSI's case study, and like PSIs elsewhere, food insecurity, housing insecurity, and the health and wellbeing of students remain pressing issues on this campus. These are complex problems to navigate, and PSIs do not bear the sole responsibility of addressing them; provincial and federal governments especially do as well, and more broadly, so does every citizen, whether affiliated with post-secondary institutions or not. However, as stated in the Okanagan Charter, PSIs have great power and responsibility to support and enhance the wellbeing of students, and they are particularly well positioned to do so.

Based on our exploration and learnings in this chapter, we have devised a list of tangible recommendations for PSIs' leadership to advance status quo approaches to promote food security, and they include the following:

1 Situate your food-security efforts within an institutional mandate – including but not limited to the Okanagan Charter.
2 Gather institutional specific evidence on student food insecurity to inform action (including prevalence data, lived experiences, current efforts, gaps, and areas for opportunities).
3 Based on institutional evidence and context, create a plan, strategy, or roadmap for action that is guided by the Okanagan Charter and specifically is
   a) cohesive, involving the whole campus;
   b) community based, including intentional efforts to better understand the diversity of intersectional lived experiences and incorporate their voices into strategies;
   c) multipronged across the food-security continuum (balancing preventative actions with more dignified short-term relief programs);
   d) holistic in framing and approach;
   e) sufficiently resourced to support institutional and student-led efforts, including projects and staff;
   f) articulate the roles and responsibilities of various levels of leadership in promoting food security (e.g., PSI vs provincial government) within your local jurisdiction;
   g) collaborate with researchers to validate a food-insecurity measurement tool specific for post-secondary students and advocate for the regular measurement of food insecurity across Canadian PSIs (e.g., the Canadian Campus Wellbeing Survey).

Although many issues have been identified in current approaches to promote food security in Canada, the lessons learned from this chapter have been synthesized into actionable recommendations that can be implemented within PSIs. Implementing these recommendations will not come without challenges, but there is great reason to believe that post-secondary leaders engaged in implementing the Okanagan Charter can inspire change within their communities, by promoting health and wellbeing.

Conclusion

In this chapter we set the following aims:

a) build knowledge on food insecurity, providing insight into the nuanced experiences of food insecurity within PSIs;
b) inspire post-secondary leaders to act on food insecurity with urgency; and
c) highlight promising practices and critical perspectives to achieving food-secure campuses, predominantly through the use of a case study focused on the University of British Columbia.

We achieved our aims by briefly exploring the topic of student food insecurity in Section 1, identifying issues with the status quo approach but also promising approaches in Section 2, and summarized areas of opportunity for PSI leadership to take action in Section 3.

When reflecting on the current state of affairs of PSI's approach to food security, the opportunity for significant change really comes from PSI's commitment to implementing the Okanagan Charter. The Okanagan Charter stands for health, and Canadian universities have an opportunity to embody the charter, demonstrating to the world that they do not stand for food insecurity and poor health and that they are willing to look after their community. PSIs fill multiple roles for students: they are educators, food providers, employers, landlords, and health care providers. This creates a unique, multidimensional relationship between institutions and students, one where institutions hold considerable power to influence students' health and wellbeing and shape their lives overall. As such, PSIs ought to be doing all that they can to care for the people whom they engage in so many ways. If they don't, can they continue to pride themselves on being health promoting campuses informed by the Okanagan Charter? Indeed, this is a privilege, but also a responsibility and an utmost necessity. The time to create flourishing campus communities is now.

REFERENCES

Ahmadi, S.M., Laban, S., & Primeau, C. (2020). *Hungry for knowledge: Assessing the prevalence of food insecurity at the University of Guelph.* Community Engaged Scholarship Institute. https://atrium.lib.uoguelph.ca/xmlui/handle/10214/2501

Batal, M., Chan, H.M., Fediuk, K., Ing, A., Berti, P.R., Mercille, G., Sadik, T., & Johnson-Down, L. (2021). First Nations households living on-reserve experience food insecurity: Prevalence and predictors among ninety-two First Nations communities across Canada. *Canadian Journal of Public Health, 112*(Suppl 1), 52–63. https://doi.org/10.17269/s41997-021-00491-x

Beam, M. (2020). Nontraditional students' experiences with food insecurity: A qualitative study of undergraduate students. *The Journal of Continuing Higher Education, 68*(3), 141–63. https://doi.org/10.1080/07377363.2020.1792254

Bessey, M., Frank, L., & Williams, P. L. (2020). Starving to be a student: The experiences of food insecurity among undergraduate students in Nova Scotia, Canada. *Canadian Food Studies/La Revue canadienne des études sur l'alimentation, 7*(1), 107–25. https://doi.org/10.15353/cfs-rcea.v7i1.375

Blundell, L., Mathews, M., Bowley, C., & Roebothan, B. (2019). Determining student food insecurity at Memorial University of Newfoundland. *Canadian Journal of Dietetic Practice and Research, 80*(1), 14–21. https://doi.org/10.3148/cjdpr-2018-026

Booth, S., Pollard, C., Coveney, J., and Goodwin-Smith, I. (2018). "Sustainable" rather than "subsistence" food assistance solutions to food insecurity: South Australian recipients' perspectives on traditional and social enterprise models. *Int J Environ Res Public Health, 15*(10, 2086.

Brescia, S.A., & Cuite, C.L. (2019). Understanding coping mechanisms: An investigation into the strategies students use to avoid, manage, or alleviate food insecurity. *Journal of College and Character, 20*(4), 310–26. https://doi.org/10.1080/2194587X.2019.1669463

Bruening, M., Brennhofer, S., van Woerden, I., Todd, M., & Laska, M. (2016). Factors related to the high ates of Fofod insecurity among diverse, urban college freshmen. *Journal of the Academy of Nutrition and Dietetics, 116*(9), 1450–7. https://doi.org/10.1016/j.jand.2016.04.004

Camelo, K., and Elliott, M. (2019). Food insecurity and academic achievement among college students at a public university in the United States. *Journal of College Student Development, 60*(3), 307–18. https://doi.org/10.1353/csd.2019.0028

Campus Health. (n.d.). *VOICE Research 4.* https://campushealth.ok.ubc.ca/voice-research/

Canadian Federation of Students. (2018). *Education justice* [White paper]. https://assets.website-files.com/6227851233f5910d2ccda042/62279dd8909984d3ba2dd94f_CFS-EducationJustice-Report-ENG-nobleed-1-1.pdf

Caron, N., & Plunkett-Latimer, J. (2022). *Canadian income survey: Food insecurity and unmet health care needs, 2018 and 2019.* Statistics Canada, Income Research Paper Series. https://www150.statcan.gc.ca/n1/pub/75f0002m/75f0002m2021009 -eng.htm

Carry, A., Szeri, A., Sadiq, R., & Mullings, D. (2022). *Student Affordability Task Force report and recommendations (affordability plan).* Finance Committee report prepared for UBC Board of Governors, University of British Columbia, Canada. https://bog3.sites.olt.ubc.ca/files/2022/03/3_2022.03_Student -Affordability-Task-Force.pdf

Carry, A., Thistle, B.M., Buszard, D., Rideout, C., Parr, A., & Dolf, M. (2019). *Addressing food insecurity at UBC.* Report prepared for UBC Board of Governors, University of British Columbia, Canada. https://bog3.sites.olt. ubc.ca/files/2019/09/3_2019.09_Addressing-Food-Insecurity.pdf

Chan, R., Cui, B., Hsu, F.Y., Kwasniak, A., Meng, K., & Perera, M. (2021). *Health equity impact assessment for UBC's Meal Share.* SEEDS Sustainability Program. https://sustain.ubc.ca/sites/default/files/seedslibrary/FNH_473 _Health%20Equity%20Impact%20Assessment%20for%20UBC%E2%80% 99s%20Meal%20Share_FinalReport.pdf

Chilton, M., & Booth, S. (2007). Hunger of the body and hunger of the mind: African American women's perceptions of food insecurity, health and violence. *Journal of Nutrition Education and Behavior, 39*(3), 116–25. https:// doi.org/10.1016/j.jneb.2006.11.005.

Choubak, M., Wilson, B., & Zivot, C. (2020). *University of Guelph Student FoodBank: A snapshot of student food security and wellbeing.* Community Engaged Scholarship Institute. https://atrium.lib.uoguelph.ca/xmlui/handle/10214/8902

Clarke, M., Kao, M., Ma, K., Zefanya, L., Quinlan, A., & Tang, I. (2019). *UBC food security: Interventions & evaluation scan.* SEEDS Sustainability Program. https://sustain.ubc.ca/sites/default/files/seedslibrary/FNH_473_Campus FoodInsecurityInterventionsScan_FinalReport.pdf

Coffino, J.A., Spoor, S.P., Drach, R.D., & Hormes, J.M. (2021). Food insecurity among graduate students: Prevalence and association with depression, anxiety and stress. *Public Health Nutrition, 24*(7), 1889–94. https://doi.org /10.1017/S1368980020002001

Coleman-Jensen, A. (2020). U.S food insecurity and population trends with a focus on adults with disabilities. *Physiology & Behavior, 220,* 112865. dc] https://doi.org/10.1016/j.physbeh.2020.112865

Coleman-Jensen, A., Rabbitt, M.P., Gregory, C.A., & Singh, A. (2019). *Household food security in the United States in 2018.* (Economic Research Report No, 270). U.S. Department of Agriculture, Economic Research Service. https://www .ers.usda.gov/webdocs/publications/94849/err-270.pdf

Collective Impact Forum. (2022). *What is collective impact.* https:// collectiveimpactforum.org/what-is-collective-impact/

Crutchfield, RM., Carpena, A., McCloyn, T. N., & Maguire, J. (2020). The starving student narrative: How normalizing deprivation reinforces basic need insecurity in higher education. *Families in Society, 101*(3), 409–21. https://doi.org/10.1177/1044389419889525

Cunningham, V. (2022). *We learn best from those with lived experience: A phenomenological study of post-secondary student food insecurity.* [Master's thesis, University of Guelph]. University of Guelph Atrium. https://atrium.lib .uoguelph.ca/xmlui/handle/10214/26936

Davison, K.M., Marshall-Fabien, G.L., & Tecson, A. (2015). Association of moderate and severe food insecurity with suicidal ideation in adults: National survey data from three Canadian provinces. *Social Psychiatry and Psychiatric Epidemiology, 50*(6), 963–72. https://doi.org/10.1007/s00127-015-1018-1

Dhunna, S., & Tarasuk, V. (2021). Black–white racial disparities in household food insecurity from 2005 to 2014, Canada. *Canadian Journal of Public Health, 112*(5), 888–902. https://doi.org/10.17269/s41997-021-00539-y

Duncan, E., Lukawiecki, J. & Bedi, G. (2022). *Campus community market.* Community Engaged Scholarship Institute. https://atrium.lib.uoguelph.ca /xmlui/handle/10214/27294

Entz, M., Slater, J., & Desmarais, A.A. (2017). Student food insecurity at the University of Manitoba. *Canadian Food Studies/La Revue canadienne des études sur l'alimentation, 4*(1), 139–59. https://doi.org/10.15353/cfs-rcea.v4i1.204

Farahbakhsh, J., Hanbazaza, M., Ball, G.D.C., Farmer, A.P., Maximova, K., & Willows, N.D. (2017). Food insecure student clients of a university-based food bank have compromised health, dietary intake and academic quality. *Nutrition & Dietetics, 74*(1), 67–73. https://doi.org/10.1111/1747-0080.12307

Fazal, Z., Featherstone, D., Gerbrandt, L., McLester, K., & Yu, B. (2022). *Thriving community food hubs: Promising practices and innovative organizational models.* SEEDS Sustainability Program. https://sustain.ubc.ca/sites/default/files/seedslibrary /LFS%20450_Project_06_CFH_GoveranceModels_FinalReport.pdf

Faulkner, G., Ramanathan, S., & Kwan, M. (2019). Developing a coordinated Canadian post-secondary surveillance system: A Delphi survey to identify measurement priorities for the Canadian Campus Wellbeing Survey (CCWS). *BMC Public Health, 19*(1), 1–11. https://doi.org/10.1186/s12889-019-7255-6.

Frank, L. (2018). "Hungry for an education": Prevalence and outcomes of ood Inisecurity among tudents at a primarily undergraduate university in rural Nova Scotia. *Canadian Journal of Higher Education/Revue canadienne d'enseignement supérieur, 48*(2), 109–29. https://doi.org/10.7202/1057106ar

Garcia, A.C., Sykes, L., Matthews, J., Martin, N., & Leipert, B. (2010). Perceived facilitators of and barriers to healthful eating among university students. *Canadian Journal of Dietetic Practice and Research, 71*(2), e28–33. https://www .proquest.com/docview/347840204/abstract/F608B35E392A4F9EPQ/1. https://doi.org/10.3148/71.2.2010.XX

Glaros, A., MacIntyre, J., Laban, S., & Maynard, M. (2021). *Student food insecurity campus readiness assessment.* Community Engaged Scholarship Institute. https://atrium.lib.uoguelph.ca/xmlui/handle/10214/2501

Government of Canada. (2022). *Studying and working in Canada as an international student.* Retrieved 18 November 2022 from https://www.cic.gc .ca/english/helpcentre/answer.asp?qnum=495&top=15

Hagedorn, R.L., Olfert, M.D., MacNell, L., Houghtaling, B., Hood, L.B., Savoie Roskos, M.R., Goetz, J.R., Kern-Lyons, V., Knol, L.L., Mann, G.R., Esquivel, M.K., Hege, A., Walsh, J., Pearson, K., Berner, M., Soldavini, J., Anderson-Steeves, E.T., Spence, M., Paul, C., ... Fontenot, M.C. (2021). College student sleep quality and mental and physical health are associated with food insecurity in a multi-campus study. *Public Health Nutrition, 24*(13), 4305–12. https://doi.org/10.1017/S1368980021001191

Hamelin, A.-M., Beaudry, M., & Habicht, J.-P. (2002). Characterization of household food insecurity in Québec: Food and feelings. *Social Science & Medicine, 54*(1), 119–32. https://doi.org/10.1016/S0277-9536(01) 00013-2

Hamilton, C., Taylor, D., Huisken, A., & Bottorff, J.L. (2020). Correlates of food insecurity among undergraduate students. *The Canadian Journal of Higher Education, 50*(2), 15–23. https://doi.org/10.47678/cjhe.v50i2.188699

Hanbazaza, M., Ball, G.D.C., Kebbe, M., Farmer, A.P., Willows, N.D., Perez, A., & Maximova, K. (2021). Food insecurity among international post-secondary students studying on a Canadian campus: A qualitative descriptive study. *The Canadian Journal of Higher Education, 51*(2), 33–45. https://doi.org/10.47678 /cjhe.vi0.188977

Haskett, M.E., Kotter-Grühn, D., & Majumder, S. (2020). Prevalence and correlates of food insecurity and homelessness mong university students. *Journal of College Student Development, 61*(1), 109–14. https://doi.org/10.1353 /csd.2020.0007

Hattangadi, N., Vogel, E., Carroll, L.J., & Côté, P. (2019). "Everybody I know is always hungry ... but nobody asks why": University students, food insecurity and mental health. *Sustainability, 11*(6), 1571. https://doi.org/10.3390 /su11061571

Heng, T.T. (2017). Voices of Chinese international students in USA colleges: 'I want to tell them that ...' *Studies in Higher Education, 42*(5), 833–50. https://doi.org/10.1080/03075079.2017.1293873

Henry, L. (2017). Understanding food insecurity among college students: Experience, motivation, and local solutions. *Annals of Anthropological Practice, 41*(1), 6–19. https://doi.org/10.1111/napa.12108

Hughes, R., Serebryanikova, I., Donaldson, K., & Leveritt, M. (2011) "Student food insecurity: The skeleton in the university closet." *Nutrition & Dietetics, 68*(1), 27–32. https://doi.org/10.1111/j.1747-0080.2010.01496.x.

Jessiman-Perreault, G., & McIntyre, L. (2017). The household food insecurity gradient and potential reductions in adverse population mental health outcomes in Canadian adults. *SSM – Population Health, 3*, 464–72. https://doi.org/10.1016/j.ssmph.2017.05.013

Knol, L.L., Robb, C.A., McKinley, E.M., & Wood, M. (2017) Food insecurity, self-rated health, and obesity among college students. *American Journal of Health Education, 48*(4), 248–55. https://doi.org/10.1080/19325037.2017.1316689

Lee, S., Ball, G.D., Farmer, A., & Willows, N.D. (2020). Exploring the experience of food insecurity among university students caring for children: A qualitative descriptive study. *Journal of Hunger & Environmental Nutrition, 15*(3), 360–71. https://doi.org/10.1080/19320248.2018.1557093

Leung, C.W., Kullgren, J.T., Malani, P.N., Singer, D.C., Kirch, M., Solway, E., & Wolfson, J.A. (2020). Food insecurity is associated with multiple chronic conditions and physical health status among older US adults. *Preventive Medicine Reports, 20*, 101211. https://doi.org/10.1016/j.pmedr.2020.101211

Linden, B., & Stuart, H. (2020). Post-secondary stress and mental wellbeing: A scoping review of the academic literature. *Canadian Journal of Community Mental Health, 39*(1), 1–32. https://doi.org/10.7870/cjcmh-2020-002

Loaded Ladle. (2022). *Our vision.* https://www.loadedladle.com/our-vision

Maroto, M.E., Snelling, A., & Linck, H. (2015). Food insecurity among community college students: Prevalence and association with grade point average. *Community College Journal of Research and Practice, 39*(6), 515–26. https://doi.org/10.1080/10668926.2013.850758

Martinez, S.M., Frongillo, E.A., Leung, C., & Ritchie, L. (2020). No food for thought: Food insecurity is related to poor mental health and lower academic performance among students in California's public university system. *Journal of Health Psychology, 25*(12), 1930–9. https://doi.org/10.1177/1359105318783028

Maynard, M.S., Meyer, S.B., Perlman, C.M., & Kirkpatrick, S.I. (2018). Experiences of food insecurity among undergraduate students: "You can't starve yourself through school." *Canadian Journal of Higher Education, 48*(2), 130–48. https://doi.org/10.7202/1057107ar

Meal Exchange. (2021). *2021 National Student Food Insecurity Report.* Retrieved 5 August 2022 from www.mealexchange.com/resources. (Site is no longer active.)

Meal Exchange. (2022). *About us.* Retrieved 5 August 2022 from https://www.mealexchange.com/about-us. (Site is no longer active.)

Men, F., Gundersen, C., Urquia, M.L., & Tarasuk, V. (2020). Association between household food insecurity and mortality in Canada: A population-based retrospective cohort study. *CMAJ: Canadian Medical Association Journal, 192*(3), E53–E53. https://doi.org/10.1503/cmaj.190385

Meza, A., Altman, E., Martinez, S., & Leung, C.W. (2019). "It's a feeling that one is not worth food": A qualitative study exploring the psychosocial experience and academic consequences of food insecurity among college students. *Journal of the Academy of Nutrition and Dietetics, 119*(10), 1713–21.e1. https://doi.org/10.1016/j.jand.2018.09.006.

Muldoon, K.A., Duff, P.K., Fielden, S., & Anema, A. (2013). Food insufficiency is associated with psychiatric morbidity in a nationally representative study of mental illness among food insecure Canadians. *Social Psychiatry and Psychiatric Epidemiology, 48*(5), 795–803. https://doi.org/10.1007/s00127-012-0597-3

Multisolving Institute. (2022). *About us.* https://www.multisolving.org/about-us/

Northern Health. (2022). *Food security.* https://www.northernhealth.ca/health-topics/food-security

Nguyen, A. (2018). *The hunger gap.* The Ubyssey. https://www.ubyssey.ca/features/hunger-food-insecurity/

Odoms-Young, A., & Bruce, M.A. (2018). Examining the Impact of Structural Racism on Food Insecurity: Implications for Addressing Racial/Ethnic Disparities. *Family & community health, 41 Suppl 2, Food Insecurity and Obesity,* S3–S6. https://doi.org/10.1097/FCH.0000000000000183

Olauson, C., Engler-Stringer, R., Vatanparast, H., & Hanoski, R. (2018). Student food insecurity: Examining barriers to higher education at the University of Saskatchewan. *Journal of Hunger & Environmental Nutrition, 13*(1), 19–27. https://doi.org/10.1080/19320248.2017.1393365

Patton-López, M.M., López-Cevallos, D.F., Cancel-Tirado, D.I., & Vazquez, L. (2014). Prevalence and correlates of food insecurity among students attending a midsize rural university in Oregon. *Journal of Nutrition Education and Behavior, 46*(3), 209–14. https://doi.org/10.1016/j.jneb.2013.10.007

Payne-Sturges, D.C., Tjaden, A., Caldeira, K.M., Vincent, K.B., & Arria, A.M. (2018). Student hunger on campus: Food insecurity among college students and implications for academic institutions. *American Journal of Health Promotion, 32*(2), 349–54. https://doi.org/10.1177/0890117117719620

Pineau, C., Williams, P.L., Brady, P., Waddington, M., & Lesley Frank, L. (2021). Exploring experiences of food insecurity, stigma, social exclusion, and shame among women in high-income countries: A narrative review. *Canadian Food Studies/La Revue canadienne des études eur l'alimentation 8*(3), 107–24. https://doi.org/10.15353/cfs-rcea.v8i3.473

Power, E., Dietrich, J., Walter, Z., & Belyea, S. (2021). "I don't want to say I'm broke": Student experiences of food insecurity at Queen's University in Kingston, Ontario, Canada. *Canadian Food Studies/La Revue canadienne des études sur l'alimentation, 8*(1). https://doi.org/10.15353/cfs-rcea.v8i1.423

PROOF. (n.d.). *Understanding household food insecurity.* Household Food Insecurity in Canada. https://proof.utoronto.ca/food-insecurity/

Reynolds, E., Johnson, C., Jamieson, J.A., & Mawhinney, H. (2018). Prevalence and correlates of food insecurity among students attending a small, rural

Canadian university. *Canadian Journal of Dietetic Practice and Research, 79*(3), 125–8. https://doi.org/10.3148/cjdpr-2018-004

Richardson, T., Elliott, P., & Roberts, R. (2013). The relationship between personal unsecured debt and mental and physical health: A systematic review and meta-analysis. *Clinical Psychology Review, 33*(8), 1148–62. https://doi.org /10.1016/j.cpr.2013.08.009

SEEDS Sustainability Program. (n.d.). *SEEDS Sustainability Program.* UBC Sustainability. https://sustain.ubc.ca/teaching-applied-learning/seeds -sustainability-program

Shankar, J., Ip, E., Khalema, E., Couture, J., Tan, S., Zulla, R. T., & Lam, G. (2013). Education as a social determinant of health: Issues facing indigenous and visible minority students in postsecondary education in Western Canada. *International Journal of Environmental Research and Public Health, 10*(9), 3908 -3929. https://doi:10.3390/ijerph10093908

Sherry, M., Thomas, P., & Chui, W.H. (2010). International students: A vulnerable student population. *Higher Education, 60*(1), 33–46. https://doi .org/10.1007/s10734-009-9284-z

Silverthorn, D. (2016). *Hungry for knowledge: Assessing the prevalence of student food insecurity on five Canadian campuses.* Meal Exchange. https://cpcml.ca /publications2016/161027-Hungry_for_Knowledge.pdf

Smith, E.A., Story, C.R., Hobbs, K.C., Bos, T., & Thareja, G. (2020). Food insecurity, Carotenoid values and coping strategies of students on a mid-sized college campus. *American Journal of Health Studies, 35*(3), 209–18. https://doi .org/10.47779/ajhs.2020.240

Statistics Canada. (2020a). *Canadian post-secondary enrolments and graduates, 2017/2018.* The Daily. https://www150.statcan.gc.ca/n1/daily-quotidien /200219/dq200219b-eng.htm

Statistics Canada (2020b). *Financial information of universities for the 2018/2019 school year and projected impact of COVID–19 for 2020/2021.* The Daily. https:// www150.statcan.gc.ca/n1/daily-quotidien/201008/dq201008b-eng.htm

Statistics Canada (2022). *Consumer Price Index, 2022.* The Daily. https://www150 .statcan.gc.ca/n1/daily-quotidien/220720/dq220720a-eng.htm

Stebleton, M.J., Lee, C.K., & Diamond, K.K. (2020). Understanding the food insecurity experiences of college students: A qualitative inquiry. *The Review of Higher Education, 43*(3), 727–52. https://doi.org/10.1353/rhe.2020.0005

Tarasuk, V., Fafard St-Germain, A.-A., & Mitchell, A. (2019). Geographic and socio-demographic predictors of household food insecurity in Canada, 2011–12. *BMC Public Health, 19*(1), 12. https://doi.org/10.1186/s12889-018-6344-2

Tarasuk, V., Fafard St-Germain, A.-A., & Loopstra, R. (2020a). The relationship between food banks and food insecurity: Insights from Canada. *VOLUNTAS: International Journal of Voluntary and Nonprofit Organizations, 31*(5), 841–52. https://doi.org/10.1007/s11266-019-00092-w

Tarasuk, V, & Mitchell, A. (2020b). *Household food insecurity in Canada, 2017–18.* Research to identify policy options to reduce food insecurity (PROOF). Retrieved from https://proof.utoronto.ca/

UBC Wellbeing. (n.d.a). *Food security initiative.* https://wellbeing.ubc.ca /foodsecurityinitiative

UBC Wellbeing. (n.d.b). *The Okanagan Charter.* https://wellbeing.ubc.ca /okanagan-charter

UBC Wellbeing. (n.d.c). *Wellbeing strategic framework.* https://wellbeing.ubc.ca /framework

United Nations General Assembly, Resolution 217 A (III). (1948). *Universal Declaration of Human Rights.* https://www.ohchr.org/EN/UDHR/Documents /UDHR_Translations/eng.pdf

United Way British Columbia. (n.d.). United for food security. https://www .uwlm.ca/foodhubs/

Vozoris, NT., & Tarasuk, V. S. (2003). Household food insufficiency is associated with poorer health. *The Journal of Nutrition, 133*(1), 120–6. https://doi.org /10.1093/jn/133.1.120.

Wattick, R., Hagedorn, R., & Olfert, M. (2018). Relationship between diet and mhealth in a young adult Appalachian college population. *Nutrients, 10*(8), 957. https://doi.org/10.3390/nu10080957

Weaver, R.R., Vaughn, N.A., Hendricks, S.P., McPherson-Myers, PE., Jia, Q., Willis, S.L., & Rescigno, K.P. (2020). University student food insecurity and academic performance. *Journal of American College Health, 68*(7), 727–33. https://doi.org/10.1080/07448481.2019.1600522

Wilcox, M., Baker, C., Burish, E., Arnold, R., Cherry, M., & Moss, T. (2021). Inequitable hunger: Scope, effects, and perceptions of college student food insecurity. *Journal of Student Affairs Research and Practice, 59*(4), 385–400. https://doi.org/10.1080/19496591.2021.1960851

Willis, D.E. (2019). Feeding the student body: Unequal food insecurity among college students. *American Journal of Health Education, 50*(3), 167–75. https:// doi.org/10.1080/19325037.2019.1590261

Willis, D.E. (2021). Feeding inequality: Food insecurity, social status and college student health. *Sociology of Health & Illness, 43*(1), 220–37. https://doi.org /10.1111/1467-9566.13212

Zigmont, V., Linsmeier, A., & Gallup, P. (2021). Understanding the why of college student food insecurity. *Journal of Hunger & Environmental Nutrition, 16*(5), 595–610. https://doi.org/10.1080/19320248.2019.1701600

9 Advancing Workplace Wellbeing within Higher Education Settings

CRYSTAL HUTCHINSON, NATASHA MALLOFF,
AND ALICIA HIBBERT

Introduction

The future of work is unfolding before us. The events of recent years have resulted in significant shifts to employees' personal and professional lives and routines on a global scale, resulting in elevated psychological stress. As workplaces continue to navigate and respond to the exacerbation of inequities resulting from the COVID-19 pandemic, climate change, and other complex societal and global issues, employee mental health and wellbeing are high priorities for organizations.

Positive mental health and resilience contribute to social connectedness, high levels of life and work satisfaction, innovation, engagement, subjective wellbeing, productivity, and enhanced performance and business outcomes (Diener et al., 2009; Harter et al., 2002; Oades et al., 2011; WHO, 2010; Youseff & Luthans, 2007). Resilient employees with positive psychological capital lead to more effective and resilient organizations (Avey et al., 2010; Malik, 2013; White, 2013; Youseff & Luthans, 2007). A growing body of evidence suggests that stressors associated with the pandemic have increased the prevalence of mental health problems (CMHA, 2020; Statistics Canada, 2020). As employers explore new and innovative ways of working through continual change and ongoing uncertainties, significant investment in workplace health promotion (WHP) efforts is critical to support employees' mental health and wellbeing, workplace psychological health and safety, and organizational resilience.

The health promoting university concept continues to be explored and theorized in the literature, along with students' mental health and wellbeing within higher education settings. This chapter focuses on the workplace as a specific context within the health promoting university movement. We examine literature on employee mental health, workplace mental health promotion, and psychological health and safety. In addition, this chapter will explore the evolution of WHP, identifying best practices, strategies, and approaches within higher education settings as it relates to the Okanagan Charter: An International Charter for Health Promoting Universities and Colleges' principles for action. We explore four case studies and make recommendations for other post-secondary institutions to consider workplace health promotion in their own contexts.

Background

The workplace is well documented as a critical setting for health promotion due to "the presence of natural social networks, the possibility of reaching a large population, and the amount of time people spend at work" (Rongen et al., 2013, p. 406). Historically, WHP efforts have focused on accident prevention, physical safety, and individual knowledge and skill-building efforts to shift health behaviours. Conversely, a large percentage of what drives our health throughout our lifetime are external factors such as our social, economic, and physical environment (Raphael et al., 2020). The social determinants of health are conditions in the environments where people live, learn, work, and play that influence quality of life and health outcomes. Providing a supportive workplace is a strategic way in which employers can reduce risk factors and promote protective factors.

Significant developments have been made in the last decade that relate to how WHP is practised and how a healthy workplace is defined. WHP once focused entirely on the physical environment and then expanded to include individual lifestyle choices. Over the last two decades, WHP grew to include critical psychosocial components such as the organization of work, workplace culture, and linkages to the broader community (Shain & Kramer, 2004; WHO, 2004). "The workplace has undoubtedly become one of the most important settings affecting the physical, mental, economic and social wellbeing of workers, and in turn the health of their families, communities and society" (Chu et al., 2000, p. 155). Health promoting workplaces can act as catalysts for positive change, impacting the overall success of the organization by enhancing knowledge and skills related to healthy behaviours and providing a supportive organizational environment that enhances wellbeing (Chu et al., 2000; Harter et al., 2002; WHO, 2010).

Mental Health and Mental Health Promotion in the Workplace

Mental health and mental illness are two separate constructs. Mental health is more than the absence of mental illness; it is "a state of wellbeing in which the individual realizes his or her own abilities, can cope with the normal stresses of life, can work productively and fruitfully, and is able to make a contribution to his or her community" (WHO, 2004, p. 12). GermAnn and Ardiles (2009) described mental health promotion as "helping people take control over their lives and improve their mental health" (p. 19) with a focus on environments that promote health and wellbeing, including workplaces.

The landscape of WHP and, more specifically, mental health promotion has significantly evolved over recent years (Samra, 2017). A decade ago, "mental health in the workplace was often considered peripheral, and certainly secondary to physical health-related illnesses and injuries" (Samra, 2017, p. 8). Four foundational documents have significantly informed and influenced the field of workplace mental health promotion. We will cover these in the sections to follow, after first introducing the concept of psychological safety. Foundational literature provides an evidence base and practical frameworks for comprehensive action.

Psychological Safety

Psychological safety has been a topic of interest over recent decades internationally in the fields of organizational behaviour, psychology, management, and leadership. The work of Dr. Amy Edmondson, a Novartis Professor of Leadership and Management at Harvard Business School, has been a driving force behind resurfacing and advancing psychological safety as a construct, particularly within the American context. In 1999, Edmondson published research that focused on the concept of psychological safety and its connection to learning behaviours in teams. She defined team psychological safety as "a shared belief that the team is safe for interpersonal risktaking" and "involves but goes beyond interpersonal trust; it describes a team climate characterized by interpersonal trust and mutual respect in which people are comfortable being themselves" (Edmondston, 1999, p. 354). Her work highlights the importance of both structural and interpersonal characteristics in influencing learning and performance in teams and identifies the critical role of team leaders in contributing to psychological safety, stating that "if the leader is supportive, coaching-oriented, and has non-defensive responses to questions and challenges, members are likely to conclude that the team constitutes a safe environment" (Edmondston, 1999, p. 356).

World Health Organization's Healthy Workplace Framework and Model (WHO, 2010)

The World Health Organization's framework calls for the development of a comprehensive approach for all workplace health promotions based on four key principles: health promotion, occupational health and safety, human resource management, and sustainable development. This approach acknowledges the importance of psychosocial wellbeing as a key component of workplace health promotion and utilizes strategies such as multisectoral partnerships, employee engagement, and inclusivity.

Guarding Minds at Work (Samra et al., 2009–20)

The 2009 launch of Guarding Minds at Work: A Workplace Guide to Psychological Health and Safety "coined the use of the term 'psychological health and safety,' and offered the first comprehensive Canadian framework for assessing and addressing workplace psychological health and safety" (Samra, 2017, p. 13). A lack of mental health or the presence of mental disorders directly results in presenteeism (loss of productivity from not being able to function on the job fully), absenteeism (regular unplanned absence from work), and poor productivity (Samra et al., 2012). Conversely, a psychologically safe workplace enhances employees' mental health and organizational outcomes (regular attendance and elevated productivity). Guarding Minds at Work established that there are thirteen evidence-informed psychosocial factors contributing to a workplace that supports mental health: an organizational culture that includes respect, recognition, and effective leadership; employee agency, engagement, and growth; balance and workload management; psychological supports; and protection of both physical and psychological safety.

National Standard of Canada for Psychological Health and Safety in the Workplace (2013)

According to Samra (2017), "one of the largest evolutionary shifts that occurred in the landscape of workplace mental health over the last decade has been the 2013 release of the National Standard of Canada for Psychological Health and Safety in the Workplace (the Standard). The Standard has provided a definition of what constitutes a psychologically safe system of work – a definition currently lacking in the law" (p. 20). The standard builds upon the thirteen factors identified by Guarding Minds at Work. It includes a complementary implementation guide for organizations. As the first standard of its kind focused on workplace psychosocial health and safety globally, it is both leading and innovative.

Kunyk et al. (2015) published a qualitative study on the acceptance of this standard in Canada, with participants across multiple industries and organizations indicating that it aligned with their organizational values. Overall, it was viewed as a "resource that could provide direction, tools, and guidance to address psychosocial elements in the workplace" (Kunyk et al., 2015, p. 44).

Okanagan Charter: An International Charter for Health Promoting Colleges and Universities (2015)

Developed in Kelowna, British Columbia, Canada, by attendees of the 2015 International Conference on Health Promoting Universities and Colleges (VII International Congress), the Okanagan Charter has galvanized action amongst higher education institutions internationally. The charter aims to inspire and mobilize international action, generate dialogue and research across health promoting universities and colleges, and integrate health into all policies and practices (Okanagan Charter, 2015). There are two calls to action:

1 Embed health into all aspects of campus culture, across the administration, operations, and academic mandates.
2 Lead health promotion action and collaboration locally and globally. (Okanagan Charter, 2015, p. 3).

With emphasis placed on whole system, campus-wide, participatory, and cross-sectoral approaches to action, the charter highlights the importance of meaningful collaboration across stakeholder groups, regardless of mandate (e.g., students, staff, faculty, administration, and community partners).

Case Studies

As momentum continues to build around the health promoting universities movement in North America, many higher education institutions are now focused on advancing health promotion action through whole systems change efforts. The following section will present case studies featuring higher education institutions implementing whole systems approaches, demonstrating WHP promising practices and leadership. The four case studies – the University of British Columbia, Queen's University, Dalhousie, and the University of Southern California (USC) – were chosen as members of the Canadian Health Promoting Campuses Network and the US Health Promoting Campuses Network. All of the Canadian institutions have made Okanagan Charter commitments, and all institutions have innovative workplace wellbeing programs and practices, representing universities of varying sizes. Following these case studies, we will explore how their actions align with the key principles of the Okanagan Charter, and provide recommendations for other post-secondary institutions to take up the calls in their own campus communities.

The University of British Columbia

The University of British Columbia (UBC) has two main campuses in Vancouver and Okanagan. It is a research university with over $775 million in research funding. There are over 71,000 students and over 5,800 faculty and 10,300 staff.

Through UBC's strategic plan, *Shaping UBC's Next Century*, UBC explicitly prioritizes wellbeing, sustainability, and Indigenous engagement, aligning with several of the Okanagan Charter's key principles for action. In addition, three themes are centred in the plan: collaboration, inclusion, and innovation. UBC commits to enhancing the wellbeing of its people while prioritizing mental health and developing a wellbeing strategic framework, taking a whole systems approach.

UBC was one of the first universities in Canada to implement a people strategy, Focus on People (FOP), in 2008, and provides funding through the Healthy Workplace Initiatives Program to support academic and administrative portfolios by developing healthy, sustainable workplaces. Beginning the following year and conducted every three years since, the Workplace Experiences Survey has helped shape FOP priorities, leading to evidence-informed action, as outlined in the Okanagan Charter. There is also an annual institution-wide mental health literacy campaign in collaboration called Thrive.

As a signatory to the Okanagan Charter: An International Charter for Health Promoting Universities & Colleges in 2015, UBC took a leadership approach in adopting the charter in 2016 with a significant funding commitment for human resources and students' administrative portfolios in partnership with UBC Wellbeing. The Charter guided the development and collaborative efforts between the Office of Wellbeing Strategy, student health promotion, and workplace wellbeing portfolios to implement and launch the Wellbeing Strategic Framework in 2019.

The Wellbeing Strategic Framework outlines six priority areas, each with its own targets and indicators, committees, and evolving milestones, leading to trans-disciplinary, whole system collaborations: Mental Health & Resilience, Food & Nutrition, Social Connection, Physical Activity, Built & Natural Environments, and Collaborative Leadership. Supported through human resources, the Workplace Wellbeing portfolio takes accountability for stewardship of workplace health promotion through an integrated and collaborative focus: mental health literacy training; mental health campaigns; the Workplace Wellbeing Ambassadors program; workplace wellbeing evaluation framework; wellbeing learning plans; embedding wellbeing in unit planning including developing toolkits, collaborative pilots with key portfolios, leadership development, coaching, performance development, and the progressive leadership development competency framework.

In support of the workplace targets and indicators articulated in the Wellbeing Strategic Framework, which focuses on people and ongoing program evaluation, the Workplace Wellbeing team monitors the following: aspects of the Workplace Experience Survey; Canadian Campus Wellbeing Survey faculty and staff results; benefit plan usage; Employee Family Assistance Program usage; sick leave averages; programming pre- and post-surveys; participation and qualitative feedback; and feedback from Workplace Wellbeing Ambassadors and Employee Affinity Groups. The measures and key performance indicators support annual reporting for mid-level strategic plans and continuous improvement opportunities for programming and initiatives.

Queen's University

Queen's University is located in Kingston, Ontario, and has almost 28,000 students and employs nearly 4,000 faculty and 5,400 staff (Queen's University, 2022b). As a large research university with over $220 million in research income, Queen's University is home to twenty-four institutional and faculty-based research centres and institutes that support interdisciplinary networks (Queen's University, 2022c).

Queen's University's organizational mission is focused on the future, an exceptional student experience, cultivating excellence and leadership, and a determination to "push the boundaries of knowledge through research – in service to an inclusive, diverse and sustainable society" (Queen's University, 2022a). Demonstrating the significance of and accountability to the health and wellbeing of the community, wellbeing is a stated core value in addition to truth, responsibility, respect, and freedom.

In 2019, Queen's adopted the Okanagan Charter. The Okanagan Charter subsequently guided the development of their Campus Wellbeing Framework. Led by the Campus Wellness Project team, a shared wellbeing vision was developed through a cross-campus and participatory approach – in keeping with the Charter's key principles for action – that involved consulting over eighteen hundred faculty, staff, and students over six months in 2019–20. The framework recognizes the importance of an inclusive culture of wellbeing. It articulates four intersecting priority focus areas that impact all of Queen's community members: culture, belonging and social connection, personal wellbeing, and places. The framework's guiding principles are values driven, campus wide, connected and inspired, participatory and strength based, and evidence based.

At Queen's, senior leaders have supported campus-wide efforts in developing a Campus Wellbeing Framework and integration of wellbeing in other mid-level strategic plans, established Student Wellness Services, and have also demonstrated commitments to a system-wide and inclusive culture of wellbeing. In 2022, they established an Employee Wellness Service, which works collaboratively with Student Wellness Services and includes financial support for programming. To ensure evidence-informed approaches, they launched an Employee Experience Survey to establish key metrics. With an approach that understands the intersections of wellbeing and inclusion, the Human Rights and Equity Office includes services related to human rights, equity, sexual violence prevention, and accessibility, in addition to ongoing university support for Employee Resource Groups and a declaration to address systemic racism. Aligned with these approaches, the Office of Indigenous Initiatives advances reconciliation to integrate Indigenous ways of knowing and being in all areas of the university. To complement these efforts in whole system change, Sustainable Queen's is a community-based movement pursuing climate action.

As part of the new Employee Wellness Services, key performance indicators and metrics to evaluate and measure workplace wellbeing systems change include results from a biannual employee and student experiences survey, post-event/initiative feedback surveys, participation levels in programs and initiatives, exit interviews, staff turnover, absenteeism rates, EFAP usage trends, and benefit plan usage. In addition to the Campus Wellbeing Framework, the Human Resources Strategic Plan names wellbeing as a key value and an Employee Wellbeing Roadmap emphasizes the importance of team culture, social connection, personal wellbeing, and wellness spaces.

Dalhousie University

Dalhousie has two campuses in Atlantic Canada (Halifax and Truro, NS) and two satellite locations (Yarmouth, NS, and Saint John, NB). It has over 20,000 students and employs 1,600 faculty and 2,900 staff, with 13 academic faculties and over $190 million of annual research income.

In 2021, Dalhousie launched a new organizational five-year strategic plan, Third Century Promise (Dalhouse University, 2021), which resulted from a comprehensive and consultative two-year planning process, including broad and cross-disciplinary inputs, nine self-study groups, caucuses for equity-deserving groups, and teams from across the university community. These participatory, comprehensive approaches align with the Okanagan Charter's principles for action. The shared plan outlines commitments to four integrated pillars: exceptional student experience, inclusive excellence (which highlights wellness as a priority), high-impact research, and civic university with global impact. Third Century Promise explicitly prioritizes equity, diversity, inclusion, accessibility, and wellness by coordinating and collaborating across units to embed these priorities throughout all efforts. This is a whole systems approach, as outlined in the Okanagan Charter.

Deepening the focus and priority on wellness in the workplace, *Work Well: Creating Space for Wellbeing*, a four-year mid-level organizational workplace wellness strategy, was launched in 2021. The strategy was developed by the Healthy Workplace Collaborative, informed by the 2019 Your Voice Workplace Survey results, an institutional Campus Health and Wellbeing self-study group, meeting the Okanagan Charter's call for participatory, comprehensive approaches. The aim of the strategy is to be responsive to workplace survey results and emerging trends, and identify immediate to long-term strategic initiatives. Included in the strategy are efforts to support managers, address workload, identify initiatives from the thirteen psychosocial workplace factors in the National Standard for Psychological Health and Safety in the Workplace, embed wellbeing into leadership competencies, and develop Equity, Diversity, Inclusion, and Accessibility (EDIA) partnerships. All of these are examples of how to enact the Okanagan Charter's principles for action.

Campus wellbeing initiatives are increasing in momentum, and they are core to the university's activities. Within human resources, the Organizational Health unit stewards the workplace wellness strategy, has a dedicated budget, and works collaboratively with Student Wellness on the Be Well Campus Wellbeing Initiative. Services and programming include support and training at the individual level, workplace level through people leaders, and roles with expertise in organizational health, equity and diversity, and accessible employment. Dating back to 2011, the Biennial Workplace Survey measures personal wellness, individual resilience, thirteen psychosocial workplace factors and, more recently, inclusion; it is being updated in alignment with the new organizational strategy. This data is analysed to build an understanding of the results across groups and time, supporting the Okanagan Charter's call for evidence-informed action.

The University of Southern California

The University of Southern California (USC) has over 49,000 students across its campuses in Los Angeles, California, USA. It is one of the world's leading private research universities with nearly $900 million in annual research expenditures, and it employs over 4,600 faculty members and over 16,000 staff.

The USC Culture Journey, an institution-wide initiative that started in 2019 and involves faculty, staff, students, and administrators, is a collective effort to explore key shared values, align supportive behaviours, and develop opportunities to improve systems and processes. This aligns with the Okanagan Charter's key principles for action that include settings-based, whole system approaches. The USC Culture Journey outlines six unifying values that support the USC's mission, guide behaviours and engagement, and create campus culture: integrity; excellence; diversity, equity, and inclusion; wellbeing; open communication; and accountability (USC Culture Journey). By aligning cross-campus efforts and leveraging the institution's shared values, USC is prioritizing changes to systems and processes to support cultural change towards wellbeing.

USC has not yet formally adopted the Okanagan Charter; however, it has provided and continues to provide an important framework that informs wellbeing efforts. USC has a long-standing history of resourcing faculty and staff mental health and wellbeing through an employee assistance program that originated in the Suzanne Dwork-Peck School of Social Work. Over time, a shift was made towards a more preventative focus, including expansion of health promotion and education programming. Such is the case with the newly launched USC WorkWell Center. The centre is the primary hub for USC faculty and staff health and wellbeing, providing cost-free, confidential counselling, coaching, workplace wellbeing consultations, critical incident management, and other health promotion and education programming. With senior leadership support, the flagship program emerging out of the new WorkWell Center is USC Healthy Campus. USC Healthy Campus is a comprehensive, collaborative, and long-term strategy to elevate faculty and staff health and wellbeing at USC. Importantly, the USC Healthy Campus initiative aligns with Okanagan Charter principles to use settings and whole system approaches, building on its own strengths to ensure health and wellbeing are part of everyday practices, intending to create a culture where wellbeing is a key priority.

Discussion

One of the most important parts of the Okanagan Charter is the key principles for action because they describe how to take action. We will examine how the four institutions described in the case studies are taking action across four of these principles, the ones that our analysis shows best align with their initiatives. We endeavour to inspire more institutions to take up the calls to embed health into all aspects of campus culture and lead workplace health promotion action in their campus communities.

Settings and Whole System Approaches

Doherty and Dooris (2006) illustrated how healthy settings efforts within the context of higher education are about more than interventions focused singularly on health behaviour, stating that settings or whole systems thinking embeds "a commitment to health into the fabric of settings – within their cultures, structures, processes and routine life" (p. 42). The settings approach provides a more effective and sustainable framework within a workplace mental health promotion context because sources of workplace stress often stem from organization-level problems instead of simply a lack of personal coping strategies (Noblet & LaMontagne, 2006). Efforts must be founded on a comprehensive understanding of the psychosocial conditions influencing employee mental health (Noblet & LaMontagne, 2006).

Employee mental health and wellbeing have a tremendous impact on organizational wellbeing and the broader community; therefore, efforts should engage students, staff, and faculty. Taken as a whole, the evidence concerning health promotion in the workplace suggests that a comprehensive approach is one in which individual and organizational interventions for health and wellbeing are targeted in a coordinated and strategic manner (Chu et al., 2000; Shain & Kramer, 2004; WHO, 2010). As Lowe (2004) pointed out, a healthy organization "requires changes in organizational cultures, systems and practices" (p. 26). Workplace health promotion efforts must be integrated not only amongst health promotion professionals but also across the institution as a deeply held value that underpins operations and everyday practices.

Dalhousie and UBC, through their organizational strategic plans, and both Queen's and USC, through their organizational values, explicitly prioritize wellbeing on an institution-wide basis. At the organizational level, it signals accountability and commitment beyond a focus on individual health behaviours.

The literature also demonstrates the important role of dedicated leadership in a whole system approach. Not only must leaders "walk the talk" in terms of modelling principles, but they must also possess mental health literacy, provide flexibility for employees, demonstrate authenticity, foster a supportive environment, and maintain open communication in addition to other behaviours that align with creating a positive organizational culture (Kahn, 1990; MacEachen et al., 2008; Noblet & LaMontagne, 2006; Oades et al., 2011). According to Kahn (1990), "supportive, resilient, and clarifying management heightened psychological safety" (p. 711), and high-quality leadership has generally been shown to enhance work performance and psychological wellbeing on and off the job (Kelloway et al., 2012).

At UBC, there is clear support from the president, and through the partnership of the Vice President (VP) Students and VP Human Resources in implementing the Wellbeing Strategic Framework (WSF) and other intersectional mid-level strategies, including key wellbeing and health promotion efforts and the WSF Mental Health & Resilience Committee. In addition, the WSF Collaborative Leadership priority area holds leadership across the organization accountable for embedding wellbeing into department and team plans.

Through the Principal and Human Resources Portfolios, Queen's senior leadership integrates wellbeing and a commitment to improve culture in their mid-level strategic plans. This led to the creation of Employee Wellness Services.

Dalhousie has a workplace wellbeing strategy stewarded through their Human Resources Organizational Health Unit. All are supported through funding and resources, increased supports, and acting on the results of institutional surveys.

The ongoing support and commitment from USC's senior VP of human resources resulted in the dedicated resources and infrastructure necessary to advance the evolution of the WorkWell Center to include more focus on health promotion efforts as well as the development of USC's (2022) Healthy Campus Strategy (led by USC's WorkWell team), which aims to advance employee and organizational health and wellbeing by infusing health into all policies, programs, services, and learning, teaching, and working environments.

Despite findings, a commonly identified gap is a lack of training, education, and support for leaders in understanding their role in impacting

employee mental health (Samra, 2017). This is an important area of recommendation for other universities to consider early in their health promotion efforts. Ultimately, those in leadership or supervisory positions
have significant potential to shape psychologically healthy and safe work
environments that enhance employees' mental health and wellbeing
through their decision-making processes and interpersonal approaches.

Participatory Approaches and Engaging Students and Others

Within the context of workplace health promotion, community
consultation and participatory approaches inform action and decision-
making (Lowe, 2004; Samra et al., 2012; WHO, 2010). Workplace health
promotion should be undertaken in partnership with all staff categories'
meaningful involvement and engagement. Participatory approaches
include forming committees, administering surveys, holding consultation
events, and leading focus groups. Work environments that include
employees in discussions on an ongoing basis related to work organization
and decision-making enhance employee mental wellbeing (Samra et al.,
2012; WHO, 2010). This is especially relevant for faculty wellbeing, which
is significantly impacted by their perceptions of involvement and influence
within their own department as well as within the broader university
(Clarke et al., 2015). Participatory processes enhance trust, mental health,
engagement, morale, worker commitment, and, ultimately, organizational
culture (Harter et al., 2002; WHO, 2010).

The University of British Columbia launched its Focus on People Strategic Framework in 2008, and priorities have been shaped and informed
by the Workplace Experiences Survey, held every three years since 2009.
Developing the Wellbeing Strategic Framework (WSF) was shaped
through focus groups, surveys, interviews, and cross-collaborative working groups, including human resources and the VP Students. The WSF
has a strong governance structure in place and priority area committees with membership across both campuses, such as the Mental Health
and Resilience Committee that has both undergraduate and graduate
student representation, HR Workplace Wellbeing staff, Student Health
Promotion and Education staff, as well as faculty members focused on
mental health and resilience research. In addition to the Workplace Experiences Survey, UBC administered the Canadian Campus Wellbeing
Survey for faculty, staff, and students, enabling global wellbeing measures. All of these perspectives are then reflected in key milestones and in
setting benchmarks for WSF targets and indicators.

At Queen's, the development of their Campus Wellbeing Framework
was led by the Campus Wellness Project Team, and through a cross-campus

and participatory approach, consulting over eighteen hundred faculty, staff, and students over six months in 2019–20, utilizing a retreat and focus group for their wellbeing project. With the resourcing of Employee Wellness Services in HR, Queen's reintroduced an Employee Experience Survey that supports an employee wellbeing roadmap.

Through a comprehensive and consultative two-year planning process that included broad and cross-disciplinary inputs, nine self-study groups, caucuses for equity-deserving groups, and teams from across the university community, Dalhousie also informed a revised organizational strategic plan. The workplace wellness strategy at Dalhousie developed by the Healthy Workplace Collaborative leveraged the 2019 Your Voice Workplace Survey results, an institutional Campus Health and Wellbeing self-study group, and other informal feedback channels that helped identify the needs of Dalhousie and its people.

Lastly, USC's Culture Journey began with a values poll of 20,000 faculty, staff, and students. This was followed by over 40 town halls that included 4,000 participants and 120 small focus group discussion sessions to gather feedback on values definitions. Survey data and Culture Sessions were synthesized to develop a consolidated list of shared values supporting the USC mission. Going forward, the USC Culture Network remains an important driver of change as it supports culture initiatives, events, and activities across schools and units at USC. The University of Southern California continues to align with these shared values while prioritizing the changes to systems and processes that will support the desired culture, including through its recent (2022) initiative, USC Healthy Campus.

We recommend that institutions looking to advance health promotion on their campuses use participatory approaches that involve a significant portion of their campus community, including faculty, staff, and students. This can occur through multipronged efforts like consultation events, focus groups, and surveys.

Local and Indigenous Communities' Contexts and Priorities

There is no one-size-fits-all approach to mental health promotion. The WHO (2010) stated that "a healthy workplace strategy must be designed to fit the unique history, culture, market conditions and employee characteristic of individual organizations" (p. 9). Local communities and Indigenous peoples' perspectives must be prioritized in action planning related to advancing workplace wellbeing and employee mental health. According to the WHO (2004), "empowerment is the process by which groups in a community … can exercise all the rights that are due to them, with a view to leading a full, equal life in the best of health" (p. 42). The Truth and Reconciliation Commission of Canada (2017) described reconciliation as a continuous process of rebuilding trust, and establishing and maintaining relationships with Indigenous peoples and communities. The importance of a Nation-specific and regional focus to this work (in opposition to pan-Indigenous approaches) is affirmed in the United Nations Declaration of the Rights of Indigenous Peoples (UN, 2007, p. 7).

Workplace health promotion leaders and practitioners should be in good relation to invite and ensure meaningful participation by Indigenous stakeholders in decision-making processes. Queen's, through the Office of Indigenous Initiatives, supports building community, advancing reconciliation/conciliation efforts, and integrating Indigenous ways of knowing and being into the fabric and life of the university. A Truth and Reconciliation Council Task Force has made several recommendations, including taking proactive steps to increase Indigenous student, staff, and faculty representation on governance bodies, raising awareness among non-Indigenous students, staff, and faculty of the complex histories and modern realities faced by Indigenous peoples, and developing Indigenous cultural awareness training, tailored to faculty, staff, senior administrators, and student leaders.

Like Queen's, UBC has an Office of Indigenous Strategy to steward the Indigenous Strategic Plan (ISP), providing planning tools and significant financial resources to advance the priorities. In addition, the WSF Mental Health and Resilience priority area focuses on a more inclusive and responsive approach to mental health literacy training and programs, considering health equity and important perspectives from community members who identify as Indigenous, Black, or People of Colour (IBPOC). Through HR's workplace wellbeing unit, a specific wellbeing survey for IBPOC faculty and staff was administered that resulted in a workplace wellbeing plan of programs and initiatives that has diversified facilitators, content, and program offerings, including an increase in Indigenous facilitators and consultants.

In developing their institutional strategy, Dalhousie engaged with Indigenous faculty and staff through their caucuses for equity-deserving groups and aligned with the institution's Indigenous Strategy and African Nova Scotian Strategy. Dalhousie has hired both a Director of Indigenous Community Engagement and a Director of African Nova Scotian Community Engagement.

Institutions looking to mobilize systemic change must engage Indigenous peoples within their campus community (Indigenous faculty, students, and staff) and the Indigenous Nations on which the campus is located. Their perspectives must be prioritized in action planning for wellbeing. This right is solidified in the United Nations Declaration of the Rights of Indigenous Peoples (UN, 2007), which is international in scope.

Acting on an Existing Universal Responsibility

Human rights, social justice, equity, and ecological health are constructs deeply interconnected with wellbeing. Organizational cultures that celebrate and appreciate diversity (of abilities, ethnicity, gender, and culture) increase productivity, employee trust, and alignment between organizational and employee values (WHO, 2010). In turn, these efforts also enhance psychosocial wellbeing. Considering the determinants of mental health, collaborative action across sectors that enhances capacity for mental health promotion is one fundamental strategy to increase awareness of and address systemic inequities. Intersectional analysis also lends insight into the complex web of power, identities, and oppression that exist within an organization and impact mental health and wellbeing. It is important to thoughtfully consider how to most strategically align WHP efforts with already existing agendas and mandates related to equity, diversity, inclusion, anti-racism, Indigenous engagement, decolonization, and sustainability.

At UBC, equity, inclusion, diversity, anti-racism, decolonization, and Indigenous engagement are prioritized through its strategic plan, intersecting mid-level strategies and task forces, and adoption of the Okanagan and Scarborough Charters. In addition, the Equity and Inclusion Office and Office of Indigenous Strategic Initiatives facilitate affinity groups and provide action planning support, toolkits, and funding opportunities. The Wellbeing Strategic Framework has priority area milestones that intersect with Inclusion Action Plan (IAP) and Indigenous Strategic Plan (ISP) identifying engagement with equity-deserving groups to involve mental health literacy training, programming, and initiatives as part of Mental Health and Resilience. The evaluation framework ensures alignment with intersecting mid-level strategies, including Focus on People for faculty and staff. Feedback through surveys and engagement with affinity groups continuously improves the Workplace Wellbeing team's offerings, programs, and training. In recent years, programming has been more diversified in content and in engagement with IBPOC facilitators and consultants. Recognizing that mental health training often does not consider intersectional identities, UBC created an intersectional mental health facilitator guide. In addition, HR has developed guidelines for managers to support 2SLGBTQ+

faculty and staff, and is evolving benefits plans to better align with an equity, diversity, and inclusion lens. Further, HR has created a Centre for Workplace Accessibility, expanding on inclusion in workplace practices with funding and a team of experts.

At Dalhousie, their new institutional strategy explicitly includes and prioritizes equity, diversity, inclusion, accessibility, and wellness, and there are efforts underway to coordinate and collaborate across units to infuse wellness and EDIA throughout all efforts and to hold themselves accountable for improvement. The institution has created the role of Vice-Provost of Equity and Inclusion to lead its existing Office of Human Rights and Equity Services. Dalhousie has also created an Accessible Employment unit in HR, completed an institution-wide Accessibility Plan, has signed on to the Scarborough Charter, and has established a pan-university committee on campus culture to hold the university accountable for the recommendations brought forward in a number of reports, including the TRC and the review of the founder of Dalhousie's involvement in slavery. The university recently announced the creation of a pan-university institute on Black Studies to serve as a centre of excellence supporting the work of established and emerging Black scholars.

Queen's has strategic commitments to equity, diversity, inclusion, anti-racism, and accessibility. To further advance its strategic commitments, Queen's has adopted the Scarborough Charter, has an Office of Indigenous Initiatives, a Human Rights and Equity Office, and supports the work of the Aboriginal Council and University Council on Anti-Racism and Equity (UCARE), and there is a Declaration to Address Systemic Racism. To advance these commitments, Queen's is providing additional anti-racism training and education for all staff and faculty, increasing mental health supports for students, staff, and faculty who are affected by racism on campus, and is undertaking, identifying, and eliminating gaps in the support and resources for 2SLGBTQ+ students, staff, and faculty.

At USC, the core value of diversity, equity, and inclusion is an essential principle that is threaded throughout faculty and staff health and wellbeing programs, and new structures and practices to promote anti-racism and inclusive excellence are under way. In order to advance equity, actions have been taken to enhance the clinical experiences of faculty and staff by placing focus on accessibility, cultural humility, and affirming care models. Working in partnership with external counsellors as part of USC's employee assistance program has supported increased access to in-community treatment, text-based psychological services, flexibility in hours of access beyond business hours, and increased inclusion by ensuring mental health services are available in multiple languages and that service providers represent diverse identities.

Health promotion is inextricably linked with social, economic, and ecological systems. More simply, conditions like poverty, climate disaster, and food insecurity will affect individual and community health. Skilled strategic thinkers are needed to ensure institutions uphold their responsibility to ensure campus community members have a right to health in the most efficient, safe, dignified, just, and equitable manner possible. Collaboration across sectors, intersectional analysis, and intra-institution alignment is key.

Conclusion

Historically, "one of the main challenges of applying a systems or whole campus approach has been to incorporate staff and faculty health and wellbeing initiatives in part because student learning outcomes are the primary focus of higher educational institutions. However, a whole campus approach necessarily involves all stakeholders, as there are benefits and consequences for staff, faculty and students" (Ardiles et al., 2017, p. 18). As hubs of innovation and learning, higher education must invest in staff and faculty wellbeing to enhance the resilience and strength of institutions (Higher Education Funding Council of England, 2009).

Institutions can take up the calls of the Okanagan Charter, using the key principles for action as a guidepost, and the case studies within this chapter as inspiration. Post-secondary institutions should carefully consider training and support for leaders in this transformation, since they have such a key role in impacting employee mental health. Second, they should use a variety of participatory approaches to engage the whole campus community in strategies, initiatives, and measurement. This includes student engagement, even when the focus is on workplace wellbeing. Indigenous peoples on campus and those whose Nations campuses are on must be consulted as part of these participatory approaches. Indigenous knowledge systems already acknowledge the inextricable links between health, social systems, economics, and the environment. Institutions need to promote external collaborations, intersectional analysis, and alignment across complex internal systems to ensure campus community members' right to health.

By increasing positive behaviours, integrating supportive organizational practices, providing resources that are aligned with the organization's health promotion vision, and encouraging shared ownership of an organization's success, "In the long run, this is what is good for the employee and the company" (Harter et al., 2002, p. 14).

FREQUENTLY USED ABBREVIATIONS/ACRONYMS

WHP – Workplace Health Promotion
WHO – World Health Organization
UBC – The University of British Columbia
FOP – Focus on People. (UBC's people plan. The Focus on People
   2025 framework speaks to how the university intends to be a first-
   choice place for faculty and staff to meet their greatest potential)
EFAP – Employee and Family Assistance Program
USC – The University of Sothern California
WSF – UBC's Wellbeing Strategic Framework
IBPOC – Indigenous, Black or People of Colour
HR – Human Resources
UCARE – Queen's University Council on Anti-Racism and Equity
IAP – UBC's Inclusion Action Plan
ISP – UBC's Indigenous Strategic Plan
2SLGBTQ+ – Two Spirit, lesbian, gay, bisexual, transgender, queer, ques-
   tioning, intersex, asexual, and other sexual or gender diverse identities.

REFERENCES

Ardiles, P., Hutchinson, C., Stanton, A., Dhaliwal, R., Aslan, M., & Black,
   T. (2017). Health promoting universities: Shifting from health education
   to social innovation. In I. Rootman, A. Pederson, K. Frohlick, & S. Dupere
   (Eds.), *Health promotion in Canada: New perspectives on theory, practice, policy, and
   research* (4th ed., pp. 268–85). Canadian Scholars.
Avey, J.B., Luthans, F.S., Ronda M., & Palmer, N.F. (2010). Impact of positive
   psychological capital on employee wellbeing over time. *Journal of Occupational
   Health Psychology, 15*(1), 17–28. https://doi.org/10.1037/a0016998
Canadian Mental Health Association (CMHA). (2020). Impact report.
   Retrieved 13 October 13 2023 from: https://cmha.ca/wp-content/uploads
   /2021/04/CMHA_ImpactReport_2020_FINAL_EN.pdf
Chu, C., Breuker, G., Harris, N., Stitzel, A., Xingfa, G., Xuequi, G., & Dwyer, S.
   (2000). Health-promoting workplaces – International settings development. *Health
   Promotion International, 15*(2), 155–67. https://doi.org/10.1093/heapro/15.2.155
Clarke, M., Kenny, A., & Loxley, A. (2015). *Creating a supportive working
   environment for academics in higher education: Country report.* Teachers and
   Teachers' Union of Ireland.
Dalhousie University. 2021. *Third century promise: Si'st Kasqimtlnaqnipunqekl
   Teli L'wi'tmasimk.* https://cdn.dal.ca/content/dam/dalhousie/pdf/about
   /Strategic-Planning/Dalhousie-University-Strategic-Plan-2021-2026.pdf

Diener, E., Wirtz, D., Biswas-Diener, R., Tov, W., Kim-Prieto, C., Choi, D.W., & Oishi, S. (2009). New measures of well-being. In *Assessing well-being: The collected works of Ed Diener* (pp. 247–66). Social Indicators Research Series 39. https://doi:10.1007/978-90-481-2354-412

Doherty, S., & Dooris, M. (2006). The healthy settings approach: The growing interest within colleges and universities. *Education and Health, 24*(3), 42–3.

Edmonston, G. (1999). Development of an IEP form for adult students. Action Research Monograph.

GermAnn, K., & Ardiles, P. (2009). *Toward flourishing for all: Mental health promotion and mental illness prevention policy background paper.* Pan-Canadian Steering Committee for Mental Health Promotion and Mental Illness Prevention.

Harter, J.K., Schmidt, F.L., & Keyes, C. (2002). *Wellbeing in the workplace and its relationship to business outcomes: A review of the Gallup studies.* American Psychological Association.

Higher Education Funding Council of England. (2009). *Creating success through wellbeing in higher education.* www.wellbeing.ac.uk

Kahn, W.A. (1990). Psychological conditions of personal engagement and disengagement at work. *Academy of Management Journal, 33*, 692–724. https://doi.org/10.2307/256287

Kelloway, E.K., Turner, N., Barling, J., & Loughlin, C. (2012). Transformational leadership and employee psychological well-being: The mediating role of employee trust in leadership. *Work & Stress, 26*(1), 39-55.

Kunyk, D., Craig-Broadwith, M., Morris, H., Diaz, R., Reisdorfer, E., & Wang, J. (2015). Employers' perceptions and attitudes toward the Canadian national standard on psychological health and safety in the workplace: A qualitative study. *International Journal of Law and Psychiatry, 44*, 41–7. https://doi.org/10.1016/j.ijlp.2015.08.030

Lowe, G. (2004). *Healthy workplace strategies: Creating change and achieving results.* Report prepared for the Workplace Health Strategies Bureau, Health Canada. https://grahamlowe.ca/wp-content/uploads/import_docs/Hlthy%20wkpl%20strategies%20report.pdf

MacEachen, E., Polzer, J., & Clarke, J. (2008). "You are free to set your own hours": Governing worker productivity and health through flexibility and resilience. *Social Science & Medicine, 66*(5), 1019–33. https://doi.org/10.1016/j.socscimed.2007.11.013

Malik, A. (2013). Efficacy, hope, optimism and resilience at workplace – Positive organizational behaviour. *International Journal of Scientific and Research Publications, 3*(10), 1–4.

Noblet, A., & LaMontagne, A.D. (2006). The role of workplace health promotion in addressing job stress. *Health Promotion International, 21*(4), 343–53. https://doi.org/10.1093/heapro/dal029

Oades, L., Robinson, P., Green, S., & Spence, G. (2011). Towards a positive university. *The Journal of Positive Psychology, 6*(6), 432–9. https://doi.org/10.1080/17439760.2011.634828

Okanagan Charter: An International Charter for Health Promoting Universities and Colleges. (2015). *Okanagan Charter.* Kelowna, BC: Author. Retrieved from http://internationalhealthycampuses2015.sites.olt.ubc.ca/files/2016/01/Okanagan-Charter-January13v2.pdf

Queen's University. 2022a. *Queen's strategy.* https://www.queensu.ca/principal/strategy

Queen's University. 2022b. *Quick facts.* https://www.queensu.ca/about/quickfacts

Queen's University. 2022c. *Research facts.* https://www.queensu.ca/research/facts

Raphael, D., Bryant, T., Mikkonen, J., & Raphael, A. (2020). *Social determinants of health: The Canadian facts.* Ontario Tech University Faculty of Health Sciences and York University School of Health Policy and Management.

Rongen, A., Robroek, S., van Lenthe, F., & Burdorf, A. (2013). Workplace health promotion: A meta-analysis of effectiveness. *American Journal of Preventative Medicine, 44*(4), 406–15. https://doi.org/10.1016/j.amepre.2012.12.007

Samra, J. (2017). *The evolution of workplace mental health in Canada: Research report (2007–2017).* https://drjotisamra.com/wp-content/uploads/2018/01/The-Evolution-of-Workplace-Mental-Health-in-Canada.pdf

Samra, J., Gilbert, M., Shain, M., & Bilsker, D. (2009–20).Guarding Minds at Work. With amendments by Stuart, H. (2022). All rights reserved. Website development and data storage by the Canadian Centre for Occupational Health and Safety (CCOHS).

Shain, M., & Kramer, D.M. (2004). Health promotion in the workplace: Framing the concept, reviewing the evidence. *Occupational and Environmental Medicine, 61*(7), 643–8. https://doi.org/10.1136/oem.2004.013193

Standards Council of Canada (2013). *Psychological health and safety in the workplace – Prevention, promotion, and guidance to staged implementation.* Bureau de normalisation du Québec (BNQ) & the Canadian Standard Association (CSA Group).

Statistics Canada. (2020). *Canadians' mental health during the COVID-19 pandemic.* The Daily. https://www150.statcan.gc.ca/n1/en/daily-quotidien/200527/dq200527b-eng.pdf?st=e0j5ghhX

Truth and Reconciliation Commission of Canada. (2017). *Homepage. National Centre for Truth and Reconciliation.* https://nctr.ca/

UBC Wellbeing. (n.d.a). *Wellbeing strategic framework.* https://wellbeing.ubc.ca/sites/wellbeing.ubc.ca/files/u9/wellbeing_strategic_framework_FINAL_0.pdf

UBC Wellbeing. (n.d.b). *UBC Wellbeing annual report 2020–21.* https://wellbeing.ubc.ca/annualreport20-21

UBC Wellbeing. (n.d.c). *Wellbeing strategic framework roadmap.* https://wellbeing
.ubc.ca/sites/wellbeing.ubc.ca/files/u1582/WSF%20Roadmap%20
Dashboard%20May%202022.pdf

United Nations (UN). (2007). *United Nations Declaration on the Rights of Indigenous
Peoples.* https://www.un.org/development/desa/indigenouspeoples
/wp-content/uploads/sites/19/2018/11/UNDRIP_E_web.pdf

University of Southern California. (2022). *USC Healthy Campus.* https://workwell
.usc.edu/wp-content/uploads/2022/01/Healthy-Campus-Overview.pdf

White, M. (2013). *Building a resilient organizational culture.* UNC Executive
Development.

World Health Organization (WHO). (2004). *Promoting mental health: Concepts,
emerging evidence, practice.* Work Health Organization Press.

World Health Organization (WHO). (2010). *Healthy workplace framework
and model: Background and supporting literature and practice.* World Health
Organization Press.

Youseff, C., & Luthans, F. (2007). Positive organizational behavior in the
workplace: The impact of hope, optimism and resilience. *Journal of
Management, 33*(5), 774–800. https://doi.org/10.1177/0149206307305562

10 Wellbeing by Design: Creating a University Built Environment to Advance Wellbeing and Sustainable Outcomes

C. OLIVER TACTO

Introduction

The academic sphere, built and designed to provide opportunities for cognitive and social development, has been the setting for emerging adults, offering an interface where learning, professional camaraderie, relationship building, and individual growth converge. On the grounds of colleges and universities, the emphasis on cultivating healthy settings becomes imperative, given the profound impact of these environments on the individuals occupying them. This chapter delves into the significant aspects of designing college campuses that are not just centres of academic learning but are also spaces where students, faculty, and staff can live, learn, work, and experience college in a sensory and meaningful manner. The importance of this venture is heightened by the principles laid out by the Okanagan Charter for Health Promoting Universities, which calls for creating a holistic learning environment and an inclusive campus culture that enhances learning about health and wellbeing while fostering resilience. This chapter navigates the diverse dimensions of creating health promoting campuses by connecting concepts of the built environment, university urbanization, biophilic design, sustainability, and the foundational tenets of the Okanagan Charter. It aims to examine the symbiotic relationship between environmental conditions and human behaviour, exploring how strategic design and system-level interventions can elevate health outcomes and enrich overall wellbeing, adhering to a "whole is greater than the sum of its parts" philosophy and underlining the overarching ambition of building vibrant, health-conducive academic communities.

Setting the Stage: The Foundations of Built Environment

The built environment has been defined differently by researchers and across various sectors. Generally, it is defined as the part of the physical environment constructed or modified by people with particular emphasis on buildings, parks, streetscapes, and other spaces that provide the setting for human activity. In one definition, the built environment consists of the following elements: land use patterns, the distribution across space of activities and the buildings that house them; the transportation system, the physical infrastructure of roads. sidewalks, and bike paths as well as the service this system provides; and urban design, the arrangement and appearance of the physical elements in a community (Handy et al., 2002).

There is a variety of terms when referring to the built environment. While these terms are often interpreted to be interchangeable, there are a few distinctions among them:

Urban design: refers to the design of the city and its physical elements, including their arrangement and appearance, and is concerned with the function and appeal of public spaces.

Land use: refers to the distribution of activities across space, including the location and density of different activities, where activities are grouped into relatively coarse categories (e.g., residential, commercial, office, industrial, and other activities).

Transportation system: includes the physical infrastructure of roads, sidewalks, bike paths, railroad tracks, bridges, etc., as well as the service provided as determined by traffic levels, bus frequencies, etc.

Built environment: comprises urban design, land use, and transportation systems and encompasses patterns of human activity within the physical environment.

The theoretical, empirical, and practical progress in built environment literature has generally demonstrated an aim to enhance the quality of life, improve system efficiency, or reduce environmental impacts.

Wellbeing in the Built Environment

The concept of quality of life, frequently equated with the inherent goodness of life, pertains to the harmonious coexistence and successful navigation of life in conjunction with the environment (Brown & Brown, 2005). For several, this quality is directly proportional to the overarching state of their wellbeing; individuals who enjoy a high quality of life are perceived to possess elevated levels of wellbeing. Extensive research underscores the influential role and substantial implications the built environment wields as a formidable determinant of an individual's and community's health and wellbeing. This section reviews the myriad outcomes discerned from investigations into the correlations between the built environment and various domains, including physical and mental health, social support, romantic relationships, and restoration.

Physical Activity

A comprehensive synthesis of twenty-one prospective cohort studies and 30 national experiments substantiates the correlation between alterations in the built environment and levels of physical activity, illustrating a significant association between enhanced objective accessibility and infrastructural amendments conducive to walking, cycling, and public transportation with augmented overall and transportation-related activity (Karmeniemi et al., 2018).

Mental Health

Over two decades of research has delved into the multifaceted interactions between the built environment and mental health across diverse populations. The impacts of various housing attributes have been linked directly to mental wellbeing, revealing instances such as residents of high-rise housing experiencing heightened psychological distress, prominently among lower-income mothers (Evans et al., 2003). Further studies align with these findings, highlighting connections between residential density and increased psychological distress (Baum & Paulus, 1987), proximity to airports correlating with elevated stress levels in children (Lercher et al., 2002), and the presence of malodorous indoor air pollutants triggering adverse behavioural manifestations (Bell et al., 2001).

Social Support

The constructed environment also indirectly influences the formation and sustenance of supportive social networks. The strategic arrangement of spaces and furniture, the introduction of focal points and activity generators such as food, and the enhancement of visual prospects were identified as influential factors in promoting social interaction within buildings and outdoor spaces (Becker, 1995; Carr et al., 1976; McCoy, 2002). However, counterproductive elements like noise can significantly inhibit communication and induce irritability and a lack of willingness to assist others (Cohen & Spacapan, 1984).

Romantic Relationships

Research at State College, Pennsylvania, reveals the importance of pedestrian and transportation infrastructure and a diverse range of affordable activities in fostering the bonds between couples (Andris & Lee, 2021).

Restoration

Empirical studies underscore the restorative capabilities of natural elements within the built environment, illustrating their potency in rejuvenating cognitive and emotional energy. Instances include natural views, landscape paintings, and indoor plants, all associated with enhanced positive affect and comfort (Kaplan & Kaplan, 1989; Larsen et al., 1998; Ulrich, 1993). Such phenomena have practical applications in health care and institutional settings, where exposure to natural elements can significantly accelerate recovery and mitigate distress (Ulrich, 1984).

The robust and well-established relationships between the built environment and myriad aspects of human life emphasize physical surroundings' pivotal role in shaping our livelihoods, energy utilization, and environmental impacts. The aforementioned classical studies poignantly delineate the detrimental consequences of adverse physical and social conditions on mental health outcomes. Although investigating the built environment's impact on human behaviour and experiences is not novel, these concepts assume high significance when considering university campus design and the interplay between the university environment and student experiences. The subsequent sections will explore the paradigms of university campus planning, evaluation metrics for the built environment, and the integrative tools linking our living experiences with the constructed environment.

Context of Higher Education

Universities and colleges worldwide serve as dynamic arenas where emerging adults navigate a complex system of academic endeavours, lifelong learning, relationship building, professional collaboration, and holistic development. In these unique ecosystems, interactions, decisions, and relationships are significantly influenced by the surrounding physical environment, which acts as a silent orchestrator of campus life.

A campus's physical design often shapes the initial perceptions and is considered pivotal by prospective students in forming their first impressions (Sturner, 1973; Thelin & Yankovich, 1987). In an observant study of campus life on twenty-nine different university campuses, Boyer (1987) observed:

> Little wonder that when we asked students what influenced them most during their campus visit, about half mentioned "the friendliness of students we met." However, it was the buildings, the trees, the walkways, and the well-kept lawns that overwhelmingly won out. The appearance of the campus is, by far, the most influential characteristic during campus visits, and we gained distinct impressions that when recruiting students, the director of buildings and grounds may be more important than the academic dean. (p. 17).

Thus, the visual presentation and architectural design of a campus thus emerge as salient factors driving students' attraction to and satisfaction with an institution.

However, universities also confront various external challenges affecting their infrastructural make-up, primarily from governmental and market pressures. These external factors resonate within the institutional framework, reflecting program availability, tuition structures, and societal research outcomes. Zusman (2005) underscored five pivotal challenges in higher education: funding (who pays for higher education?), beneficiary identification (who benefits?), beneficiary selection (who decides who benefits?), curriculum determination (what should be offered?), and outcomes definition (what should the outcomes be?).

Colleges and universities continue to grapple with these and additional challenges related to the overall wellbeing of students, faculty, staff, and the surrounding community, especially underscored by the emergence of the global coronavirus (COVID-19) pandemic in 2020. The pandemic accentuated existing vulnerabilities and challenges within student health and wellbeing, leading to increased stress and anxiety, and a concomitant decline in academic experiences (Son et al., 2020). Today's administrators perceive these public health issues as multifaceted, impacting students' physical, mental, emotional, and social wellbeing, necessitating significant modifications to academic engagement and overall quality of life.

Reflecting on the Okanagan Charter's principles, it is crucial to consider the built environment's ramifications on the holistic college experience, including the health and wellbeing of the university community. The Charter emphasizes the creation of health promoting universities that integrate wellbeing into every aspect of campus culture and lead health promotion action and collaboration locally and globally. This emphasis on holistic wellbeing aligns with the pressing need for universities to address complex public health issues and their impact on the various facets of student life.

In such a scenario, envisioning a paradigm where prospective students prioritize institutions that diligently incorporate health promoting designs into their campuses seems imperative. Here, the emphasis would transition from merely seeking esteemed and reputable institutions to opting for campuses where all members can live, learn, work, and experience college in a thriving and meaningful way. Applying the Okanagan Charter in this context would encourage universities to embed wellbeing into the fabric of institutional culture, fostering a supportive environment conducive to the multilayered development of students, faculty, staff, and the wider community.

Built Environment: A Settings Approach to Health Promotion

The approach to health promotion through a settings approach underlines the importance of understanding and addressing the various contexts where people live, learn, work, and play. This strategy accentuates the holistic consideration of individual and community-level environments and their intersectionality, especially within the dynamic ecosystems of higher education institutions. These institutions are distinctive hubs where the union of leadership, policy, practices, and locale creates many intervention opportunities, presenting both prospects and challenges in coordinating health promotion and wellbeing initiatives. Several attempts were conducted to systematize the impact and effectiveness of interventions in various settings (e.g., school-based health promotion and community development). However, only a few organizations and institutions have successfully developed a practical framework where the setting approach is nested to guide and promote a health promoting campus. The essence is to go beyond mere program implementation to enrich the holistic experience and wellbeing of students on college campuses.

The Ottawa Charter for Health Promotion (WHO, 1986) stipulated that health is a cumulative experience lived by and manifested within the everyday settings of learning, working, and nurturing relationships. The Ottawa Charter illuminated and revealed five health promotion action areas (building healthy public policy, creating supportive environments, strengthening community action, developing personal skills, and reorienting all sectors towards prevention) to achieve "health for all," underlining the integral connections between individual, community, and environmental determinants, incorporating cultural norms, social structures, ecosystems, and built environments. Universities serve as pivotal settings, hosting many learning and developmental activities for students and staff alike. This charter emphasized the seamless integration of physical, mental, and social wellbeing, echoing the ethos of self-realization, needs satisfaction, and environmental adaptability.

This seminal charter was further enhanced by the Okanagan Charter (2015), which is revered as the gold standard for higher education institutions to actualize health and wellbeing through integrative strategies in social and environmental domains. The Charter calls for two actions: infusing health into the everyday aspect of campus culture and spearheading health promoting collaborations at local and global spaces. The Okanagan Charter, thus, serves as a comprehensive framework, providing actionable pathways and catalysing health-centric transformations within academic environments and beyond.

This progressive approach aligns succinctly with the Geneva Charter for Wellbeing (WHO, 2021), which proposes the inception of "sustainable wellbeing societies" and delineates five key areas, including 1) nurturing a healthy planet, 2) constructing equitable economic structures, 3) developing holesome public policies, 4) achieving universal health coverage, and 5) mitigating the repercussions of digital transformations. The synergy of these charters fosters a conducive atmosphere, optimizing the holistic wellbeing of individuals within the larger society.

To actualize these principles, a comprehensive approach is desired to focus on individual wellbeing and the environmental and planetary contexts. The conceptual shift by the work of Aaron Antonovsky towards salutogenic and ecological approaches underscores the multifaceted aspects of settings – the implicit social norms, power hierarchies, moral cultures, and broader sociopolitical contexts (Hancock, 1985; Kickbusch, 1996; Richard et al., 1996).

Moreover, this chapter navigates the intricate significance of physical and built environment processes, presenting a pivotal discourse for health promotion practitioners to address the various challenges and pathways for institutional wellbeing. By embedding the principles of the Okanagan Charter, it lays down a foundational scaffold to explore and implement innovative solutions, intending to foster resilient, inclusive, and sustainable learning environments that resonate with the collective aspirations and wellbeing of the university community.

Built Environment and Wellbeing in Higher Education

The relationship between the built environment and wellbeing is pivotal in urban planning discussions, particularly within higher education settings where health promotion practitioners and university campus master planners are primary stakeholders. However, detailed assessments and evaluations drawing the relationships between the built environment and the holistic wellbeing of students, staff, faculty, and the surrounding community are surprisingly rare. While efforts to understand this connection have often centred on individual behavioural changes and happiness (Gibbs, 2017; LaFountaine et al., 2006; Myers & Sweeney, 2008), a discernible gap exists in students focusing on environmental interventions.

In alignment with the principles of the Okanagan Charter, there is an academic need to investigate the built environments and the implications of setting approaches within higher education institutions (Dooris, 2006). During the last two decades, health promotion practitioners and university administrators were increasingly joined by others in taking a more careful look at the built environments and implications of the settings approach. The Charter elucidates the need to embed health into every aspect of campus culture, emphasizing the creation of supportive environments and the cultivation of community wellbeing. Health promotion practitioners are thus adopting a proactive stance, addressing individual and community needs through a whole systems approach.

Historically, wellbeing initiatives have predominantly concentrated on augmenting individual capacities. However, the recent shift towards environmental and systemic interventions is vital, resonating with various leading public health models and international resolutions such as the United Nations General Assembly's *Happiness: Towards a Holistic Approach to Development* (2013). These paradigms prioritize environmental factors and interventions as pivotal global strategies for enhancing collective and societal wellbeing (Helliwell et al., 2020).

Higher education institutions are microcosms reflecting the broader societal structures. Thus, the impetus to actualize community wellbeing within college campuses is essential to ensure optimal learning environments that foster holistic health and wellbeing for every individual – including students, staff, and faculty. The American College Health Association (ACHA) has pioneered movements to guide the Healthy Campus framework (ACHA, 2020), a manifestation of the principles embodied in the Okanagan Charter. These frameworks aim to elevate one's quality of life, cultivate healthy behaviours, and augment the capacities of students, faculty, and staff by surpassing conventional approaches focused primarily on diagnosis and treatment.

Considering the context of higher education, a pertinent enquiry arises: "How can universities leverage built environment and healthy settings approaches to yield positive wellbeing outcomes?" The Okanagan Charter provides a viable framework to explore this question, promoting campus design planners, landscape architects, campus master planners, and social scientists to delve into human interactions with their encompassing environments and expertise. As the National Intramural Recreational Sports Association (NIRSA) (2000) highlights, this multifaceted perspective underscores wellbeing as a collective aspiration and a shared responsibility, encompassing the campus-wide community, educational experience, and individual entities. By collectively integrating the Okanagan Charter's tenets, universities can adopt a more nuanced and holistic approach to designing their campuses. This method fosters a sense of community wellbeing. It advances the discourse on the intricate relationship between the built environment and wellbeing, contributing to the development of sustainable and health promoting academic settings.

University Urbanization and Wellbeing

Throughout the twentieth century, higher education institutions have witnessed an exponential expansion characterized by increasingly diverse student communities, surging enrolments, and a pivot towards on-campus residential education. As a result, student affairs departments have evolved into vast entities, striving to reinforce and augment academic and extracurricular learning environments (Schwartz & Stewart, 2017). This escalation has resulted in pronounced urbanization within university campuses, transforming once verdant expanses (e.g., green and open spaces) into densely populated built environments (e.g., buildings and parking structures).

A pressing consequence in response to urbanization is the objective and subjective experiences that caused students to become less connected with their natural counterparts and living elements. Historically, humans evolved in tandem with the natural world. However, the contemporary urban framework ensconces individuals, especially students, predominantly within indoor confines, resulting in 90 per cent of their daily experiences unfolding in such environments. This dramatic transition from natural settings is posited to impede their wellbeing and academic trajectories (Srivastava, 2009).

Implementing sustainable and nature-inclusive designs on university campuses is a multifaceted challenge. The systemic dilemmas many universities face are characterized by the decline of green spaces due to the construction of modern buildings to accommodate the growing population and diverse needs (Seymour, 2016). This unplanned and unreflective urbanization disturbs human-to-nature connections and raises concerns about sustainability and wellbeing. While there is a pressing need to provide sufficient infrastructure such as living spaces, classrooms, and socializing areas, the inadvertent sidelining of nature and open spaces leads to a detrimental disconnect between university community members and their environment. Such conditions are comparable to students' experiences to animals in outdated zoos, living and learning under conditions with limited access to natural light, ventilation, and other elements (e.g., raw materials, vegetation, natural views, and other natural shapes) integral to wellbeing (Roös, 2017).

If not mitigated, the rise in university urbanization can herald long-term micro- and macro-level negative consequences, including unsustainable energy consumption, unhealthy indoor and outdoor environments, and a decline in overall student wellbeing. Drawing insights from the Okanagan Charter, realizing and adopting health promoting environmental designs and sustainable practices that reconcile the growing needs of university communities with the innate human need for nature is imperative. University urbanization, driven by the demand to meet various infrastructural needs, has unintentionally neglected the inherent human connection with nature, significantly impacting student wellbeing and sustainability. By aligning the principles of the Okanagan Charter with university planning and architecture, institutions can reconstruct the lost harmony between humans and nature within academic settings, thereby fostering a culture of health, happiness, and overall wellbeing amidst the evolving landscape of higher education.

Connecting with Nature through Biophilia and Biophilic Design

There are several strategies and tools university that campus master planners and designers can utilize to create a built environment that enhances the health and wellbeing of all. Acknowledging that humans have an inborn tendency to focus on and affiliate with other living things, one of several approaches includes designing college campuses by connecting the entire university community with nature and the natural environment. Biophilic Design is a design strategy that seeks to create a good, healthy, and cultivating habitat for people to advance their health and wellbeing. Biophilic design's premise and overarching goal is to encourage using and applying natural elements and processes as intentional and inspirational designs in the built environment. The concept of connecting and exposing humans to natural elements and features has positive effects on overall health, wellbeing, and quality of life, as supported in extensive bodies of research. Bridging the gap between students and nature, for instance, posits the opportunity to foster a safe learning community and built environment, promotes healthy behaviour choices, and increases overall wellbeing.

The biophilia hypothesis by Kellert and Wilson (1993) states that the attraction to life and lifelike processes is further understood through the complex perspective of human evolution when humans lived and interacted in the natural environment to survive. Over time, our ancestors' survival behaviours and patterns consisted of finding suitable food, water, and shelter, keeping track of time and spatial location, and reacting to predators while paying detailed attention to their natural surroundings and environments. As a result, humans highly connected with nature would have a tremendous evolutionary advantage over others who were not as connected. Biophilia originated with the understanding that 99 per cent of the human species' history was developed in the adaptive response to natural (not artificial) or human-created forces. Moreover, the idea that there is an association between the biological bond between humans and nature is captured in two theories developed by Environmental Psychology researchers – Attention Restoration Theory and Stress Recovery Theory (Joye & van den Berg, 2012; Kaplan & Kaplan, 1989). Both theories support the idea that specific environments are stressful, while others evoke positive moods. These theories suggest that environments have specific attributes and qualities that can draw attention and help people recover from mental and emotional stress at expedited rates. Furthermore, biophilia is identified as the inherent human inclination to affiliate with nature that, even in the modern world, continues to be critical to people's physical and mental health and wellbeing (Kellert, 1997; Kellert, 2012; Kellert & Wilson, 1993; Wilson, 1986).

Differences between the past and present among populations are surfacing in the literature that supports the changes in time spent with nature and natural environments. The problem with modern society is the widening gap between humans and nature. According to Clements (2004), children, for example, spend less time outside and in natural environments than previous generations. Studies also have shown differences in contact with nature based on geographic location and where one grows up and lives. One study found that individuals in developed countries spend most of their time indoors (MacKerron & Mourato, 2013). More humans live away from natural environments and urban settings than in rural areas. This gap brings significant concerns and may significantly impact how humans connect and how minimal exposure to nature limits individuals' health, happiness, and wellbeing. Within university settings, a compelling need exists within university settings to investigate and integrate biophilic design's implications meticulously. While substantial evidence corroborates the positive impact of natural elements on health outcomes, an in-depth exploration of biophilic interventions in universities is pertinent. These interventions can offer insights into mitigating the effects of nature prevalent in modern societal structures and thus align with the holistic and ecological visions of the Okanagan Charter. The convergence of biophilic design with the tenets of the Okanagan Charter provides an opportunity to incorporate health into all aspects of campus culture, weaving the learning environment with nature. The Charter underlines the need for an ecological and sustainable approach, integral to biophilic design, to foster holistic wellbeing and sustainable practices within universities.

Integrating biophilic design within universities is a transformative strategy to enhance the health and wellbeing of the academic community, correlating with the principles of the Okanagan Charter. The innate human connection with nature, shaped by evolutionary patterns, implies that designing learning environments interconnected with natural elements can open pathways to enhanced mental health, reduced stress, and holistic wellbeing. The modern challenge remains in effectively bridging the burgeoning gap between humans and nature, reaffirming the need for sustainable, ecological, and health promoting designs in universities, thus contributing to the global dialogue on health, sustainability, and environmental symbiosis.

The Symbiosis of Nature Connectedness and Wellbeing

When considering the built environment on a college campus, one must investigate biophilia's direct and indirect impacts on people's physical and mental health, performance, and wellbeing. The literature reveals evidence that there is a strong relationship between nature connectedness and wellbeing, and close contact with nature can be beneficial, for example, leading to improvement in mood, cognition, and health and other benefits for humans (Browning et al., 2014; Nisbet & Zelenski, 2011). Likewise, philosophers and psychologists have conceptualized wellbeing as one's connection with nature and determined that to attain wellbeing, there are two perspectives: *hedonic* and *eudaimonic* approaches.

The philosophical conceptualizations of wellbeing, underscored by psychologists and philosophers, pivot around the intricate alignment with nature. Within this contextual framework, wellbeing is perceived through the lenses of hedonic and eudaimonic philosophies. The hedonic viewpoint epitomizes wellbeing as the culmination of pleasurable experiences and desire fulfilment, resonating with subjective wellbeing and encompassing the emotional experiences of the absence of negativity (i.e., evaluating one's life as satisfying) (Diener, 2009; Kahneman, 1999). Examples of widely used measurement scales to assess hedonic wellbeing include the Positive and Negative Affect Schedule (Watson et al., 1988), the Subjective Happiness Scale (Lyubomirsky & Lepper, 1999), and the Satisfaction with Life Scale (Diener et al., 1985),

On the other hand, the eudaimonic perspective focuses on one's deeply held values and realizations for one's full potential (Ryff, 1995). Ryff and Keyes (1995) proposed that wellbeing consists of six actualization facets: mastery, life purpose, autonomy, self-acceptance, positive relatedness, and personal growth. While there are distinct differences between the hedonic and eudaimonic perspectives, individuals with hedonic and eudaimonic motives tend to have higher wellbeing. They are considered to flourish at high levels (Forgeard et al., 2011).

In addition to attaining wellbeing through hedonic and eudaimonic approaches, researchers also examined nature's direct and indirect exposure to people's wellbeing and happiness (Bowler et al., 2010). Researchers are discovering many areas where exposure to nature significantly affects physical and mental health, performance, and wellbeing. While data is limited, a growing body of research observes nature's impact on health and wellbeing outcomes in various sectors – education, health, recreation, housing, and community. For instance, health care settings have witnessed remarkable improvements in patient recovery, stress alleviation, and overall staff morale through integrative nature interactions (Kuo, 2010; Louv, 2012; Marcus & Sachs, 2014; Taylor, 2001; Ulrich, 2008; Wells & Rollings, 2012). These profound interactions signify the intrinsic relationship between nature connectedness and pro-environmental attitudes, subsequently influencing subjective wellbeing (Nisbet & Zelenski, 2013).

The developing trends in biophilic research spotlight the necessity of meticulously curating university environments aligned with biophilic design principles. Such an approach is not merely an architectural endeavour but a holistic strategy to improve student health, happiness and overall wellbeing. It demands a call for systemic considerations of the architectural impacts on the collective wellbeing of the campus community. Within this scenario, implementing biophilia and biophilic designs emerges as foundational elements for connecting campus communities to natural elements, orchestrating a multisensory experience that nurtures exploration, curiosity, and growth.

The comprehensive integration of biophilic design within university campuses transcends architectural innovations, embarking to foster sustainable wellbeing in alignment with the Okanagan Charter. Universities can harness the symbiotic relationship between nature connectedness and holistic wellbeing by fostering an environment enriched with natural elements. It realizes the significance of engendering an educational ecosystem resonating with the harmonious principles of biophilia, thereby illuminating pathways for enhanced physiological, psychological, and environmental wellbeing within the academic community.

Nature Connectedness in Action: Principles of Biophilic Design

Suppose biophilic design is a human-centred approach and emergent potential strategy to bridge the gap between university urbanization and achievement of community wellbeing. In that case, certain principles must be considered to guide campus master plan designs and strategic planning at the university-wide level. The beauty and challenge of biophilic design is identifying the long-term impacts and applications of such a dynamic approach. Since the surfacing of the biophilia hypothesis, researchers and practitioners in environmental and building design fields have identified fundamental principles and a framework for satisfying nature experiences in the built environment (Browning et al., 2014; Kellert et al., 2008).

Principles and Guiding Frameworks for Authentic Experiences

Biophilic design necessitates unwavering adherence to established principles to manifest impactful and coherent interventions. As Kellert (2018) has indicated, these principles act as cardinal conditions and advantages, guiding campus master planners in the integrative biophilic transformation of university landscapes. The principles emphasize the following:

1 Human Adaptations: Enhancing physiological and psychological wellbeing through nature-induced adaptations.
2 Ecological Integration: Emphasizing the ecological whole over its segmented components.
3 Natural Engagement: Promoting immersive interactions with nature's features and processes.
4 Intrinsic Value Realization: Acknowledging the diversity of human values connected to the natural environment.
5 Emotional Connectivity: Fostering emotional bonds with structures and landscapes, evoking communal affiliations encompassing both human and non-human environments.
6 Multi-Setting Incorporation: Applying biophilic experiences embedded across various settings, including interiors, exteriors, and transitional landscapes.

Table 10.1. Experiences and Attributes of Biophilic Design by Kellert and Calabrese (2015)

Direct Experience of Nature	Indirect Experience of Nature	Experiences of Space and Place
Light	Images of natures	Prospect and refuge
Air	Natural materials	Organized complexity
Water	Natural colours	Integration of parts to
Plants	Simulating natural light	wholes
Animals	and air	Transitional spaces
Weather	Naturalistic shapes and	Mobility and wayfinding
Natural landscapes and	forms	Cultural and ecological
ecosystems	Evoking nature	attachment to place
Fire	Information richness	
	Age, change, and the	
	patina of time	
	Natural geometries	
	Biomimicry	

7 Authenticity of Experience: Prioritizing genuine natural interactions over artificial and constructed representations.
8 Eco-Conscious Relationships: Enhancing human affiliations to natural systems while mitigating adverse environmental impacts.

The evolutionary trajectory of biophilic principles and characteristics culminates in delineating three core "experiences" and twenty-four "attributes" outlined by Kellert and Calabrese (2015) (see table 10.1). While research in biophilic design is still relatively rare, especially within higher education environments, academic literature is advancing to reference these experiences and attributes as patterns to build a healthy and restorative environment. When considering applying biophilic design to campus learning environments, these experiences and attributes represent the basic categories of the biophilic design framework.

The direct experience of nature refers to contact with environmental features in the built environment, including light, air, plants, animals, water, landscapes, and others. On the other hand, the indirect experience of nature refers to contact with the representation or image of nature, the transformation of nature from its original condition, or exposure to particular patterns, processes, and characteristics of the natural world. These may include pictures and artwork, natural materials such as wood furnishings, configured ornaments inspired by shapes and forms occurring in nature, and processes that have been significantly important in human evolution, such as aging, natural geometries, and others. Finally, the experience of space and place refers to spatial features characteristic of the natural environment that have advanced human health and wellbeing. Examples include prospect and refuge, organized complexity, mobility and way of finding, and more.

The Okanagan Charter, focusing on health promotive and sustainable academic environments, provides an overarching framework to integrate biophilic design principles within higher education institutions. While reflecting upon the biophilic framework, health promotion practitioners must ponder the contemporary applicability of these experiences and attributes within colleges and universities. How can these meticulously curated experiences and attributes seamlessly be embedded within learning environments to cultivate healthy and restorative atmospheres while aligning with the Okanagan Charter's objectives? By incorporating biophilic design principles within the strategic fabric of university planning and design, institutions can actualize the vision aspired by the Okanagan Charter, fostering holistic symbiosis between individuals and their environment. This endeavour to instill nature connectedness within the academic ecosystem signifies a paradigmatic shift towards sustainable wellbeing and ecological consciousness, underpinning the journey of universities towards becoming sanctuaries of learning, health, and sustainability.

Evaluative Frameworks for Built Environments and Human-Nature Interactions

Understanding and assessing the dimensions of the built environment that influence health-related behaviours such as walking and biking are paramount in advancing public health goals and enhancing individual quality of life. These assessments align with the Okanagan Charter's vision of integrating health, wellbeing, and sustainability into everyday living environments, fostering physical activity and connectedness to nature. Many validated tools have been developed to measure the health impacts of community-built environments, yet a limited number have garnered widespread application.

Categorization of Traditional Assessment Tools

Brownsen et al. (2009) performed a comprehensive review of surveys and tools, categorizing them traditionally into the following:

1 Interview or Self-Administered Questionnaires: Primarily measure perceptions of the environment.

2 Archival Data Collection Tools: Utilize existing data often through Geographic Information Systems (GIS).
3 Systematic Observation Audit Tools: Structured evaluations of environmental characteristics.

Utilization of the Built Environment Assessment Tool

The Built Environment Assessment Tool employed by the Centers for Disease Control and Prevention (CDC, 2015) serves to evaluate the fundamental features of the built environment impacting health, focusing on infrastructure, walkability, bikeability, and related physical activities. It assesses the holistic aspects and quality of built environments, correlating them to behaviours influencing individual health within those spaces. However, the scope of such tools needs broadening to include the multifaceted personal relationships and connections individuals maintain with their environment, especially within the context of universities.

Enhancing Measurement of Human-Nature Relationships

To bridge the identified gaps, universities must explore innovative measurement techniques to scrutinize the intersections between physical learning environments, human-nature relationships, and holistic wellbeing. Several conceptual frameworks and measures exist to assess human-nature relationships: commitment to nature (Davis et al., 2009); connectedness to nature (Mayer & Frantz, 2004); connectivity with nature (Dutcher et al., 2007); emotional affinity toward nature (Kals et al., 1999); environmental identity (Clayton, 2003); inclusion of nature in self (Schultz, 2001); nature relatedness (Nisbet et al., 2009).

Progress in Higher Education Institutions

Emerging studies underscore the mental health benefits of interactions with natural environments, emphasizing the importance of green and blue spaces in wellbeing (Gascon et al., 2015). Researchers and practitioners within higher education institutions are working alongside national associations like the American College Health Association, the NASPA, and the American College Health Foundation, to name a few, to develop new ways to measure these relationships and embed such assessments to track key performance indicators associated with the health and wellbeing of students, staff, and faculty. Travia et al. (2021) collaborated with the American College Health Foundation in the development of *Measuring Wellbeing in a College Campus Setting*, a survey instrument to

measure mental health and emotional wellbeing across campus communities. This tool incorporates evaluations of "institutional environments"
and perceptions of environmental factors impacting mental health and
emotional wellbeing. Pursuing standardized measures continues as
higher education institutions strive to refine assessment methodologies
related to wellbeing and built environments.

The evolving assessment frameworks within built environments and
human-nature interactions present an opportunity to align more closely
with the Okanagan Charter's principles. The collective endeavour to refine and standardize measures is critical in bolstering wellbeing across
university campuses, ensuring a balanced integration of health, nature,
and learning environments. The commitment to fostering environments
conducive to wellbeing, mental health, and inclusive, sustainable living is pivotal in the evolution of holistic education and public health
paradigms.

Advancing Wellbeing through Design

Incorporating biophilic designs into university master planning and
campus design necessitates the participation of the entire university
community, aligning with the holistic and inclusive perspectives of the
Okanagan Charter. Dooris and Doherty (2010) advocated for a whole system
approach, emphasizing its indispensability in achieving comprehensive
and effective implementation. This approach aligns with the Okanagan
Charter's call for embedding health into all aspects of campus culture
across administration, operations, and academic mandates.

The Fundamental Role of Multilevel Collaboration and Stakeholder Engagement

Realizing such a transformative approach requires extensive, multilevel
collaboration to orchestrate substantial change involving senior university leadership. Such collaborations are instrumental in fostering a collective ethos where health is perceived as a shared responsibility. This
principle resonates with the Okanagan Charter, reinforcing the commitment to cultivating wellbeing within campus environments and emphasizing the collective action of all university constituents and stakeholders.

A pivotal factor in the seamless execution of wellbeing-focused design
is resilient institutional support and stakeholder engagement. Universities must bring together various stakeholders and gather additional
information to determine the willingness of universities to learn and
improve such wide-scale efforts in design and planning. This effort is in

sync with the Okanagan Charter's emphasis on creating supportive environments, acknowledging the intricate interplay between individual, societal, and environmental components.

Critical Considerations for Institutional Transformation

Poland et al., (2009) developed salient queries when determining institutional changes in health care settings, and they are similarly applicable in higher education institutions:

1 Identification of Stakeholders: Who are the primary stakeholders influencing or impacted by this setting?
2 Evaluation of Agendas and Resources: What agendas, stakes in change or the status quo, and resource accessibility do they hold?
3 Functions of the Settings: What are the varied functions of this environment for different stakeholders (students, staff, faculty, and local community members)?
4 Analysis of Absentees: Who is absent from this environment and why?
5 Perceptions of Health: How do different stakeholders perceive health and its significance?
6 Understanding and Action on Determinants of Health: How are the determinants of health and wellbeing interpreted and addressed in this setting?

Exploring the answers to these questions involves a thorough exploration and collaboration across various university domains, presenting substantial challenges in assembling stakeholders, overseeing progress, and fostering a common agenda. Universities must consider the implications of building a sustainable infrastructure to administratively support pursuing university-wide holistic change in designing health promoting environments. Coherent organizational structures are vital to support the institutional and cultural modifications essential for embedding health and wellbeing. The early identification and implementation of such structures are crucial for enduring sustainability, reflecting the Okanagan Charter's principles of sustainability, health, and wellbeing.

As the Okanagan Charter highlights, the endeavour to holistically integrate wellbeing through design involves multilevel collaborations, institutional support, and the incorporation of varied perspectives. The commitment to this extensive, inclusive approach ensures the longevity and efficacy of health promoting biophilic designs within university environments, contributing to the overarching objective of fostering holistic wellbeing and sustainability.

Conclusion

Significance of Learning Environments in Higher Education

College and university environments are unique places with a particular purpose: student learning. Student learning encompasses the holistic experiences of human development, social engagement, and wellbeing. The Okanagan Charter accentuates the integration of health and sustainability in post-secondary institutions, and these environments, inherently complex and varied in scale, can epitomize these principles. This variation in built environments, spanning from the intricate design of classrooms to the expansive layouts of entire campuses, necessitates comprehensive, systems-level approaches to manifest learning environments' ideals, as Strange and Banning (2001) emphasized. Common themes from the literature include access to natural and circadian electrical lighting, views, connections to nature (biophilia), indoor air quality, control of one's environment, and spatial layout.

A Harmonious Interplay of Design and Wellbeing

The built environment serves a dual role, optimizing learning processes and fostering essential skills and experiences paramount for achieving holistic wellbeing. This dual nature, grounded in the settings approach to health promotion as posited by Poland, Krupa, and McCall (2009), substantiates the creation of supportive environments as a foundation for promoting health and wellbeing. Furthermore, the physical environment contributes to college students' learning wellbeing in two fundamental ways. First, the essential features of the physical environment can encourage or discourage learning processes, ways in which students engage with each other, and decisions that impact behavioural outcomes. Second, designing college and university campus physical environments can also promote acquiring skills and experiences necessary to learning and achieving greater wellbeing. Supported by Poland, Krupa, and McCall (2009, 513), "a settings approach is an attractive and eminently feasible route to health promotion," and creating supportive environments is a building block of health promotion.

Biophilic Design: A Strategy to Enhanced Wellbeing

Biophilic design is the "deliberate attempt to translate an understanding of the inherent human affinity with natural systems and processes – known as biophilia – into the design of the built environment" (Kellert et al., 2008, p. 1989). It is emphasized that "the positive experience of natural systems and processes in our buildings and constructed land-scapes remain critical to human performance and wellbeing" (Kellert et al., 2008, p. 1981). This design philosophy has evolved with diverse applications, particularly within health care settings, lending empirical evidence to its benefits on human health and wellbeing. However, there remains an opportunity to explore the impact of integrating biophilic design and natural elements within academic learning environments, especially in higher education and among colleges and university settings.

Forging Collaborative Partnerships for Sustainable Impact

Improving the built environment is a challenging task and requires the contributions of various stakeholders within a community, especially when making decisions about improving health. There is a gap and need for more work to understand and measure the impact of the built environment in higher education, especially when linking the built environment to the health, safety, and wellbeing of faculty, staff, and students. The synergies between university health promotion and student affairs practitioners, campus planners, and senior executive leaders can bring forth transformative changes across the university community, influencing various domains such as planning, infrastructure, transportation, recreation, and building design. Additionally, the convergence of diverse partnerships, including community organizations, public health departments, and local businesses, can significantly enhance the measurement and enhancement of built environments in higher education settings. Finally, these entities must engage with other aspects of social justice, equity, fairness, diversity, inclusion, and access to all resources, programs, and services related to wellbeing.

Advancing Health Promotion within Colleges and Universities

This imperative for transformative change aligns with the Okanagan Charter's call to action to embed health into all aspects of campus culture, academic mandates, and operational practices. The Charter provides a strategic framework, urging institutions to strive for excellence in promoting the health and wellbeing of people and the planet. It thus becomes a beacon guiding the holistic advancement of learning environments in colleges and universities, reinforcing the advancement of learning environments that are conducive to learning, holistic development, and the wellbeing of all stakeholders, thereby reflecting a profound understanding and application of health promotion and sustainability principles in higher education settings.

REFERENCES

American College Health Association. (2020). *American College Health Association-National College Health Assessment III: Reference Group Executive Summary Spring 2020.* American College Health Association.

Andris, C., & Lee, S. (2021). Romantic relationship and the built environment: A case study of a US college town. *Journal of Urbanism: International Research on Placemaking and Urban Sustainability, 17*(1), 47–68. https://doi.org/10.1080 /17549175.2021.2005117

Baum, A., & Paulus, P.B. (1987). Crowding. In D. Stokols & I. Altman I. (Eds.) *Handbook of environmental psychology* (pp. 533–70). Wiley.

Becker, F.D. (1995). *Workplace by design.* Jossey-Bass.

Bell, I.R., Baldwin, C.M., & Schottenfeld, R.S. (2001). Psychological sequelae of hazardous materials exposure. In J.B. Sullivan & G.R. Krieger, G.R. (Eds.) *Clinical environmental health and toxic exposures* (2nd ed., 404–12). Lippincott Williams and Wilkins.

Bowler, D.E., Buyung-Ali, L.M., Knight, T.M., & Pullin, A.S. (2010). A systematic review of evidence for the added benefits to health of exposure to natural environments. *BMC Public Health, 10,* 456. Retrieved from https://link .springer.com/content/pdf/10.1186/1471-2458-10-456.pdf

Boyer, E. (1987). *College: The undergraduate experience in America.* HarperCollins.

Brown, R.J., & Brown, I. (2005). The application of quality of life. *Journal of Intellectual Disability Research, 49*(10), 718–27. https://doi.org/10.1111 /j.1365-2788.2005.00740.x

Browning, W.D., Ryan, C.O., & Clancy, J.O. (2014). 14 patterns of biophilic design: Improving health & wellbeing in the built environment. Terrapin Bright Green. https://www.terrapinbrightgreen.com/wp-content /uploads/2014/04/14-Patterns-of-Biophilic-Design-Terrapin-2014e.pdf

Brownson, R.C., Hoehner, C.M., Day, K., Forsyth, A., & Sallis, J.F. (2009). Measuring the built environment for physical activity: State of the science. *American Journal of Preventive Medicine, 36*(4), S99-S123. https://doi.org /10.1016/j.amepre.2009.01.005.

Capaldi, C.A., Dopko, R.L., & Zelenski, J.M. (2014). The relationship between nature connectedness and happiness: A meta-analysis. *Frontiers in Psychology,* 976. https://www.frontiersin.org/journals/psychology/articles/10.3389 /fpsyg.2014.00976/full

Carr, S., Francis, M., Rivlin, L.G., & Stone, A.M. (1976). *Public space.* Cambridge University Press.

Centers for Disease Control and Prevention. (CDC). (2015). *The built environment: An assessment tool and manual.* National Center for Chronic Disease Prevention and Promotion, Division of Community Health. https:// www.cdc.gov/nccdphp/dnpao/state-local-programs/built-environment -assessment/pdfs/BuiltEnvironment-v3.pdf

Clayton, S. (2003). Environmental identity: A conceptual and operational definition. In S. Clayton and S. Opotow (Eds.), Identity and the natural environment: The psychological significance of nature (pp. 45–65). MIT Press.

Clements, R. (2004). An investigation of the status of outdoor play. *Contemporary Issues in Early Childhood, 5*, 68–80. https://doi.org/10.2304/ciec.2004.5.1.10

Cohen, S., & Spacapan, S. (1984). The social psychology of noise. In D.M. Jones, & A.J. Chapman (Eds.), Noise and society (pp. 221–45). Wiley.

Davis, J.L., Green, J.D., & Reed, A. (2009). Interdependence with the environment: Commitment, interconnectedness, and environmental behavior. *Journal of Environmental Psychology, 29*(2), 173–80. https://doi.org/10.1016/j.jenvp.2008.11.001

Diener, E. (2009). Subjective wellbeing. In E. Diener (Ed.), *The science of wellbeing: The collected works of Ed Diener* (vol. 37, pp. 11–58). Springer.

Diener, E., Emmons, R., Larsen, J., & Griffin, S. (1985). The satisfaction with life scale. *Journal of Personality Assessment, 49*(1), 71–5. https://doi.org/10.1207/s15327752jpa4901_13.

Dooris, M. (2006). Health promoting settings: future directions. *Promotion & Education, 1*(1), 2–4. https://doi.org/10.1177/10253823060130010101

Dooris, M. (2009). Holistic and sustainable health improvement: The contribution of the settings-based approach to health promotion. *Perspect Public Health, 129*(1), 29–36. https://doi.org/10.1177/1757913908098881

Dooris, M., & Doherty, S. (2010). Healthy universities – time for action: A qualitative research study exploring the potential for a national programme. *Health Promotion International, 25*(1), 94–106. https://doi.org10.1093/heapro/daq015

Dutcher, D.D., Finley, J.C., Luloff, A.E., & Buttolph Johnson, J. (2007). Connectivity with nature as a measure of environmental values. *Environment and Behavior, 39*(4), 474–93. https://doi.org/10.1177/0013916506298794

Evans, G.W., Wells, N.W., & Moch, A. (2003). Housing and mental health: A review of the evidence and a methodological and conceptual critique. *Journal of Social Issues, 59*(3), 475–500. https://doi.org/10.1111/1540-4560.00074

Forgeard, M.J.C., Jayawickreme, E., Kern, M.L., & Seligman, M.E. (2011). Doing the right thing: Measuring wellbeing for public policy. *International Journal of Wellbeing, 1*(1), 79–106. https://doi.org/10.5502/ijw.v1i1.15

Gascon, M., Triguero-Mas, M., Martinez, D., Dadvand, P., Forns, J., Plasencia, A., & Nieuwenhuijsen, M.J. (2015). Mental health benefits of long-term exposure to residential green and blue spaces: A systematic review. *International Journal of Environmental Research and Public Health, 12*(4), 4354–79. https://doi.org/10.3390/ijerph120404354

Gibbs, T.A. (2017). *Striving for wellness: An exploration of motivation, goal pursuits, and wellbeing in an online educational environment* [Doctoral dissertation, Ohio State University].

Hancock, T. (1985). Beyond health care: From public health policy to healthy public policy. *Canadian Journal of Public Health, 76*(Suppl 1), 9–11.

Handy, S.L., Boarnet, M.G., Ewing, R., Killingsworth, R.E. (2002). How the built environment affects physical activity: Views from urban planning. *American Journal of Preventive Medicine, 32*(2, Suppl 1), 64–73. https://doi.org/10.1016/S0749-3797(02)00475-0

Hayes, N., & Joseph, S. (2003). Big 5 correlates of three measures of subjective wellbeing. *Personality and Differences, 34*(4), 723–27. https://doi.org/10.1016/S0191-8869(02)00057-0

Helliwell, J., Layard, R., Sachs, J., & De Neve, J.E. (2020). *World happiness report 2020.* New York: Sustainable Development Solutions Network. https://worldhappiness.report/ed/2020/

Joye, Y., & van den Berg, A.E. (2012). Restorative environments. In S. Clayton (Ed.), *The Oxford handbook of environmental and conservation psychology* (pp. 57–66). Oxford University Press. https://onlinelibrary.wiley.com/doi/10.1002/9781119241072.ch7

Kahnemann, D. (1999). Objective happiness. In D. Kahneman, E. Diener, and N. Schwarz (Eds.), *Wellbeing: The foundations of hedonic psychology* (3–25). Sage

Kals, E., Schumacher, D., and Montada, L. (1999). Emotional affinity toward nature as a motivational basis to protect nature. *Environment and Behavior, 31*(2), 178–202. https://doi.org/10.1177/00139169921972056

Kaplan, R., & Kaplan, S. (1989). *The experience of nature.* Cambridge University Press.

Karmeniemi, M., Lankila, T., Ikaheimo, T., Koivumaa-Honkanen, H., & Korpelainen, R. (2018). The built environment as a determinant of physical activity: A systematic review of longitudinal studies and natural experiments. *Annals of Behavioral Medicine, 52*(3), 239–51. https://doi.org/10.1093/abm/kax043

Kellert, S. (1997). *Kinship to mastery: Biophilia in human evolution and development.* Island Press.

Kellert, S. (2018). *Nature by design: The practice of biophilic design.* Yale University Press.

Kellert, S., & Calabrese, E.F. (2015). The practice of biophilic design. https://www.biophilic-design.com/_files/ugd/21459d_81ccb84caf6d4bee8195f9b5af92d8f4.pdf

Kellert, S.R., Heerwagen, J., & Mador, M.L. (2008). *Biophilic design: The theory, science, and practice of ringing buildings to life.* Wiley.

Kickbusch, I. (1996). Tribute to Aaron Antonovsky – "What creates health." *Health Promotion International, 11*(1), 5–6. https://doi.org/10.1093/heapro/11.1.5

Kuo, F. (2010). *Parks and other green environments: Essential components of a health human habitat.* National Recreation and Parks Association.

LaFountaine, J., Neisen, M, & Parsons, R. (2006). Wellness factors in first year college students. *American Journal of Health Studies, 21*(3/4), 214–18.

Larsen, L., Adams, J., Deal, B., Kweon, B.S., & Tyler, E. (1998). Plants in the workplace. *Environmental Behavior, 30*(3), 261–81. https://doi.org/10.1177/001391659803000301

Lercher, P., Evans, G.W., Meis, M., & Kofler, W. (2002). Ambient neighborhood noise and children's mental health. *Occupational Environmental Medicine, 59*, 380–6. https://doi.org/10.1136/oem.59.6.380.

Louv, R. (2012). *The nature principle: Reconnecting with life in a virtual age.* Algonquin Press.

Lyubormirsky, S., & Lepper, H. (1999). A measure of subjective happiness: Preliminary reliability and construct validation. *Social Indicators Research, 46,* 137–55. https://doi.org/10.1023/A:1006824100041

MacKerron, G., and Mourato, S. (2013). Happiness is greater in natural environments. *Global Environmental Change, 23*(5), 992–1000. https://doi.org/10.1016/j.gloenvcha.2013.03.010

Marcus, C.M., & Sachs, N.A. (2014). *Therapeutic landscapes: An evidence-based approach to designing healting gardens and restorative outdoor spaces.* Wiley.

Mayer, F.S., & Frantz, C.M. (2004). The connectedness to nature scale: A measure of individuals' feelings in community with nature. *Journal of Environmental Psychology, 24*(4), 503–15. https://doi.org/10.1016/j.jenvp.2004.10.001

McCoy, J.M. (2002). Work environments. In R.B. Bechtel, & A. Churchman (Eds.), *Handbook of environmental psychology* (2nd ed., pp. 443–60). Wiley.

Myers, J.E., & Sweeney, T.J. (2008). Wellness counseling: The evidence base for practice. *Journal of Counseling and Development, 86*(4), 482–93. https://doi.org/10.1002/j.1556-6678.2008.tb00536.x

NIRSA: Leaders in Collegiate Recreation, NASPA-Student Affairs Administrators in Higher Education & ACHA-American College Health Association (2020, November). Inter-association definition of wellbeing.

Nisbet, E.K., & Zelenski, J.M. (2011). Underestimating nearby nature: Affective forecasting errors obscure the happy path to sustainability. *Psychology and Science, 22*(9), 1101–6. https://doi.org/10.1177/0956797611418527

Nisbet, E.K., & Zelenski, J.M. (2013). The NR-6: A new brief measure of nature relatedness. *Frontier Psychology, 4,* 813. https://doi.org/10.3389/fpsyg.2013.00813

Nisbet, E.K., Zelenski, J.M., & Murphy, S.A. (2009). The nature relatedness scale: Linking individuals' connection with nature to environmental concern and behavior. *Environment and Behavior, 41*(5), 715–40. https://doi.org/10.1177/0013916508318748

Okanagan Charter: An International Charter for Health Promoting Universities and Colleges. (2015). *Okanagan Charter.* Kelowna, BC: Author. Retrieved from http://internationalhealthycampuses2015.sites.olt.ubc.ca/files/2016/01/Okanagan-Charter-January13v2.pdf

Oswalt, S.B., Lederer, A.M., Chestnut-Steich, K., Day, C., Halbritter, A., & Ortiz, D. (2020). Trends in college students' mental health diagnoses and utilization of services, 2009–2015. *Journal of American College Health, 68*(1), 41–51. https://doi.org/10.1080/07448481.2018.1515748

Poland, B., Krupa, G., & McCall, D. (2009). Settings for health promotion: An analytic framework to guide intervention design and implementation. *Health Promotion Practice, 10*(4), 505–16. https://doi.org/10.1177/1524839909341025

Richard, L., Potvin, L., Kischuk, N., Prlic, H., & Green, L.W. (1996). Assessment of the integration of the ecological approach in health promotion programs. *American Journal of Health Promotion, 10*(4), 318–28. https://doi.org/10.4278/0890-1171-10.4.318

Roös, P. (2017). *Regenerative-adaptive design for coastal settlements: A pattern language approach to future resilience* [Doctoral dissertation, Deakin University]. Retrieved from https://dro.deakin.edu.au/articles/thesis/Regenerative-adaptive_design_for_coastal_settlements_a_pattern_language_approach_to_future_resilience/21111577/1/files/37454746.pdf

Ryff, C.D. (1995). Psychological wellbeing in adult life. *Current Directions in Psychological Science, 4*(4), 99–104. https://doi.org/10.1111/1467-8721.ep10772395

Ryff, C.D., & Keyes, C.L. (1995). The structure of psychological wellbeing revisited. *Journal of Personality and Social Psychology, 69*(4), 719–27. https://doi.org/10.1037//0022-3514.69.4.719

Schultz, P.W. (2001). The structure of environmental concern: Concern for self, other people, and the biosphere. *Journal of Environmental Psychology, 21*(4), 327–39. https://doi.org/10.1006/jevp.2001.0227

Schwartz, R., & Stewart, D.-L. (2017). The history of student affairs. In V. Torres., S. Jones, & J.H. Schum (Eds.), *Student services: A handbook for the profession* (6th ed., pp. 20–38). John Wiley & Sons.

Seligman, M. (2011). *Flourish: A visionary new understanding of happiness and wellbeing.* Free Press.

Seymour, M. (2016). *Nature and environment in modern architecture.* Routledge.

Son, C., Hegde, S., Smith, A., Wang, X., & Sasangohar, F. (2020). Effects of COVID-19 on college students' mental health in the United States: Interview survey study. *Journal of Medical Internet Research, 22*(9), e21279. https://doi.org/10.2196/21279

Srivastava, K. (2009). Urbanization and mental health. *Industrial Psychiatry Journal, 18*(2), 75–6. https://doi.org/10.4103/0972-6748.64028

Strange, C.C., & Banning, J.H. (2001). *Educating by design: Creating campus learning environments that work.* Jossey-Bass Higher and Adult Education Series. Jossey-Bass.

Sturner, W.F. (1973). The college environment. In D.W. Vermilye (Ed.), *The future in the making* (pp. 71–86). Jossey-Bass.

Taylor, A. (2001). Coping with ADD: The surprising connection to green places. *Environment and Behavior, 33*(1), 54–77. https://doi.org/10.1177/00139160121972864

Travia, R.M., Larcus, J.G., Thibodeau, K.R., Hutchinson, C.R., Wall, A., & Brocato, N. (2021). *Measuring wellbeing in a college campus setting.* American College Health Foundation. Retrieved from https://www.acha.org/documents/Resources/Guidelines/Measuring_Wellbeing_In_A_College_Campus_Setting_White_Paper.pdf

Thelin, J.R., & Yankovich, J. (1987). Bricks and mortar: Architecture and the study of higher education. In J.C. Smart (Ed.), *Higher education: Handbook of theory and research* (vol. 3, pp. 57–83). Agathon Press.

Ulrich, R.S. (1984). View through a window may influence recovery from surgery. *Science, 224*(4647), 420–1. https://doi.org/10.1126/science.6143402

Ulrich, R.S. (1993). Biophilia, biophobia, and natural landscapes. In S.R. Kellert & E.O. Wilson (Eds.), *The biophilia hypothesis* (73–137). Island Press.

Ulrich, R.S. (2008). Biophilic theory and research for health care design. In S.R. Kellert et al. (Eds.), *Biophilic design* (87–106). Wiley.

United Nations General Assembly. (2013). *Happiness: Towards a holistic approach to development.* Retrieved from https://www.un.org/esa/socdev/ageing/documents/NOTEONHAPPINESSFINALCLEAN.pdf

Watson, D., Clark, L.A., & Tellegen, A. (1988). Development and validation of brief measures of positive and negative affect: The PANAS scales. *Journal of Perspectives in Social Psychology, 54*(6), 1063–70. https://doi.org/10.1037//0022-3514.54.6.1063

Wells, N., & Rollings, K. (2012). The natural environment: Influences on human health and function. In S. Clayton (Ed.), *The Oxford handbook of environmental and conservation psychology* (pp. 509–23). Oxford University Press.

World Health Organization (WHO). (1986). *Ottawa Charter for Health Promotion, 1986* (No. WHO/EURO: 1986-4044-43803-61677). WHO. Regional Office for Europe.

World Health Organization (WHO). (2016). *Shanghai Declaration on Promoting Health in the 2030 Agenda for Sustainable Development.* Paper presented at 9th Global Conference on Health Promotion, 21–4 November, Shanghai.

World Health Organization (WHO). (2021). *Geneva Charter for Wellbeing.* WHO 10th Global Conference on Health Promotion.

Wilson, E.O. (1986). *Biophilia: The human bond with ther species.* Harvard University Press.

Zusman, A. (2005). Challenges facing higher education in the twenty-first century. *American Higher Education in the Twenty-first Century: Social, Political, and Economic Challenges, 2,* 115–60.

11 Considerations for Developing a Healthy Campus Model: Adoption, Formulation, Implementation, and Evaluation

CHAD LONDON AND VICKI SQUIRES

Introduction

There is no disputing the pressing need to improve wellbeing on post-secondary campuses. The COVID-19 global pandemic has put wellbeing under a microscope, shining a light with newfound brightness on historical concerns around mental health, physical inactivity, food insecurity, inequality, substance abuse, environmental degradation, and the complexity and intersectionality of wellbeing (e.g., Dooris et al., 2020). The World Health Organization (1986) offered the following comment on wellbeing: "To reach a state of complete physical, mental, and social wellbeing, an individual or group must be able to identify and to realize aspirations, to satisfy needs, and to change or cope with the environment" (p. 1). Wellbeing is a holistic term encompassing all aspects of life and is comprised of multiple dimensions that need to be addressed (Dodge et al., 2012; Hayes & Joseph, 2003; Seligman, 2011).

More people with pre-existing mental health challenges are choosing to enrol in universities and colleges, which coincides with the onset of some mental disorders that occur during the ages (15–25) when many youths are enrolling (Mackean, 2011). The National College Health Assessment–Canadian Consortium (American College Health Association, 2016) conducted a survey with students on forty-one Canadian campuses, and results pointed to many alarming statistics. For example, 53.9 per cent of students reported feeling overwhelmed with the demands they were feeling in their lives at the time the survey was administered (American College Health Association, 2016). Although approximately 79 per cent of students felt that their campus had a sincere interest in their wellbeing, close to 18 per cent disagreed with that statement. Approximately 42 per cent of the students expressed that stress had negatively impacted their academics within the last twelve months (American

234 Chad London and Vicki Squires

College Health Association, 2016); 21 per cent felt that depression was having a negative impact on their academics within the same time frame, and 33 per cent noted the negative impact that anxiety had on their academic performance (American College Health Association, 2016). Perhaps most alarming was that 13 per cent had seriously considered suicide within the previous twelve months, including 3 per cent who had considered suicide within the previous two weeks (American College Health Association, 2016).

While mental health has been given the most attention in recent years, other dimensions of wellbeing have proven to be lacking in post-secondary students. Food insecurity is shockingly high among students, with 35 per cent reporting that as a crucial concern (Entz et al., 2017), and financial insecurity and employment status are also key issues (Britt et al., 2016; Qenani et al., 2014). Physical health has suffered because of the sedentary lifestyles of students (Herman, 2017; Tremblay et al., 2010), and lack of sleep and poor sleep quality are also contributing to poor health outcomes (Chaput et al., 2017).

Despite the need to address these health challenges, the work of embedding wellbeing into the daily life of campuses and communities has had difficulty gaining traction (Canadian Mental Health Association, 2020; Squires & London, 2022). Over the past thirty-five years there have been several attempts to provide wellbeing frameworks that governments, civil society, and post-secondary institutions can use to organize and inspire their efforts to improve wellbeing of their members and surrounding communities. From the Ottawa Charter for Health Promotion (WHO, 1986) and the Edmonton Charter for Health Promoting Universities and Institutions of Higher Education (WHO, 2006) to the Okanagan Charter: An International Charter for Health Promoting Universities and Colleges (Okanagan Charter, 2015), and more recently the United Nations 2030 Agenda for Sustainable Development (and its 17 Sustainable Development Goals) (UN, 2018) and the Geneva Charter for Wellbeing (WHO, 2021), post-secondary institutions have had decades of opportunity to transform themselves into health promoting campuses. While the scope and audience of those frameworks vary, each has served as a policy development model that universities and colleges can consider as they advance health, wellbeing, and sustainability on their campuses.

Dr. Mark Dooris and colleagues in the UK Health Promoting Universities Network (Dooris et al., 2010) developed a framework that was founded on many aspects of the various health promotion charters as a whole systems and settings-based approach for universities and colleges to promote wellbeing. A healthy settings approach was seen as a way to connect all of the higher education institutions and its community into a "whole," recognizing that the institution does not exist in isolation; rather, it is part of a system, located in a particular place, influenced by multiple sectors, and in part served by health-supporting organizations external to the university. Affecting human and ecological wellbeing are values underpinning the community, along with drivers of public health and the broader higher education system. Higher education institutions are encouraged to view wellbeing holistically, rather than as a disconnected set of services and programs, and to recognize the intersection of health determinants across social, economic, and environmental dimensions. The ultimate goal is to develop an ethos or way of being as a campus that embeds health promotion within the environment operationally and organizationally. This model is further described in Dolf and Dooris's chapter in this volume.

The Okanagan Charter

At the 2015 International Conference on Health Promoting Universities and Colleges held in Kelowna, British Columbia, participants developed a series of commitments and Calls to Action for post-secondary education institutions interested in promoting wellbeing (Okanagan Charter, 2015). Charter purposes include 1) guiding and inspiring action using a framework aligned with principles of Health Promoting Universities and Colleges; 2) generating dialogue and research that connects networks at all levels and that accelerates action; and 3) mobilizing action across sectors to integrate health in the policies and practices across organizations (Okanagan Charter, 2015, p. 3). Further details on the Calls to Action can also be found in Dolf and Dooris's chapter.

Building on the momentum realized in Kelowna at the 2015 international conference, the Canadian Health Promoting Campuses Network (CHPCN) was established in 2016 with the purpose of engaging post-secondary education institutions to advance the health promoting campuses movement across Canada (CHPCN, 2022). The network established a process whereby Canadian institutions of higher education could formally adopt the charter to strengthen their commitment to wellbeing and activate the calls to action. Institutions were encouraged to have a dialogue about the Okanagan Charter at all levels within their organization, engage senior leadership in developing Charter commitments tailored to their setting, and develop a written statement declaring those institutional commitments and have it signed by the top executive in their university. Those statements of adoption were reviewed by the CHPCN, and adoption of the Okanagan Charter was confirmed for the respective institution. The Okanagan Charter was initially formally adopted by six campuses, followed shortly thereafter by four others.

Examining Progress

We wanted to know how different campuses have applied the principles and the Calls to Action of the Okanagan Charter. We were curious about the different approaches signatory campuses had taken to implement the Charter. To better understand the stages of adoption and implementation, we organized the findings along the lines of policy development. However, there are differences between charters and policies. The use of the word "Charter" signals it is a "formal document describing the rights, aims, or principles of an organization or group of people" (Collins Dictionary, n.d.) Although a charter is not truly a policy, the framework suggested by Howlett et al. (2020) for studying policy cycles is helpful in structuring our conceptions of the implementation and evaluation of the Okanagan Charter commitments.

For the purposes of this study, we thought of the policy cycle as having four stages, based on the work of Howlett et al. (2020). The first stage is Policy Adoption, whereby a problem is recognized, possible solutions are proposed or examined, and a solution is determined using the tools or policy instruments available (Howlett et al., 2020). The second stage is Policy Formulation, where the solution is better articulated and a plan of action is crafted. The specific initiatives are then enacted in the Policy Implementation stage. The Policy Evaluation stage may occur at different times during implementation, and results can inform further action (Howlett et al., 2020).

Although the policy cycle model may suggest that the process is linear, it is most often iterative (Howlett et al., 2020). Squires (2010) proposed the process may be better conceived of as staged incremental transformation, with steady progress towards an end goal that can include transformative change. The process occurs through a series of intentional, incremental steps including ongoing evaluation and course correction where required (Squires, 2010). Using the policy cycle as a research framework, we explored the process followed by the first signatories of the Okanagan Charter; these campuses are identified in table 11.1. The institutions varied in geographic location from the west coast of British Columbia (UBC and Simon Fraser) to the east coast (Memorial University in St. John's, Newfoundland), the prairies (Universities of Lethbridge, Calgary, Saskatchewan, and Mount Royal University), and in central Canada (University of Guelph, and Western University and King's University College in London, Ontario). Some were in large metropolitan cities and others in smaller centres closely connected to rural communities. They varied in terms of total enrolment and demographics, mandate (comprehensive or undergraduate), and research intensity.

Campus websites, publicly available documents, and specific campus resources were explored to determine how their health promotion

Table 11.1. Two Stages of Signatory Campuses

First Stage of Signatory Campuses (2015)	Second Stage of Signatory Campuses (2016 – 2017)
University of British Columbia	University of Saskatchewan
Simon Fraser University	University of Guelph
Mount Royal University	King's University College
University of Lethbridge	Western University
University of Calgary	
Memorial University	

efforts were communicated to internal and external audiences. Institutional vision and mission statements, and strategic plans, were examined to look for references to wellbeing, health, and the Okanagan Charter. Only two of the ten featured wellbeing prominently in their strategic plans, although all ten made reference to wellbeing as a value or priority. Even though the institutions had formally adopted the Okanagan Charter within the two years preceding data collection, there was limited publicly available information related to the charter, other than press releases and announcements promoting the signing ceremony itself. Primarily, we relied on conversations with people on these campuses, and our discussions revealed a lot more about the journey to sign the Charter and the actions that followed. We believe the conversations we had provide some very important insights that may assist other campuses in the future with designing fulsome health promotion plans. First, we will provide an overview of our review of documents and then relate it to our conversations with key leaders and champions from signatory campuses.

Documents and Websites

A few key themes became apparent. First, we discovered that the term "Okanagan Charter" was not commonly used. Wellbeing and wellness generated many topics, and if the Okanagan Charter was mentioned, it was within the context of the university's wellness strategy. Most often, searching the terms "wellbeing" and "wellness" brought up the services and programs available. These initiatives and services were primarily for serving students and were aimed at treatment and intervention rather than promotion of health and wellbeing and prevention of issues. While there may be well-planned and implemented initiatives focused on health promotion on campuses, they are not usually highlighted in a central website location.

Second, most strategic planning documents did not explicitly refer to the Okanagan Charter. In only one institution's case, the Okanagan Charter was described within the plan and linked to a major strategic goal for the university. Furthermore, initiatives linked to this strategy were articulated more fully and targets and indicators for measuring progress on these goals were identified. Additionally, specific actions were described as examples of that strategy and links to associated plans and strategies were provided. However, this approach was the exception. Most often, there were separate wellness plans not explicitly tied into the campus-wide strategic plan. For example, one campus had posted a Wellness Strategy, another campus had developed a document for their mental health strategy, and another had conducted an audit of all wellness services, programs, and initiatives on their campus.

Third, most campuses had a media announcement when they became signatories of the Charter. For most, the story figured prominently on their campus website, and for a few campuses the local news outlets carried an item about signing the Okanagan Charter. Interestingly, entering the search term "Okanagan Charter" on a search engine platform currently results in many news releases about campuses signing the Charter, including the recent flurry of activity in the United States with more than thirty-two campuses signing on since August 2021. However, there were no publicly posted updates on campus progress towards achieving the commitments articulated in the Okanagan Charter.

Fourth, senior leaders did not appear to comment on the Okanagan Charter or wellbeing strategies. The one exception was that same campus that had a well-articulated strategy connected to the Charter. The president alluded to the Okanagan Charter in several documents and communications. He emphasized the importance of wellbeing for all students, staff, and faculty and reiterated the campus's commitment at any opportunity he had, including in strategic plan updates, president's office blogs, and even convocation addresses.

Overall, one campus had communicated the commitment of the university to implementing the Okanagan Charter, explicitly connecting it to strategic goals as well as indicating targets and indicators to measure progress. Only through our semi-structured interviews were we able to generate much information about the campus-level work being conducted to address the commitments outlined in the Okanagan Charter.

Our Conversations

We talked to thirteen participants who provided various perspectives on the adoption and implementation of the Okanagan Charter. We are using pseudonyms for the participants' names and have numbered the campuses as there were four campuses where we interviewed two people (see table 11.2). Of the ten campuses, there was one campus where we

Table 11.2. Pseudonyms of Our Campus Leaders

Campus	Pseudonyms
1	Richard
2	Luke
	Celeste
3	Elise
	Claire
4	Paul
	Blair
5	Lori
6	Thomas
7	Jennifer
8	Andrea
9	Katherine
	Stephanie
10	No respondents

struggled to find someone who would be able to have a conversation with us. As a result, the data represent our conversations with people from nine out of the ten campuses.

We used the stages of the policy cycle to organize the data generated from our discussions; key themes emerged as outlined in table 11.3 and will be described in more detail in subsequent sections.

Adoption

In describing our findings, it is important to note that in Canada, provincial governments have jurisdiction over both health and education. The federal government has some influence through funding of capital projects and financial support of research and government priorities, but the provincial governments set priorities and fund the post-secondary systems. Some campuses were already invested in wellbeing work, including programs such as Healthy Campus, and several provincial governments were particularly supportive of wellbeing and mental health programs. Specifically, the Alberta and British Columbia governments had invested in mental health initiatives and health promotion programming, and at the time of the study, both provincial ministries of advanced education identified several wellbeing priorities that they expected post-secondary institutions to address, and the ministries aligned financial resources to support work on those priorities.

Table 11.3. Key Themes Generated from Our Conversations

Adoption		
Initial interest	Support from leaders	Executive leadership were interested in the Charter
	Connection to the International Union for Health Promotion and Education congress	Key champion attended the 2015 conference where the Okanagan Charter was developed
Formulation		
Determination to become a signatory	Calls to Action and Commitments examined	Determination of campus-specific initiatives that address the Charter commitments and Calls to Action
	Signing of the charter	News release and celebration of signing
	Develop plan and responsibilities	
	Inclusion of commitments in institutional strategic plans	
Implementation		
Focus on all	Coordinated efforts across students, staff, and faculty	Joint work on initiatives that connect to all constituents, complemented by work on constituent specific initiatives
Leadership	Supportive leadership and engaged champions	Authentic engagement in planning and implementation
	All levels of the institution represented	Steering committee includes leadership and representatives from administrative and academic units, student groups
	Collaborative leadership	Well-articulated leadership structure
	Joined up approach	Each group knows what the others are doing, and they work collaboratively on many initiatives
Resources	Dedicated financial resources	Funds for ongoing work and for grassroots initiatives
	Dedicated human resources	Director or office charged with coordination
		Part of someone's accountabilities
Communication	Embedded in key documents	Inclusion in strategic plans
	Topic visible across institution	Wellbeing strategy is evident on website, is referred to at speeches, events
	Intentional and strategic	Planned messages to units and to all constituents

Evaluation	
Plan contains detailed goals and milestones	Timeline and specific goals are well articulated
	Progress is noted; goals revised if necessary
Periodic review of progress	Score cards or progress reports are constructed

Challenges	
Change of leaders	Priorities as chosen by executive leadership can change especially with sudden change
	Loss of champions
Lack of resources	Everything done off the sides of people's desks
	Key connecting people or departments not identified
Continued siloed approaches	No mechanism to join up approaches
Poorly articulated goals	Goals may be vague or not well described
Focus on students only	Minimal attention to employee wellbeing

Because of this context, some institutions were part of the organizing of the 2015 International Conference on Health Promoting Universities and Colleges in Kelowna, where the Okanagan Charter was developed. Several executive leaders on campus had heard about the conference and supported key people to attend the conference. Moreover, a few of the executive senior leaders (presidents and provosts) also attended the conference and were involved in the crafting of the plan. The attendees then returned to their campuses and communicated the progress. Six institutions were the initial signatories to the charter with four more campuses signing the next year. In one case, a champion of the Charter moved from one of the original signatory campuses to another campus that subsequently signed the Charter in the next round.

For example, Paul noted that the IUHPE coincided with the development of a Wellness Strategy for University 4, so it was easy to consider the commitments of the Okanagan Charter as the strategy was being developed. For Stephanie, the campus leadership was already engaged in conversations about elevating wellbeing as a priority and embedding it in their work campus-wide; they happened to hear about the conference and sent a delegate to participate in the development of the Charter. Among the participants of this study, Jennifer, Luke, Andrea, Celeste, and Lori attended the IUHPE conference and were part of the development of the Okanagan Charter.

Luke pointed out that the Charter was a "powerful document" because it is a "simple framework, something that people can understand and implement relatively easily." Richard articulated that "The principles of the Charter were speaking towards environment, setting conditions that are positive rather than always this focus on eradicating issues and then shifting the responsibility... I just saw so much more potential for having this shift of policy towards wellness." In signing the Charter, Richard believed that the institution was accountable rather than any individual directors or leaders.

Thomas stated that at University 6, the principles of the Okanagan Charter and the approach to promoting wellbeing within a campus "very much aligned with my beliefs and where we aligned as an organization." Furthermore, on their campus, the former principal "was a big champion of mental health and wellness, so there was a significant senior buy-in to this as something that was critical to its adoption." For University 9, Katherine recounted the involvement of the Associate Vice President of Student Affairs who spearheaded the effort to gain commitment across campus and sign the Charter.

Jennifer reiterated this sentiment, noting that signing the Okanagan Charter demonstrated their "commitment to the wellbeing of our campus community. They saw it as a tool to further some of the work on the campus." Furthermore, according to Jennifer, University 7 had "a strong focus on the student experience and supporting the whole student as well as the campus community at large. So I think it just resonated with our campus and with our culture here." The timing worked well, as Jennifer explained:

> [W]hen we initially signed on, we had listed five different commitments that we had been making, so there was firstly a commitment to support the inclusion of wellbeing in the University strategic planning processes. Secondly, a commitment to promote wellbeing and priority areas identified by the healthy campus steering committee. Thirdly, a commitment to invest new and ongoing funds into wellbeing through allocations to campus programs, services and process to support and foster campus wellbeing. Fourth, a commitment to evaluate and report on health promotion outcomes. And fifth, a commitment to convey conversations and share best practices across Canadian and International campuses.

The Okanagan Charter provided a framework for their wellbeing work on their campus. Interestingly, most of their strategic plans and action plans did not explicitly name the Okanagan Charter commitments as being linked to the goals and initiatives; the academic plan was the exception and referred to the commitments of the Okanagan Charter.

For several participants, the Charter was refreshingly about whole campus approaches rather than health promotion in isolated silos; Celeste mentioned that it was a broader approach to wellbeing and there was "still space for contributions from the broader community" in crafting the final Charter language. From her perspective, "health promotion needs to be rooted in the local context of wherever it is you're doing that work"; she was pleased that the idea of connection to the local context was embedded in the final draft.

Formulation

According to the participants, once executive leadership determined that they wanted to be a signatory of the Okanagan Charter, they needed to determine how the campus would connect the programming, plans, and initiatives in alignment with the commitments and Calls to Action of the Charter. Once they had developed a plan, they organized a formal signing of the Charter. Most often, the signing was heralded through a media release that described the Okanagan Charter and how the campus was going to support the implementation of the Charter commitments within their context.

Designing the campus plan to address the Charter commitments was a crucial step in establishing the enthusiasm, energy, and motivation for addressing campus goals. Richard posited that the Charter was "a highly abstract document that has tremendous power if you can get some design people around it with a good sense of implementation strategy but also with a courage to risk and fail because if they are too careful you might not do anything that grabs attention or excites people or activates this and it can become vanilla. So part of what has to be built into this is a kind of energy filled with hope and inspiration and conviction that we can always do better." The positive framing was an important element of the Charter.

Stephanie noted that the Calls to Action informed how they framed their wellbeing efforts; however, the campus leaders were also constructing their campus-specific actions and targets based on standards from different organizations and commissions such as Healthy Workplace Standards. Katherine added that the focus was on supporting the wellbeing of the whole person, which has implications for the range of actions being considered. At Elise and Claire's campus, the Okanagan Charter was tightly connected to their development and framing of a campus mental health strategy. The recently crafted strategic plan at their campus also embedded the Charter and wellbeing into the plan, making wellness a foundational priority for the whole campus.

Several campuses embedded wellbeing into their strategic plans. Andrea, Luke, Celeste, Lori, Katherine, and Jennifer made this point; Andrea added that the press release about signing the Charter was important, but "where it started to impact more was when it got added to the Strategic Plan and the measures of our strategic plan." Lori noted that they had been engaged in work "which had very similar principles and themes that are outlined in the Charter, but it was important to us that our university sign onto the Charter because it gave greater weight in terms of the importance of work that we were doing." She emphasized that the principles were all about "systemic and collaborative action" and the whole campus approach was essential. Interestingly, Luke stated that people attending community consultations held prior to the work of the Charter strongly identified wellbeing as one of their top priorities. They also developed commitments to support the plan, including one which was "a commitment to collaborate with community members to embed wellbeing into all organizational plans, policies, practices and strategies." There had been ongoing work in different units on campus, according to Luke, but the framework drew together all of this work into a more coherent and comprehensive approach.

In crafting their own institutional commitments to align with the Okanagan Charter, most campuses focused on the campus community.

However, several campuses included the broader community; for example, Jennifer noted that their plans identified how they were "strategically partnering with external community agencies to support wellbeing on campus." Lori, Katherine, Stephanie, and Luke added that they were working with community connections, the city, and the provincial ministry on furthering these initiatives. Additionally, Lori had connections with several other organizations that were signatories to or interested in the work of the Charter. Being liaisons with the national and international networks was also a significant linkage to the broader health promoting campus community. Lori, Luke, Jennifer, and Andrea all identified that they were part of these two larger networks.

Moreover, when developing their institutional commitments, Celeste believed it was less important for constituents such as students to know where the commitment was coming from, but it was more important to focus on what the university was doing. The strategic plan and the associated targets needed to be explicit. For example, University 2 had developed a target around decreasing food insecurity. Celeste referred to the Charter instead as a "set foundation piece, like this is something the university has committed to, and I always share the calls to action, especially the Call to Action Number One about talking about embedding wellbeing across the institution and putting in academic mandates and so I do use it as almost like a bit of a rationale if you will for the work that we're doing." Lori supported this idea and noted that the Charter was a tool for helping people work towards wellbeing. Referring to the Charter adds a lot of credibility to the work, according to Lori, so it provides a rationale and a set piece.

Implementation

The focus of this study was the journey that each campus had as they began working on the initiatives. While some campuses had crafted a specific wellness or mental health strategy that was expressed as a "whole of campus" approach, most were focused on student-specific initiatives and strategies and were aimed at intervention rather than promotion. Even when speaking of employee wellness, Blair identified that the strategies were most often aimed at interventions and helping employees to get "back to optimal health sooner." He believed that on the prevention side, "there is a lot of work to do or a lot of discovery to happen there." Additionally, for prevention programs, campuses had to be careful that the participants were not only people who were healthy members of campus but that the program also appealed to others who were not at or close to optimal health, whether the programs are aimed at financial health, physical health, or mental health. Katherine noted that a key action item for their campus was to conduct "more research around how to embed wellness concepts and principles into policies and create and promote a wellness policy tool kit for employees."

In most cases, the senior executive leadership were not identified as champions of the approach; however, Andrea, Elise, Richard, and Luke all pointed out that their presidents were firm champions of the Charter. In one case, a particular office and director were obviously the connection point for all wellbeing initiatives; however, those champions were less obvious. Furthermore, some of the original champions, whether they were presidents or provosts or directors of the wellbeing offices, were no longer at that campus. In one such case, the work had completely stalled, according to one participant, and health promotion strategies were not evident on institutional websites or documents.

As was mentioned, for one campus we could not identify anyone at the time of our study who would have the information required to serve as a participant. In contrast, at Lori's campus, they intentionally built up and celebrated champions from across campus, profiling them on their website and highlighting what the champions were doing to create wellbeing within the learning environment. Interestingly, Stephanie pointed out that leadership matters; leaders set the tone and can model responses to challenges such as provincial government funding cuts with a calming approach. They can demonstrate a problem-solving approach to worrying (and sometimes quickly emergent) issues. Katherine added that "collaborative leadership is an important facilitator of health promotion success. I think it's really important in terms of collaborative leadership to have the students, faculty, and staff aligned going forward." There were several research collaborations and partnerships as well on Elise and Claire's campus, where faculty engaged in wellbeing focused research with service units and community organizations as well.

On campuses that were moving ahead with the work, a leader of the strategy or the unit was connected to the specific programs and initiatives. As Celeste pointed out, "you need someone on the ground to coordinate, facilitate, kind of that secretariat role to bring things forward." Furthermore, there was a structure that connected the various leaders in a coordinated mechanism to share ideas and progress to date. The wellbeing leadership was structured into collaborative teams with identified leaders and members of the campus drawn together into a steering committee to guide the work. Additionally, the collaborative leadership structure helped coordinate action into a joined-up approach where the intents and actions of wellbeing initiatives were communicated.

Students were seen by many participants as key champions of the wellbeing work on campus; Richard, Paul, Luke, Thomas, Jennifer,

Stephanie, Elise, and Lori all mentioned the central role students played in leading the wellbeing work. Students were also vocal advocates for promoting further initiatives and resources to support wellbeing. In fact, Luke mentioned that students had led the call for new developments regarding mental health. Claire remarked that the student peer mentors could connect with their fellow students more effectively and had had significant success with upstream initiatives such as campaigns targeted on sleeping well. At several campuses, though, students were less involved.

As noted in our discussion of key communications on websites and documents, some campuses had continued to build awareness of the Okanagan Charter and had strived to build engagement with the initiatives through targeted communication and inclusion of the message in core institutional documents such as strategic plans. Moreover, progress on those initiatives was described periodically. The Okanagan Charter was elevated in importance by inclusion in these documents. Messages about wellbeing needed to be communicated often. As Paul said, "You just keep on doing it but with a focus on quality that we don't just keep relentlessly pounding stuff out, but we do it in a coordinated way with the services but also the strategy." Thomas pointed out that the campus viewbooks included information about the Okanagan Charter and the university website was updated periodically "to help promote awareness." Blair also believed that the messages had to be thoughtfully created and distributed. Campuses needed to bring the message together in a "very coherent and compelling way"; furthermore, Blair said that "it is of great significance of how people react and actually act in response to messaging." Katherine emphasized that it was especially important to communicate to the employees and students what specifically the campus was doing to support their wellbeing. Elise contended that they were including social media strategies among their communication tools.

Thomas reiterated this point. He said that they needed to continue to educate people "about the importance of the Charter, the importance of how this links to our campus community and our overall strategic plan. We believe wellness is the foundation; health and wellness and promoting that is the foundation of any community." Luke also supported this notion and said that the Charter led to university-wide communication and engagement on this priority, leading to a "much bigger level of visibility than we ever had." Key to this growing awareness was having a centralized wellbeing website that drew information from all parts of campus together into one website that also highlighted the targets, milestones, tools, and resources. The website served as a way to connect the dots. Stephanie also pointed out that their campus was developing a website to update the campus and invite input; however, the website was under development at the time of this study. One thing their campus had done was develop a branding process for any employee wellness initiatives. The branding helped build awareness and engagement; Stephanie noted that the brand is recognizable among employees at that university.

Importantly, on campuses where progress on the work of the Okanagan Charter was evident, the participants spoke of the crucial support for the work through human and financial resources. Celeste said that University 2 made a substantial financial commitment to the area, and importantly, included wellbeing as part of their operational funding. Furthermore, the university learned through a consultative process that there should be "greater investment in prevention and upstream kind of approaches at the university," according to Celeste. Having a specific office to coordinate the work was tremendously important to maintain momentum, and having an identifiable connector or leader who was steering this work was equally critical. The campus community could connect with the office or the leader of this work. Specific accountabilities for the work were embedded not only in this campus leader's profile but also in the accountabilities of the campus senior leaders. For example, the president publicly reaffirmed his commitment to this work at every public opportunity and then followed up the commitment with resources. The people or offices tasked with implementation had a steering group to guide the work; often the steering group included senior leaders on campus.

Jennifer confirmed that their campus also had a steering committee; this committee was "responsible for working to create a campus environment that focuses on facilitating wellbeing, respect, and safety." The committee examined the Okanagan Charter and helped to align the Charter commitments with their work and priority areas. Representatives on this committee come from all over campus and include senior leaders, faculty, staff, and students. They also needed to ensure that everyone was aware "where people are doing this work, that there is connection," even though the committee was not "the keeper of everything that is happening." This structure was very similar to the one described by Katherine where there was wide representation from across campus on the Healthy Campus Advisory Committee. There was also an operational committee that gathered information and data to inform the development of goals. Elise and Claire identified that their campus had a similar implementation committee. Additionally, they had a programs subcommittee and an evaluation subcommittee. They also noted that they had alumni representation on the implementation committee, which was a unique comment in this study; they were starting conversations on how alumni engagement can be more meaningful for these individuals.

Evaluation

As researchers, we also wanted to know how campuses were measuring progress. We asked questions about what goals and targets were established for the campus and how they were going to report the progress to the campus. Most often, specific targets or milestones were not identified and no timelines were given for when the campus would review the commitments or their progress against their campus-specific goals.

However, there were leaders in evaluation and specific evaluation activities. At University 2, the campus articulated in detail on the website what the specific initiatives and actions were, the targets for that initiative, and the indicators that would be evident when progress had been made; this evaluation plan was publicly available on the website. However, the mechanism for measuring progress and reporting back was not as obvious, and there were no publicly available documents that marked progress in yearly intervals since the signing of the Charter. At University 1, Richard identified that they had developed a scorecard to display progress made on certain initiatives but that work was on hold for the time being. Lori noted that their campus was in the process of constructing targets and conducting evaluation; they had been communicating progress to the campus community via yearly reports, but lately had not produced these comprehensive statements.

Jennifer also described the detailed targets for their divisional plan, which was aligned with their campus strategic plan, and she pointed out that the government also had expectations that certain metrics were tracked. She said that there was an "eclectic mix of data sources" that their campus used. Similarly, Blair noted that their ICT (Information and Communication Technologies) unit was "actually creating dashboards in a variety of areas" and that periodic reporting against measures and metrics was an obligation as outlined in their wellness strategy. Much of the reporting would be aggregate measures in order to ensure privacy and confidentiality.

The measuring and the metrics used need to be intentional and meaningful so they can inform decision-making regarding next steps or programs, according to Paul. Richard supported this idea and said that "your evaluation is meaningless unless you have a goal that is meaningful. It's principled and is based on some sort of theoretically based solution." In so doing, he added that the focus is on supporting "the whole community to share responsibility for wellness." Luke agreed and said that they had to make decisions about which data to report on, with considerations of validation, strategic connections to initiatives, and usefulness of the data for future action; the data had to be "useful and translatable." The campus needed to focus on the most relevant data and then they had to do "a really good job of measuring regularly and reporting back regularly." Claire noted that their evaluation subcommittee was still working on which metrics to focus on and which metrics to include in the annual report that would be distributed to the Provost's committee and then the Board of Governors.

Intervention services such as numbers of visits are easy to track, but outcomes are harder to measure. Celeste also agreed with this point, saying that assessing impact and culture change is difficult. Additionally, the student population changes yearly, so campuses will need to monitor trends more than changes in individual students. She went on to explain, though, that it was "great to have some clear targets that we can collectively work towards ... it does help at the operation level to have some shared priorities, again just to help break down some of those existing silos." Claire added that they were going through a messy phase in evaluation trying to determine what metrics to include. For example, some measures are "really complex ... like how do you measure changed behaviours or changed feelings, awareness, and things like that." Elise also pointed out that showing the impact of an initiative was extremely difficult.

Thomas pointed out that their campus conducted a yearly audit of the programs and initiatives undertaken and identified any progress towards their wellbeing commitments. This audit was then used as a foundation for a yearly report to the governing bodies on campus, and it was also used to inform some budgetary decisions. The document also helped the campus identify that they needed to "be thinking about specialized populations on campus" and how to support their wellbeing. That process had led Thomas to wonder whether campuses could be certified publicly for enacting the Okanagan Charter, similar to the program used to certify energy sustainability of buildings.

In terms of evaluation, most activity seemed to concern outcomes and programs focused on students. Most participants pointed out the anticipated launch of the Canadian Campus Wellbeing Survey that had been developed. Luke described in more detail the development of the survey, led by a team of researchers from across the country, and the support of the provincial ministry that dedicated resources to the development and the piloting of the survey. Richard was especially appreciative that it had a positive focus as opposed to a deficits focus. (For more information on this survey, please see chapter 3 in this book, which focused on the CCWS.)

Challenges

Essentially, all the strengths seen in some campuses were mirrored opposites to the challenges experienced by several campuses. Thus, where the leading campus had engaged leadership and champions who knew how to be influential in galvanizing action, campuses that had shown little progression had changed leadership or lost their champions. For instance, according to Luke, on one campus one of the first leaders of the effort had died suddenly and the campus struggled to regain traction with the work of the Okanagan Charter. On Richard's campus, the president, who was very supportive of the work on wellbeing, was about to retire and the strategic planning had been put on hold, as had any planning for a specific wellness strategy. As a result, any kind of progress was slowed to a halt. Also, students played a large role in advocating for wellbeing programs and initiatives, but most students are there for only four or five years, and student leaders such as presidents hold their positions for only a year or two. The strength of the student voice on campus is dependent on the students who become involved in the wellbeing programs and who the student leaders on campus are.

Although some campuses had dedicated resources for both student and employee initiatives, other campuses were not so fortunate. In fact, Paul characterized the wellbeing initiatives as being run off the sides of their desks. Blair also noted the number of people who had turned over in the key positions responsible for leading particular employee or student programs. It seemed that the sense of urgency for addressing the wellbeing of staff and faculty was not as prevalent as it was for students at University 4. Although all campuses are facing fiscal constraints, some campuses were more challenged financially because of the funding and policies of the provincial governments, such as at University 1, which had a multi-year freeze on tuition levels.

Several participants pointed out that there needed to be further work on how to engage more faculty from across the campus in these conversations. Although some faculty were involved in steering committees and may be included in the planning, they often were from faculties traditionally connected to health and wellbeing. Moreover, campuses needed to determine how to further connect the Okanagan Charter commitments to the classrooms, with implications for both students and faculty, a point made by Jennifer and Paul.

Additionally, on campuses that struggled, there were no structures set in place to connect the work or share ideas. There were no opportunities for cross-unit discussions regarding the calls to action. There may be pockets of excellence in parts of the campus, but they were not necessarily highlighted or communicated to the rest of campus. Wellbeing was not elevated to the level of a strategic priority for these campuses. Even with campuses that had shown some progress, choosing to not include it in the strategic plan was seen as a missed opportunity; according to Paul, this was the case at his university.

For those campuses who had not progressed much in their work, there was not a road map evident. More specifically, the campuses may have completed an audit of their services and programs, but they had not determined goals or targets and thus did not have a way to describe any progress made. Also, Celeste noted that "the Charter and what it stands for is fundamentally in opposition to how universities work"; furthermore, "there has to be a cross campus coming together around this, again going back to that idea of health promotion needs to be rooted in the local context."

At some campuses, there had been a real focus on student supports, programs, and initiatives; employees and staff may be connected to wellbeing resources through employee resources. However, there were very few campuses where the campuses had strategies that were explicitly for all campus community members and that were focused on health promotion rather than health prevention initiatives or interventions.

As Jennifer noted, there may be many departments and programs focused on wellbeing, but doing this work at a cross-institutional level was very difficult. Furthermore, there may be competing priorities across the campus that added to the challenge of keeping this work at the forefront and engaging the whole campus. That was the issue at Andrea's campus, where funding a new building for a college had taken precedence in terms of attention and financial resources.

From the findings then, there were several outstanding themes that underpin this study. Even though all ten campuses were early signatories to the Okanagan Charter, there was huge variance among the universities regarding their progress in fulfilling their Charter commitments. Much of the variance could be attributed to the way the work was operationalized and communicated among the units on campus. The most critical element though, was the leadership for this priority area. The executive senior leadership needed to recognize the value of the work by elevating wellbeing to a strategic priority and then resourcing the priority area so that there were hubs of the work where ideas and initiatives could be connected and operationalized. In addition, there needed to be champions who could galvanize action and campus commitment through their dedication and passion for embedding wellness in everything the campus did. The leaders and champions should come from all constituents (staff, faculty, students) and should include formal and informal leaders throughout the organization.

Putting It into Context

The elements of Dooris et al.'s (2010) model for Health Promoting Universities were discussed in our conversations. Some people discussed the way the Charter framed the foundational underpinnings of health promotion. The values, the classroom environment, the need for leadership at all levels, the supporting policies and practices, the provincial context of their campuses, and the need to examine the whole campus community as part of the systems approach to promoting health were described in various ways by participants. The emphasis on leadership as a key driver of these efforts was identified by Dooris et al. (2021); they stated that "effective, authentic and credible senior-level leadership was understood to be a prerequisite for the successful implementation of a health promoting university initiative" (p. 305). Having wellbeing embedded in strategic plans was also essential for success. The focus on wellbeing was boosted by "finding appropriate entry points and windows of opportunity for agenda-setting; engaging with strategic planning cycles; utilizing the potential offered by organizational change; advocating for health to be both named as a responsibility within a senior leader's role and embedded in multiple roles across the university and learning to navigate the largescale and complex nature of universities" (Dooris et al., 2021, p. 305). Wellbeing needs to be embraced as a priority and embedded in the organizational systems. However, there is the "ongoing challenge of finding ways to translate the rhetoric of whole university and whole system approaches into meaningful action within large, complex and culturally diverse organizations" (Dooris et al., 2020, p. 739). Even with good intent, engaged leadership, and an organizing framework of the Okanagan Charter, most campuses still struggle with operationalization.

A key theme from our discussions was the need for culture change, from siloed pockets of excellence regarding health promotion to a connected and coherent framework. This structure would exemplify a whole campus approach where there are shared commitments and bridges are built between academia and operations to actualize those commitments and meet those targets. The framework galvanizes the action, and the connections inspire more actions and ideas. Luke captured this key foundation well, saying,

> There's a lot of opportunity to advance health promotion theory and how it's tailored to a campus setting. More and more researchers actually want to look at that specifically, so I think that's exciting, because we are a very unique context. Our size, our scope, our mandate allows for quite powerful change. That's one of the reasons that the World Health Organization was excited about the Charter, because they thought cities and campuses were an ideal scale to leverage change, so to prove that out and actually see whether that's the case would be interesting. So yeah, health promotion theory, campus scale and also I think a lot of the work that we've been

doing is Call to Action one, like changing our policies, practices, culture on campus, but what about the outreach with the broader community, engagement with them, change in international (engagement) maybe such as the Sustainable Development Goals.

The path forward is suggested by this quote. How do campuses and health promotion networks engage in 'joined up' approaches to improve the health and wellbeing outcomes on our campuses and then work with our communities to broaden the social impact? Furthermore, how do the national networks then work together globally to amplify the outcomes of the International Union for Health Promotion and Education in trying to achieve the United Nations SDGs?

Conclusion

Despite broad understanding and support for the expectation that higher education institutions need to do more to enhance wellbeing on their campuses, they seem to be struggling more than ever to address issues such as the mental health crisis of students. Wellbeing of faculty and staff is also a struggle, particularly through the COVID-19 pandemic.

However, insights provided through the health promoting universities model (Dooris et al., 2010) and the Okanagan Charter (2015) are gaining attention in the post-secondary education sector as efforts increase to improve wellbeing in holistic ways. Higher education institutions across the world can learn from leading universities that have extensive experience and success in implementing holistic wellbeing efforts and measuring their success. Exemplar universities in Canada have demonstrated the positive impact of adopting the Okanagan Charter; these campuses keep the importance of wellbeing visible and consistently present, support the crucial role of wellbeing champions and collaborative leadership, and invest human and financial resources into healthy campus initiatives. Higher education institutions can break down silos and create structures that facilitate collaboration and increase integration.

Through regional and global networks of health promoting universities, evidence-based resources are being shared and collaborative strategies are being developed. The emergence of a pan-national framework for Canadian universities (the Okanagan Charter) highlights promising practices and the role of policy development in promoting systemic change. While emerging from a global pandemic seems daunting, health promoting universities cannot merely survive, but flourish, by embedding wellbeing in all they do.

REFERENCES

American College Health Association. (2016). *American College Health Association–National College Health Assessment II: Canadian Reference Group Data Report Spring 2016.* American College Health Association.

Britt, SL., Mendiola, M.R., Schink, G.H., Tibbetts, R.H., & Jones, S.H. (2016). Financial stress, coping strategy, and academic achievement of college students. *Journal of Financial Counseling and Planning, 27*(2), 172–83.

Canadian Mental Health Association. (2020). *COVID 19 national survey dashboard.* Retrieved from: https://www.camh.ca/en/health-info/mental-health-and-covid-19/covid-19-national-survey

Chaput, J., Wong, S.L., & Michaud, I. (2017). Duration and quality of sleep among Canadians aged 18 to 79. *Health Reports, 28*(9), 28–33. Retrieved from www150.statcan.gc.ca

Dodge, R., Daly, A., Huyton, J., & Sanders, L. (2012). The challenge of defining wellbeing. *International Journal of Wellbeing, 2*(3), 222–35. https://doi.org/10.5502/ijw.v2i3.4

Dooris, M., Cawood, J., Doherty, S., & Powell, S. (2010). *Healthy universities: Concept, model and framework for applying the healthy settings approach within higher education in England.* Final project report http://www.healthyuniversities.ac.uk/wp-content/uploads/2016/10/HU-Final_Report-FINAL_v21.pdf

Dooris, M., Powell, S., & Farrier, A. (2020). Conceptualising the 'whole university' approach: An international qualitative study. *Health Promotion International, 35*(4), 730–40. https://doi.org/10.1093/heapro/daz072

Dooris, M., Powell, S., Parkin, D., & Farrier, A. (2021). Health promoting universities: Effective leadership for health, wellbeing and sustainability. *Health Education, 121*(3), 295–310. https://doi.org/10.1108/he-12-2020-0121

Entz, M., Slater, J., & Desmarais, A.A. (2017). Student food insecurity at the University of Manitoba. *Canadian Food Studies, 4*(1), 139–59. https://doi.org/10.15353/cfs-rcea.v4i1.204

Hayes, N., & Joseph, S. (2003). Big 5 correlates of three measures of subjective wellbeing. *Personality and Individual Differences, 34*(4), 723–7.

Herman, K.M. (2017). How did we get so sedentary? Sedentary behaviours among Canadian adults. *Alberta Centre for Active Living, 28*(4), 1–5. Retrieved from https://www.centre4activeliving.ca/media/filer_public/21/cc/21ccbb90-7210-4d43-973a-1ce5e70d542d/2017-apr-sedentary.pdf

Howlett, M., Ramesh, M., & Perl, A. (2020). *Studying public policy: Policy cycles & policy subsystems* (4th ed.). Oxford University Press.

MacKean, G. (2011). *Mental health and wellbeing in post-secondary education settings: A literature and environmental scan to support planning and action in Canada.* Canadian Association of College & University Student Services and Canadian Mental Health. https://www.athabascau.ca/mental-health/documents/mental_health_postsecondary_education.pdf

Okanagan Charter: An International Charter for Health Promoting Universities and Colleges. (2015). *Okanagan Charter*. Kelowna, BC: Author. Retrieved from http://internationalhealthycampuses2015.sites.olt.ubc.ca/files/2016/01/Okanagan-Charter-January13v2.pdf

Qenani, E., MacDougall, N., & Sexton, C. (2014). An empirical study of self-perceived employability: Improving the prospects for student employment success in an uncertain environment. *Active Learning in Higher Education, 15*(3), 199–213. https://doi.org/10.1177/1469787414544875

Seligman, M.E.P. (2011). *Flourish – A new understanding of happiness and wellbeing – and how to achieve them*. Nicholas Brealey Publishing.

Squires, V. (2010). *A policy study of the emergence of a joint interdisciplinary school* [Unpublished doctoral dissertation]. University of Saskatchewan.

Squires, V., & London, C. (2022). The Okanagan Charter: Evolution of health promotion in Canadian higher education. *Canadian Journal of Higher Education, 51*(3), 100–14. https://doi.org/10.47678/cjhe.vi0.189109

Tremblay, M.S., Colley, R.C., Saunders, T.J., Healy, G.N., & Owen, N. (2010). Physiological and health implications of a sedentary lifestyle. *Applied Physiology, Nutrition, and Metabolism, 35*(6), 725–40. https://doi.org/10.1139/h10-079

United Nations (UN). (2018). *The 2030 agenda and the sustainable development goals: An opportunity for Latin America and the Caribbean*. Retrieved from https://repositorio.cepal.org/bitstream/handle/11362/40156/25/S1801140_en.pdf

World Health Organization (WHO). (1986). *Ottawa charter for health promotion*. Retrieved from http://www.who.int/healthpromotion/conferences/previous/ottawa/en/index.html

World Health Organization (WHO). (2006). *The Edmonton Charter for Health Promoting Universities and Institutions of Higher Education*. World Health Organization. https://healthycampuses.ca/wp-content/uploads/2015/01/2005_Edmonton_Charter_HPU.pdf

World Health Organization (WHO). (2021). *The Geneva Charter for Wellbeing*. Retrieved from https://www.who.int/publications/m/item/the-geneva-charter-for-well-being

Conclusion: The Future of Health Promotion: Moving from Local and National to Global Wellbeing

VICKI SQUIRES

As evidenced in this book's chapters, a health promotion orientation can build capacity across the higher education sector to address complex problems such as climate change, colonialism, racism, food insecurity, sedentary behaviour, and mental illness, which are determinants of poor health and wellbeing outcomes. Health promotion also addresses inequities in health outcomes, which we saw become even more pronounced when the world experienced a global pandemic. Gaining traction with this agenda is difficult for many reasons, including the difficulty of explaining the dimensions of wellbeing and their interrelated impacts on overall health. Additionally, systems- and settings-based approaches require a shift of culture from thinking about the issue in siloed and discrete ways. For example, researchers have traditionally explored wellbeing from disciplinary perspectives, leading to numerous definitions and conceptual models. Structures for grants, tenure and promotion standards, disciplinary framing of research problems, and venues for dissemination all encourage exploration of wellbeing from specific viewpoints rather from joined-up or multi-disciplinary approaches. Universities are complex and expensive organizations, and as governments reduce their proportion of financial support, universities rely more on the market, adopting neo-liberal approaches. This competition for dollars and students reinforces disciplinary divisions rather than collaborative and interdisciplinary work (Eastman et al., 2022). The structure that supports academic self-governance "relies heavily on peer mechanisms and collegial control and tends to be unresponsive to demands for utility, applicability, and economic or social benefits" (Eastman et al., 2022, p. 333). Moreover, the structures inhibit interdisciplinary exploration even though the complex, multifaceted issues of our time are best served by multiple perspectives. Climate change, water and food security, and poverty are several examples of global challenges that cannot be investigated through one discipline.

Higher education is a critical setting in and "*through* which to promote health and wellbeing by harnessing and maximizing their wider potential to exert influence and serve as catalysts for societal change" (Cawood et al., 2010, p. 259). This notion of campuses being a catalyst setting to drive healthy communities is reiterated in the Okanagan Charter (2015): "health promoting universities and colleges transform the health and sustainability of our current and future societies, strengthen communities and contribute to the wellbeing of people, places and the planet" (p. 2). This volume of chapters argues that post-secondary campuses must act as that catalyst and that the Okanagan Charter provides a promising framework to organize that work at institutional, local, national, and global levels. More scholarship is needed to understand how health promoting universities can do that effectively. While there are many "pockets of excellence" within campuses, few successfully galvanize that into the strategic whole of a university approach with staying power. Nevertheless, there is strong agreement that the aspirational vision of the Okanagan Charter is crucial to promote the wellbeing of our people and planet today and in the future.

Throughout this book, the authors made connections to how we can move the health promotion agenda forward. In their contributions, most authors focused on specific health promotion topics, settings, or areas of implementation related to wellbeing, demonstrating that health promotion is a complex process requiring an interdisciplinary and joined-up approach. The first chapters laid the foundations for systems- and settings-based approaches. Dolf and Dooris described the history and development of the Okanagan Charter, key underpinning health promotion and sustainability concepts, and the current state of global, regional, and national health promoting university networks that are mobilizing the Charter. The next chapter by Squires and colleagues emphasized the key role of collaborative leadership in developing a systems approach and sustaining interdisciplinary efforts across campus. The chapter contributed by Faulkner and his colleagues identified that an assessment of the current state of wellbeing on post-secondary campuses is essential in defining health promotion goals, in measuring progress, and in ensuring that this work continues to be prioritized.

The next section includes an elaboration of key elements of a systems approach to health promotion, anchored in experiences and perspectives of specific demographic groups. Foulds and Ferguson examined Indigenous wellbeing on campuses and how campuses need to consider how wellbeing initiatives can support Indigenous students, staff, and faculty. Kumaran and Kalagnanam focused on equity, diversity, and inclusion on campuses and how those principles need to underscore our efforts. Carry provided a senior leadership perspective emphasizing that campuses have a responsibility to ensure the wellbeing of students.

The third section includes examples of specific health promotion initiatives or considerations for policy and practice. London and Forneris described the contribution that academic units can play in health promotion efforts, and Kozicky and colleagues identified how campuses can apply health promotion principles to promoting a food-secure campus for students. This chapter is followed by a contribution from Hutchinson and colleagues describing how workplace health promotion not only focuses on physical environment but also health literacy and psychosocial factors. Tacto provided an overview of how US colleges are creating healthy settings by designing campuses with built and natural environments where students, faculty, and staff can live, learn, work, and experience college in a meaningful way. The last contribution by London and Squires presented how signatory campuses to the Okanagan Charter are progressing (or not) towards achieving the commitments that they made in signing the Charter. Together, the chapters provide an overview of promising practices and key considerations for expanding health promotion efforts on campuses.

In addition to the ideas described by the authors of this volume, there are other possibilities for expanding these efforts. Two examples follow with the understanding that there are other ways that we can support our health promotion efforts. The two pathways I will expand upon are connecting health promotion efforts with the work of addressing the Sustainable Development Goals and leveraging our existing networks to build a stronger global advocacy coalition championing systems approaches in health promotion.

The United Nations Sustainable Development Goals and the Okanagan Charter

Interestingly, in the same year as the development of the Okanagan Charter (2015), world leaders at the United Nations adopted Transforming Our World: The 2030 Agenda for Sustainable Development. Fundamental to the 2030 Agenda are the Sustainable Development Goals (SDGs), which are a set of priorities that guide countries in addressing the most urgent challenges that the world is facing. These challenges include "ending poverty and hunger; protecting the planet from degradation and addressing climate change; ensuring that all people can enjoy prosperous, healthy and fulfilling lives; and fostering peaceful, just and inclusive societies free from fear and violence" (SDSN Australia/Pacific, 2017, pp. 5–6). The priorities are organized into seventeen goals, and each goal is supported by a series of actions aligned with achieving that goal. Germane to the topic of this book, SDG #3 focuses on Good Health and Wellbeing.

There are several important differences between the two frameworks. The Okanagan Charter focuses on health promotion in the post-secondary sector because of the research function of these institutions and the ability to teach members of the community who will then go on to become contributing members and engaged leaders in the communities. Although the Charter identifies the intersectionality of sustainability and the health of the planet and its people, the specific actions aligned with achieving the calls to action of the Charter are not articulated; signatory campuses and organizations must determine for themselves which goals and initiatives that they will engage in to address their Charter commitments. The scope of the work is also different, in that the Okanagan Charter focuses on local systems approaches and working through national and international networks, whereas the SDGs are anchored in global systems approaches.

However, there are many similarities. As noted in the Okanagan Charter, the higher education sector is uniquely positioned to play a vital role in catalysing societal and ecological wellbeing towards the achievement of SDGs. For example, universities not only search for solutions to challenges that arise due to climate disruption (Leal Filho, 2010), but they also play a critical part in getting society ready to adapt to the effects of climate change by providing research and education on adaptation strategies (ACUPCC, 2018). Zhou et al. (2020) claimed that the role of the universities is to teach "game-changers of the future" (p. 88) who can operate in a way that contributes to creating a sustainable world.

Neary and Osborne (2018) also emphasized that collaboration is one of the key factors to achieve the "third mission" of the university. According to the authors, the "third mission" means engaging in activities that are "beyond the research and teaching remit of the university" (Neary & Osborne, 2018, p. 341) that contribute to a positive outcome for the wider public, notably the cooperation among universities, government, industry, and civil society. The authors highlighted that more effective execution of SDG initiatives requires a strong connection among universities, local businesses, policymakers, and society. This collaboration promotes the importance of using different perspectives, which is crucial not only for obtaining a comprehensive understanding of the problem but also for creating sustainable solutions to challenges that SDGs aim to solve. Importantly, collaboration within the university is a place to start, drawing together the interdisciplinary expertise and perspectives.

The connection between the health promotion framework of the Okanagan Charter and the SDG goal on global health and wellbeing is clear. Indeed, the Okanagan Charter (2015) identifies a transformative vision: "Health promoting universities and colleges transform the health and sustainability of our current and future societies, strengthen communities and contribute to the wellbeing of people, places and the planet" (p.2). Universities and colleges have a responsibility to examine promising avenues to galvanize our efforts and amplify our impact. How to connect our work in a global effort, though, remains a challenge. The next section identifies one possibility.

Leveraging Capacity-Building Networks

As described in Dolf and Dooris's chapter, national and international health promoting university networks have been established over the last two decades. Among their responsibilities is the stewardship of the adoption and implementation of the Okanagan Charter. There is variability across networks regarding how they are structured, how often they meet, and how active they are as a network. Similar to campus efforts, networks require resources and champions to be more effective in achieving their health promotion goals. National contexts matter, including the amount of government support, the types of grants available to fund this type of work, the infrastructure in place for networking, and the priorities of governments and campuses.

Most national networks are connected to the International Health Promoting Campuses Steering Group. It is at this level that global health promotion can be realized through knowledge sharing, capacity building, and convening regional perspectives to advance global agendas together. The same challenges apply at the national level, and, in addition, languages can be a barrier for ensuring that all voices and insights are being heard at the international level. Ensuring that the international network has an inclusionary environment can be a challenge, but it is a crucial part to establish and cement global connections and combined efforts.

Previous collaborations include several international health promoting university symposia and, at the most recent event, a pre-conference symposium organized by many of the contributing authors of this book. For the pre-conference symposium, we focused on the adoption and implementation of the Okanagan Charter. Although the pandemic has been challenging in countless ways, the familiarity we now have with virtually connecting for meetings and conferences meant that the spread of the full-day pre-symposium reached across twenty-three countries. The last international conference, originally planned to have a hybrid delivery approach, moved to be fully online for several reasons. However, the ability to be flexible and inclusive by leveraging online platforms provides promising opportunities to expand our efforts internationally.

Moreover, several different health promotion charters have been developed over the last forty years, as noted by Dolf and Dooris. As we approach the ten-year anniversary of the development of the Okanagan Charter, there is an opportunity to engage once again in an international launch of the Charter. The alignment of the next International Health Symposium scheduled for 2025 provides a venue for some of that work. Representatives from the World Health Organization will participate in those discussions, as they have in the past. Additionally, this venue may be important for determining further links with the SDG goals and for exploring ways in which the work of the International Health Promoting Campuses Steering Committee and the United Nations can be more closely aligned in a global advocacy coalition for health and wellbeing.

Future Directions

Achieving the transformative vision outlined in the Okanagan Charter has many layers of complexity. The core business or mandate of higher education includes teaching and research rather than health promotion. To build commitment for health promotion, campuses must construct a case that illustrates how resources (human and financial) invested in wellbeing can have a positive impact on the teaching and research goals of the campuses (Dooris et al., 2017).

Furthermore, higher education institutions need to change the narrative of how we discuss and conceive of health. Illnesses and interventions are more top of mind when describing health rather than the promotion of wellbeing by engaging in positive and health-forward types of actions and strategies (Dooris et al., 2017). Promotion and prevention strategies take fewer resources than interventions and will result in fewer illnesses and poor health outcomes, which in turn frees up even more resources to invest in promotion and prevention as well as resources to further support the teaching and research missions of the post-secondary sector. This positive cycle can then change the narrative around health and wellbeing. The strategies intentionally must be broad-based and "supported by all aspects of the college or community: academic policies and practices, physical and social environments, access to health food and recreational facilities and various work and volunteer opportunities" (Mirwaldt, 2010, p. 140).

An additional challenge for health promoting campuses is that many health determinants are beyond the control of universities (Dooris et al.,

2017). However, we can work with our community partners to improve conditions; these partnerships include municipal governments and committees, the Indigenous communities of that land, the health region and other local organizations. For example, child care centres, food-security supports, addiction centres, spiritual centres, and community sports clubs can all work with universities in linking students, staff, and faculty to those supports in a respectful manner. Hancock (2017) and Dooris et al. (2017) advocated strongly for working closely with communities in health promotion and noted that the collaboration needed to go beyond the municipal government.

Additionally, we potentially can have a huge impact on the health promotion agenda through our research and teaching agendas. Through our research and our engagement with communities, we can advocate for change in the broader community and collect evidence that supports the systems- and settings-based approach to health promotion. Through our teaching mission, we can educate our students as the next leaders of our campuses and communities on the positive impacts of health promotion for society. By promoting awareness of the intersections of the many determinants of good health, we can further the sustainability, social justice, and inclusion goals; essentially, achieving a broad understanding of health promotion has an impact on many of the other SDGs in addition to the advancement of global health and wellbeing. However, to determine progress and impact of health promotion efforts, we need to develop a robust and meaningful set of indicators that can be broadly communicated and implemented.

Evaluating the outcomes of healthy settings initiatives and collecting evidence that the actions positively impact campuses are especially challenging for several reasons (Dooris et al., 2022). Students only remain connected to the university for the duration of their program; it is very difficult to gather longitudinal data that can prove effectiveness in the long term. Additionally, whole system approaches are complex; the determination of what to measure and how to measure it depends on particular perspectives. Campuses in Canada are guided by provincial government funding and priorities, and these can vary significantly from government priorities in other countries. Furthermore, higher education institutions and the faculty within those campuses tend to be rewarded for individual rather than collective successes. However, as Dooris (2022) pointed out, "a transdisciplinary approach to research is most likely to lead to innovation by focusing on synergy generated at the interface of different subject disciplines and that interprofessional approaches to learning and working are most likely to address societal needs and challenges" (p. 161).

Transdisciplinary approaches will support collective action and capitalize on multiple perspectives; these collaborative opportunities will more likely lead to innovative solutions for the complex global challenges and thereby work towards achieving the SDGs and galvanizing global health promotion efforts.

Conclusion

We cannot ignore the need for global wellbeing of people, places, and planet. The pandemic highlighted how different local, national, and global communities do not have access to the same resources for health promotion nor access to the needed prevention and intervention supports such as health education and vaccines. As Dooris et al. (2021) posited, there is "an opportunity for higher education to use the disruptive impact of COVID-19 as a catalyst to 'build back better' – harnessing its leadership to effect visionary change both within universities and in society as a whole" (p. 307). We need to work collectively, focusing on the upstream strategies such as health promotion in a broad and collaborative way. We cannot afford to invest our energies and resources in just one piece of the puzzle. We require a collaborative, joined-up effort that coalesces our collective knowledge, strengths, and efforts to engage in research and implementation of health-forward approaches to global wellbeing.

REFERENCES

American College & University President's Climate Commitment (ACUPCC). (2018). *Higher education's role in adapting to a changing climate*. American College & University President's Climate Commitment.

Cawood, J., Dooris, M., & Powell, S. (2010). Healthy universities: Shaping the future. *Perspectives in Public Health, 130*(6), 259–60. https://doi.org/10.1177/1757913910384055

Dooris, M. (2022). Health-promoting higher education. In S. Kokko & M. Baybutt (Eds.), *Handbook of settings-based health promotion* (pp. 151–65). https://doi.org/10.1007/978-3-030-95856-5_8

Dooris, M., Doherty, S., & Orme, J. (2017). The application of salutogenesis in universities. In M.B. Mittlemark & G.F. Bauer (Eds.), *The handbook of salutogenesis* (pp. 237–45). https://doi.org/10.1007/978-3-319-04600-6_23

Dooris, M., Kokko, S., & de Leeuw, E. (2022). Evolution of the settings-based approach. In S. Kokko & M. Baybutt (Eds.), *Handbook of settings-based health promotion*, pp. 3–22. https://doi.org/10.1007/978-3-030-95856-5_1

Dooris, M., Powell, S., Parkin, D., & Farrier, A. (2021). Health promoting universities: Effective leadership for health, wellbeing and sustainability. *Health Education, 121*(3), 295–310. https://doi.org/10.1108/HE-12-2020-0121

Eastman, J., Jones, G.A., Trottier, C., & Begin-Caouette, O. (2022). *University governance in Canada: Navigating complexity.* McGill-Queen's University Press.

Hancock, T. (2017). Healthy cities and communities: Urban governance for health and wellbeing. In I. Rootman, A. Pederson, K.L. Frohlich, & S. Dupere (Eds.), *Health promotion in Canada: New perspectives on theory, practice, policy, and research* (4th ed., pp. 220–45). Canadian Scholars Press.

Leal Filho, W. (2010). Climate change at universities: Results of a world survey. In W.L. Filho (Ed.), *Universities and climate change* (pp. 1–19). Springer.

Mirwaldt, P. (2010). Health and wellness services. In D. Hardy Cox & C.C. Strange (Eds.), *Achieving student success: Effective student services in Canadian higher education* (pp. 124–40). McGill-Queen's University Press.

Neary, J., & Osborne, M. (2018). University engagement in achieving sustainable development goals: A synthesis of case studies from the SUEUAA study (2018). *Australian Journal of Adult Learning, 58*(3), 336–64.

Okanagan Charter: An International Charter for Health Promoting Universities and Colleges. (2015). *Okanagan Charter.* Kelowna, BC: Author. Retrieved from http://internationalhealthycampuses2015.sites.olt.ubc.ca/files/2016/01/Okanagan-Charter-January13v2.pdf

Sustainable Development Networks Solutions (SDSN). (2020). *Accelerating education for the SDGs in universities: A guide for universities, colleges, and tertiary and higher education institutions.* Sustainable Development Solutions Network.

Sustainable Development Networks Solutions (SDSN) Australia/Pacific. (2017). *Getting started with the SDGs in universities: A guide for universities, higher education institutions, and the academic sector.* Sustainable Development Solutions Network–Australia/Pacific.

Zhou, L., Rudhumbu, N., Shumba, J., & Olumide, A. (2020). Role of higher education institutions in the implementation of sustainable development goals. In G. Nhamo & V. Mjimba (Eds.), *Sustainable development goals and institutions of higher education* (pp. 87–96). Springer.

Contributors

Ainsley Carry, University of British Columbia

Vanessa Cunningham, University of Guelph

Matt Dolf, University of British Columbia

Mark Dooris, University of Central Lancashire

Michael Fang, University of British Columbia

Guy Faulkner, University of British Columbia

Leah J. Ferguson, University of Saskatchewan

Tanya Forneris, University of British Columbia

Heather J.A. Foulds, University of Saskatchewan

Alicia Hibbert, University of British Columbia

Crystal Hutchinson, University of British Columbia

Suresh Kalagnanam, University of Saskatchewan

Maha Kumaran, University of Saskatchewan

Min-Jung King, University of Guelph

Sara Kozicky, University of British Columbia

Sam Laban, University of Guelph

Chad London, Mount Royal University

Philip A. Loring, University of Guelph

Natasha Malloff, University of British Columbia

Olena Shakhova, University of Saskatchewan

Vicki Squires, University of Saskatchewan

C. Oliver Tacto, University of Saskatchewan

Caroline Wu, University of Marysville

Kelly Wunderlich, University of British Columbia

Index